Essential
Epidemiology

Essential Epidemiology

PRINCIPLES AND APPLICATIONS

William A. Oleckno
Northern Illinois University

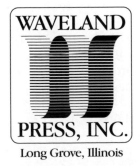

WAVELAND
PRESS, INC.
Long Grove, Illinois

For information about this book, contact:
Waveland Press, Inc.
4180 IL Route 83, Suite 101
Long Grove, IL 60047-9580
(847) 634-0081
info@waveland.com
www.waveland.com

To
Barbara R. Oleckno
(1921–2001)
mother and friend

About the Author

William A. Oleckno is a distinguished teaching professor and the coordinator of the Public and Community Health Programs at Northern Illinois University. He earned his Master of Public Health degree from the University of Pittsburgh and his doctorate from Indiana University at Bloomington. His research interests are in environmental health and epidemiology, and he has authored or coauthored over fifty publications related to these areas. He was formerly an assistant professor and the coordinator of the Environmental Health Sciences Program at Indiana University School of Medicine in Indianapolis. Dr. Oleckno has taught introductory courses in epidemiology at the undergraduate and graduate levels for approximately twenty-five years.

Contents

Preface

This book was made possible because of a Presidential Teaching Award I received in spring 1998 from Northern Illinois University, where I have been a professor and the coordinator of the Public and Community Health Programs for over two decades. Among other benefits, this prestigious award provided a sabbatical leave to develop a project related to the improvement of teaching. I chose to take my sabbatical in spring 2000 to begin writing this text, which I hoped to use in my Principles and Methods of Epidemiology class. This has been a long-standing aspiration of mine because of my passion for epidemiology, a subject I have taught now for almost 25 years.

Essential Epidemiology: Principles and Applications is intended to be a textbook and general reference on basic epidemiology. It is suitable for use in introductory epidemiology courses in undergraduate and graduate programs in the health professions, including public health, community health education, environmental health, and health administration, as well as allied health, nursing, medicine, dentistry, and related fields. It should also be useful to health professionals seeking a general reference on the basic principles, concepts, and methods of epidemiology.

In writing *Essential Epidemiology* I have sought to avoid two contrasting pitfalls of many introductory textbooks—oversimplification and convolution. Oversimplification can have the unfortunate consequence of concealing important exceptions to the rules and other nuances that are vital to understanding epidemiology in a more than superficial way. Convolution, on the other hand, can result from trying to integrate overly complex subject matter into an introductory textbook when it is more suited to advanced works on the topic. My goal has been to produce an engaging textbook that is clearly written and easy to follow, but one that provides sufficient depth and breadth for a comprehensive understanding of the essentials of epidemiology. I am aware that I stand on the shoulders of many individuals who have written introductory textbooks in this field, but I am hopeful that *Essential Epidemiology* will not only fulfill my goal but will find a place in the classroom and on the shelves of practicing health professionals because of its intrinsic value and user-friendly features. Some of these include:

- Comprehensive learning objectives for each chapter that can be used by students and instructors to assess whether the subject matter has been mastered
- Chapter overviews that provide a brief synopsis of the chapter contents
- Use of boldface to identify important new terms in each chapter

- A list of new terms at the end of each chapter
- Use of italics to emphasize key words and phrases
- Tables and figures to summarize, clarify, or add to important content in the text
- Boxed exhibits to present supplementary material
- Use of easily remembered mathematical symbols, such IR_C for cumulative incidence rate and IR_{P-T} for person-time incidence rate
- Sample problems with detailed step-by-step solutions and additional commentary
- Bulleted summaries highlighting the main contents of each chapter
- Practical problems and exercises at the end of each chapter
- A comprehensive glossary of common terms used in epidemiology
- A list of the formulas cited in the text with reference to where they appear in the text
- Appendices describing useful resources in epidemiology and selected answers to the chapter problems and exercises

In addition, an instructor's guide containing detailed answers to all the chapter problems and exercises is available to instructors from Waveland Press, Inc., and a CD-ROM containing applets for solving epidemiologic problems using formulas in the textbook is available directly from the author. The CD-ROM allows instructors and students to calculate basic rates, confidence intervals, tests of significance, and other epidemiologic measures discussed in the text, while minimizing the need to perform the sometimes-tedious algebra.

Epidemiology is a dynamic and important field that is fundamental to the health sciences. For some students, however, it can be a difficult subject to master because it requires a fair amount of deductive and inductive reasoning and because of its quantitative aspects. *Essential Epidemiology* is written so that students with a rudimentary understanding of statistics (usually a prerequisite for courses in epidemiology) should be able to comprehend the important principles, concepts, methods, and analytical techniques pertaining to epidemiology. The text is designed to help students understand and apply the fundamentals of epidemiology and to use this knowledge to evaluate studies in the epidemiologic and biomedical literature.

Chapters 1–3 focus on the nature and uses of epidemiology, its historical foundations, and important disease-related concepts. Chapter 4 summarizes the major epidemiologic study designs and how to recognize them in the literature. Chapters 5 and 6 describe the most common biostatistical measures used in epidemiology and methods of comparing rates, including rate adjustment and measures of association. Chapters 7 and 8 discuss association and causation and methods for assessing the accuracy of epidemiologic findings, including how to recognize and control bias, confounding, and sampling error. Chapter 9 discusses screening for disease detection, and chapters 10–13 deal with the basic design, conduct, analysis, and interpretation of the more common analytic and experimental epidemiologic study designs. Finally, chapter 14 discusses the investigation of disease outbreaks, the identification of disease clusters, and the nature of public health surveillance, including sources of data and practical uses. The result is a comprehensive introductory textbook of epidemiology that is both informative and practical.

Acknowledgements

Writing and publishing a textbook is never a solitary effort. Many individuals contribute in direct or indirect ways to the final product. I am particularly grateful to Larissa Simon Brouwers, who served as a graduate assistant under my direction in the fall and summer of 2000. Larissa read the first draft of the manuscript and among other things provided many helpful suggestions and criticisms that I believe resulted in better organization and clarity throughout the text. She was a diligent reviewer and was never shy about sharing her ideas for improvement.

I would also like to acknowledge the assistance of the staff at Waveland Press, Inc. Tom Curtin, who oversaw the project, showed an immediate enthusiasm that buoyed my interest in completing this book in a timely manner. I will never forget the call I received from him following the submission of a prospectus, outline, and sample chapters. He was genuinely excited about the high quality of the materials he had received and eager to proceed with the text. Jeni Ogilvie was responsible for the excellent in-house editing of the manuscript. We shared numerous e-mails and correspondence during this project and met on a couple of occasions. She was always very professional and extremely gracious, and I must say that it was a delight working with her. Gayle Zawilla assisted with the development of the book's index, for which I am very appreciative, and Katy Murphy did an excellent job of typesetting during the comprehensive reviews of the galley proofs and the final typescript.

I also want to thank Northern Illinois University and the students and faculty who supported my nomination for a presidential teaching award, which provided me with the support I needed to complete this book. I am especially grateful to Sherilynn F. Spear, chair of the School of Allied Health Professions, who prepared the original nomination package. She has been a continuing source of encouragement for much of my tenure at Northern. Finally, I owe a deep debt of gratitude to my wife, Karen, who gave up my company for too many evenings and weekends as I struggled to keep this book moving forward.

William A. Oleckno
epiresources@yahoo.com

CHAPTER ONE

Scope and Significance of Epidemiology

Learning Objectives

▸ Describe the importance of epidemiology.

▸ Describe applications of epidemiology.

▸ Define and give examples of risk factors, epidemics, and the disease iceberg concept.

▸ Discuss the meaning and scope of epidemiology.

▸ Define temporal pattern of disease and compare and contrast short-term fluctuations, cyclic patterns, and secular trends.

▸ Distinguish between descriptive and analytic epidemiology.

▸ Distinguish between efficacy and effectiveness.

Overview

Epidemiology is the study of the distribution, determinants, and deterrents of morbidity or mortality in human populations. It provides the basis for describing and explaining disease occurrence in a community and for developing, prioritizing, and evaluating public health programs. It is also useful in identifying risk factors and causes of disease, evaluating the efficacy of various treatments, and investigating disease outbreaks. Because of these applications, epidemiology is often referred to as the cornerstone or foundation of public health.

Introduction

Epidemiology is a dynamic field concerned with the occurrence of disease and other health-related problems in human populations. Its scope covers the description of disease patterns, the search for causes of disease, and practical applications related to disease surveillance and control. Epidemiology has been referred to as the cornerstone of public health practice and provides the basis for our understanding health-related problems, including their distribution, natural history, antecedents, and prevention. Epidemiology is also important to the practice of medicine as increased knowledge of disease occurrence aids in diagnosis and treatment. Before defining epidemiology in greater detail, we will first take a closer look at its importance and applications.

Importance of Epidemiology to Public Health

Epidemiology provides the *basis for describing and explaining disease occurrence in a community*. A typical epidemiologic question might be, "How many new cases of acquired immune deficiency syndrome (AIDS) were reported among teenagers in the United States last year?" If 300 new cases were reported, this tells us something about the occurrence of AIDS. We need a reference point, however, to make sense of this number. We might, for example, want to compare the number of reported cases to numbers in prior years to get a sense of whether AIDS is increasing or decreasing in this age group. It would be better, however, to compare the *rates* of AIDS since the population of teenagers may have changed from one year to the next. Rates allow us to make comparisons that account for differences in the sizes of the groups being compared. The importance of using rates instead of raw numbers to make comparisons is discussed in chapter 5.

Describing public health problems from an epidemiologic perspective helps us to understand their potential significance and impact. Through comparisons of epidemiologic measures such as incidence, prevalence, and mortality rates we can identify potentially high-risk groups and perhaps begin to explain the reasons behind differences in disease occurrence. For example, the incidence of AIDS is almost three times higher in young adults, 20–24 years of age, compared to teenagers.[1] This suggests that the occurrence of AIDS varies by age. In seeking an explanation for the difference, one might want to examine behaviors or other factors that differ between the age groups and that might therefore account for the apparent difference in the risk of contracting the human immunodeficiency virus (HIV), which has been implicated as the cause of AIDS. Greater promiscuous sexual activity and intravenous drug use, for example, are two factors that explain the higher rate of AIDS in young adults compared to teenagers in the United States.

Epidemiology is also important to public health because it provides a *basis for developing, prioritizing, and evaluating public health programs*. Public health programs should be developed based on need, and the epidemiologic approach is helpful in needs assessment. As a prelude to developing new programs in public health, one might ask such questions as, "What problems are present in the community?" "What problems have the greatest public health impact?" and "Are adequate health services available and accessible?" These questions, and related ones, can be answered epidemiologically. Public health surveillance, a tool of epidemiology, and epidemiologic surveys can be used to assess the frequency and scope of particular public health problems. Measures of morbidity, mortality, years of potential life lost, as well as other epidemiologic measures (see chapter 5), can be used to characterize the impact of public health problems. Finally, epidemiology can be used to evaluate the success of public health programs. Significant reduction in risk-taking behaviors, incidence of disease, or mortality may all be useful measures of a program's long-term success. Some other applications of epidemiology are discussed in the section that follows.

Some Applications of Epidemiology

Identifying Risk Factors for Disease

A major objective of epidemiology is identifying risk factors for disease. This is a step toward understanding disease causation. John Last defines a **risk factor** as a behavior, environmental exposure, or inherent human characteristic that is associated with an important health-related condition.[2] Specifically, risk factors are associated with an increased probability of a particular health-related outcome (i.e., disease). However, risk factors do not always cause disease. The criteria for establishing causation are discussed in chapter 7. Perhaps the most well known risk factor today is cigarette smoking, which the Surgeon General of the U.S. Public Health Service has determined to be a cause of lung cancer, heart disease, certain chronic lung diseases, and other conditions. A high serum cholesterol level is a risk factor for coronary heart disease, since high cholesterol levels have been shown through epidemiologic studies to be associated with an increase in the incidence of the disease. Interestingly, the term *risk factor* was popularized after its repeated use in research papers based on the Framingham Heart Study, one of the most well-known and enduring studies in epidemiology.[2]

The Framingham Heart Study, which began in 1948, is a 30-year-plus longitudinal study, which was originally designed to identify risk factors associated with cardiovascular disease (CVD). The study began with a representative sample of approximately 5,200 adult men and women residing in Framingham, Massachusetts, a town of about 28,000. The subjects were tracked throughout the years by monitoring hospital admissions and other sources and examining subjects biennially for the presence of CVD. The Framingham Heart Study has contributed significantly to our understanding of the risk factors that predispose individuals to CVD, including hypertension, diabetes, cigarette smoking, and blood cholesterol levels.[3, 4, 5]

Evaluating the Efficacy of Various Treatments

Is vitamin C efficacious in treating the common cold? Should individuals at high risk for heart disease take an aspirin a day to prevent a first or second heart attack? Is chemotherapy with Taxotere (docetaxel) efficacious in treating advanced lung cancer? Each of these questions is best answered epidemiologically by a randomized controlled trial (see chapter 4), which has become the gold standard for determining the efficacy* of various preventive and therapeutic procedures. The Hypertension Detection and Follow-Up Program, for example, evaluated two approaches to treatment using a randomized controlled trial involving 10,940 subjects with hypertension. Subjects were randomly assigned to either stepped care or referred care. Those assigned to stepped care received progressive increases in their prescribed blood pressure medications or additional antihypertensive medicines so as to achieve desired blood pressure levels. Those in the referred care group were advised to see their usual health care providers for treatment. The study found that the five-year mortality was 17% lower for those receiving stepped care compared to those receiving referred care.[7] The implication was for more aggressive treatment of hypertension.

Investigating Disease Outbreaks

When routine vaccination for adenovirus types 4 and 7 was suspended at Fort Jackson, South Carolina, in 1997 because of a vaccine shortage, an outbreak of adenovirus type 4-associated acute respiratory disease began. The victims of the outbreak were soldiers completing their basic training at the fort. In all, 1,018 men and women trainees were hospitalized from May through December of 1997 with fever and other acute respiratory symptoms consistent with the disease. The majority of these patients tested positive for adenovirus type 4. Fortunately, in this case, reinstitution of the vaccine was effective in preventing further spread of the disease, and the epidemic quickly subsided.[8]

Disease outbreaks or **epidemics**, like that at Fort Jackson, are circumstances where there is a clear increase in the number of cases of a disease compared to what is normally expected for the particular time and place. Epidemics are investigated to identify their causes so as to minimize their immediate impact and, most important, prevent similar outbreaks from occurring in the future. Epidemic investigation is a challenging dimension of epidemiology and one that is important to the maintenance of public health.[9] The investigation of epidemics is discussed in chapter 14.

Other Uses of Epidemiology

In addition to the applications already discussed, there are several other areas where epidemiology is useful. As implied in the section on the importance of epidemiology, the epidemiologic approach can be very helpful in the health planning process, particularly in needs assessment, objective setting, and program evaluation. Epidemiology is also useful in health policy formulation since it can answer vital questions about the benefits or harm resulting from specific interventions.[10]

---

* **Efficacy** refers to the benefits of a treatment, procedure, or service among those who use it compared to those who do not. A related term is **effectiveness**, which refers to the benefits among those to whom a treatment, procedure, or service is offered, whether or not they use it.[2, 6]

Epidemiology also increases our understanding of the natural history or life cycle of specific diseases (see chapter 3). Furthermore, it can help us estimate an individual's risk of specific diseases based on epidemiologic findings from populations with characteristics similar to the individual. This is the basis for health risk appraisals for cancer and heart disease based on personal risk factors, such as age, sex, and family medical history. Epidemiology also aids us in completing the clinical picture of a disease by filling in the gaps for health care providers, who ordinarily have an inaccurate view of the severity and distribution of disease in the community due to the fact that not everyone who is ill seeks treatment. This illustrates the **disease iceberg concept**.[11] When physicians, for example, see influenza patients in their offices during the "flu season," they often overestimate the severity of the disease since they tend to see only the sicker patients (those requiring medical treatment). Also, if we were to rely on the number of patients seeking medical assistance to measure the extent of influenza in a given community, we would inevitably underestimate the true frequency since many patients rely on self-treatment at home. The disease iceberg concept derives from the fact that four-fifths of an iceberg is submerged or out of view. Table 1–1 summarizes some of the common applications of epidemiology.

Table 1–1 Common Applications of Epidemiology

- Describing and explaining disease occurrence in a community
- Assisting in developing, prioritizing, and evaluating public health programs
- Identifying risk factors and causes of diseases
- Evaluating the efficacy of various treatment options
- Investigating disease outbreaks or epidemics
- Assisting in health planning and health policy formulation
- Understanding the natural history of diseases
- Estimating individual risks of diseases
- Completing the clinical picture of disease

Definition of Epidemiology

By now, you should have a fairly good idea of what epidemiology is and why it is important to public health and medicine. It would be helpful, however, to have a good, concise definition of this field of study. For those who are interested in the origin of terms, epidemiology is derived from the Greek words "epi" (on or upon), "demos" (people), and "logos" (word or statement). Literally, it translates as "a statement of what is upon the people."[12] A more practical definition is offered below. This definition can be thought of as the 3-D definition of epidemiology, where each of the "D" words in the definition has special significance:

> *Epidemiology is the study of the distribution, determinants, and deterrents of morbidity or mortality in human populations.*

The term *distribution* refers primarily to how **morbidity** (illness, disease, injury, etc.) or **mortality** (death)* is distributed in a given population or community. Specifically, we are interested in describing the frequency and patterns of morbidity or mortality in terms of *person, place,* or *time* variables. Person variables relate to *who* is affected; place variables relate to *where* they are affected; and time variables relate to *when* they are affected. Table 1–2 lists some of the more common person variables that may be used to describe the distribution of morbidity or mortality. As an example, we might describe the distribution of lung cancer in the United States by age group, sex, race, smoking status, and occupation. This description would yield a fairly good picture of who is afflicted with lung cancer in the United States and would suggest what groups appear to be at greatest risk for this disease.

Table 1–2 Commonly Used Person Variables

• Age	• Religion
• Sex	• Marital status
• Race/ethnicity	• Health status
• Socioeconomic status	• Immunization status
• Occupation	• Lifestyle or behavioral practices (e.g., smoking)
• Education	• Environmental exposures

Place variables include specific geographic areas (e.g., census tracts, neighborhoods, cities, counties, states, regions, countries) and general locations (urban or rural areas, schools or other institutions, indoors or outdoors, at home or at work, along the river, etc.). Time variables may include the time of onset of a given disease (i.e., hour of the day, day of the week, month of the year, etc.) or the time of diagnosis, especially for those health-related problems where it is virtually impossible to know the actual time of onset (e.g., depression, arthritis, prostate cancer). Infectious diseases are usually classified by when the first symptoms of disease appear. Chronic diseases tend to be classified by the date of diagnosis. Classifying morbidity or mortality by time can also reveal **temporal patterns of dis-**

---

* Morbidity is defined as any departure from physiological or psychological well-being, and may include objective and subjective states.[2] It is commonly used interchangeably with disease and refers to nonfatal conditions. In addition to morbidity and mortality, epidemiology may also focus on other health-related attributes or outcomes, such as cholesterol levels, cigarette smoking, drug abuse, and violence, as explained in subsequent chapters.

ease, which are illustrated in figure 1–1. Common temporal patterns of morbidity and mortality include:

- Short-term fluctuations
- Cyclic patterns
- Secular trends

Generally, **short-term fluctuations** represent relatively brief, unexpected increases in the frequency of a particular disease. Short-term fluctuations are commonly manifested in epidemics. The sudden outbreak of cryptosporidiosis in Milwaukee, Wisconsin, in the spring of 1993 represents a short-term fluctuation. In this example over 400,000 people were afflicted with a parasitic infection causing diarrhea and abdominal pain over the course of several weeks. The source of the infection was traced to the protozoan *Cryptosporidium parvum*, which was spread through the public water supply. Once improvements were made in the water treatment system, the incidence of cryptosporidiosis dropped dramatically.

Cyclic patterns represent periodic, often predictable, increases in the frequency of a particular cause of morbidity or mortality. For example, each year over the Labor Day weekend we expect that the number of traffic deaths will increase by an anticipated amount. Also, influenza tends to show a seasonal variation in frequency each year with the number of cases peaking in the late fall and winter months.

Secular trends represent long-term changes in morbidity or mortality patterns. The U.S. mortality rate for septicemia, for example, showed a steady increase between 1951 and 1988. During the same time period, the mortality rate for cerebrovascular disease declined significantly and only recently has begun to level off.[13] Caution must be exercised, however, in associating secular changes with external influences. Sometimes changes in diagnostic criteria, completeness of reporting, demographics, and other factors may explain part or all of a secular trend. See figure 1–1 on page 8.

Describing the distribution of morbidity or mortality by person, place, or time variables is a major focus of **descriptive epidemiology**. This aspect of epidemiology is concerned with the variations of morbidity or mortality in a community. This information is not only useful in health care planning but can provide clues to the potential causes of disease. The characteristics of descriptive epidemiologic studies are discussed in chapter 4.

While the term *distribution* in the definition of epidemiology refers to the who, where, and when of morbidity or mortality, the term *determinants* refers to why morbidity or mortality occur. The goal of this dimension of epidemiology, known as **analytic epidemiology**, is to identify the causes of morbidity and mortality. Uncovering the causes of morbidity and mortality is usually accomplished by testing hypotheses using a variety of epidemiologic research designs. Initial steps are usually directed at identifying and confirming suspected risk factors for disease. Judgments about causation are then based on the weight of accumulated evidence (see chapter 4). Discovering the causes of morbidity and mortality is one of the most challenging aspects of epidemiology.

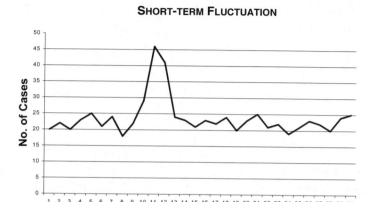

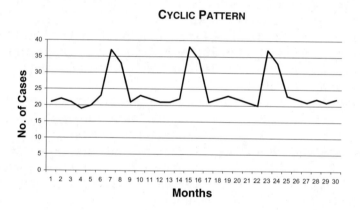

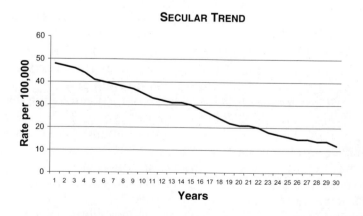

Figure 1–1 Temporal patterns of disease

The third "D" in the "3-D" definition of epidemiology refers to *deterrents*. From a practical point of view, the ultimate goal of epidemiology is to prevent, reduce, or control morbidity and mortality in human populations. In a sense, describing the distribution and identifying the determinants of morbidity or mortality are a prelude to seeking deterrents. Morbidity and mortality can sometimes be controlled without fully understanding their distribution or determinants, as history has shown (see chapter 2), but knowledge of these aspects often leads to more effective strategies for their prevention or reduction.

Finally, epidemiology is concerned with *human populations*. As a branch of public health, epidemiology is a human science, and it seeks to understand and explain health-related problems in defined groups of people or communities (e.g., the population of a state or region, African Americans, women between 45 and 54 years of age). **Clinical epidemiology**, an offshoot of classical epidemiology, is patient oriented; it seeks to use epidemiology to aid decision making about clinical cases of disease, such as in the diagnosis, prognosis, and treatment of disease.[6] Clinical epidemiology can be defined as "the application of epidemiologic principles and methods to problems encountered in clinical medicine."[6(p2)] Unlike classical epidemiology, which is a branch of public health, it is most appropriate to view clinical epidemiology as a branch of medicine.

Summary

- Epidemiology is the study of the distribution, determinants, and deterrents of morbidity or mortality in human populations. It seeks to describe, explain, and prevent public health problems that plague our society. It also provides a basis for developing, prioritizing, and evaluating public health programs.

- Some of the specific applications of epidemiology include identifying risk factors and causes of diseases, evaluating the efficacy of various treatment options, explaining the natural history of diseases, estimating an individual's risk of a specific health problem, and completing the clinical picture of disease for health care practitioners.

- Depending on its purpose, epidemiology may be classified as descriptive epidemiology or analytic epidemiology. Descriptive epidemiology describes morbidity or mortality by person, place, or time variables. Analytic epidemiology seeks to identify the causes of morbidity and mortality.

New Terms

analytic epidemiology	effectiveness	mortality
clinical epidemiology	efficacy	risk factor
cyclic pattern	epidemic	secular trend
descriptive epidemiology	epidemiology	short-term fluctuation
disease iceberg concept	morbidity	temporal pattern of disease

Study Questions and Exercises

1. Human immunodeficiency virus (HIV) infection is a significant public health issue in the United States and abroad. Untreated, an estimated 90% or more of those infected with HIV will develop acquired immune deficiency syndrome or AIDS. Research has identified a number of risk factors for HIV infection. Identify and discuss four distinct risk factors and rank them in relative order of importance in the spread of HIV infection in the United States.

2. Planning public health programs at the community level typically involves six major steps: (a) assessment of needs, (b) determination of priorities, (c) development of goals and objectives, (d) design of activities to achieve objectives, (e) implementation of the program, and (f) evaluation of processes and outcomes. Describe how epidemiology can contribute to each of these steps. In which steps is epidemiology likely to make the greatest contributions and in which the least?

3. Because of the disease iceberg concept physicians often have a distorted view of the true nature of a disease in the communities they serve. Since those who seek treatment from physicians often differ from those who do not, a physician's view of the severity or distribution of a disease in the community may not be characteristic of the disease as a whole. Identify three diseases or conditions that are likely to exhibit the disease iceberg concept and indicate why. Also, name three diseases or conditions that are unlikely to demonstrate the disease iceberg concept and again indicate why.

4. Epidemiology has been referred to as the cornerstone of public health practice. Other than its role in health planning, how is epidemiology fundamental to the practice of public health?

References

1. Health Resources and Services Administration, Maternal and Child Health Bureau (1999). *Child Health USA 1999.* Washington, DC: The Bureau.
2. Last, J. M., ed. (1995). *A Dictionary of Epidemiology.* New York: Oxford University Press.
3. Brink, S. (1998). Unlocking the Heart's Secrets. *U.S. News & World Report* (On-Line). Available: http://www2.usnews.com.usnews/issue/980907/7fram.htm (Access date: January 5, 1999.)
4. Woodward, M. (1999). *Epidemiology: Study Design and Data Analysis.* Boca Raton, FL: Chapman and Hall/CRC.
5. Hennekens, C. H., and Buring, J. E. (1987). *Epidemiology in Medicine.* Boston: Little, Brown and Company.
6. Fletcher, R. H., Fletcher, S. W., and Wagner, E. H. (1988). *Clinical Epidemiology: The Essentials,* 2nd ed. Baltimore: Williams and Wilkins.
7. Meinert, C. L. (1986). *Clinical Trials: Design, Conduct, and Analysis.* New York: Oxford University Press.
8. McNeill, K. M., Hendrix, R. M., Lindner, J. L., Benton, F. R., Monteith, S. C., Tuchscherer, M. A., Gray, G. C., and Gaydos, J. C. (1999). Large, Persistent Epidemic of Adenovirus Type 4-Associated Acute Respiratory Disease in U.S. Army Trainees. *Emerging Infectious Diseases* 5(6): 798–801.
9. Reingold, A. L. (1998). Outbreak Investigations—A Perspective. *Emerging Infectious Diseases* 4(1): 21–27.
10. Ibrahim, M. A. (1985). *Epidemiology and Health Policy.* Rockville, MD: Aspen.
11. Duncan, D. F. (1988). *Epidemiology: Basis for Disease Prevention and Health Promotion.* New York: Macmillan.

12. Markellis, V. C. (1986). Epidemiology: Cornerstone for Health Education. *Health Education* 16:14–17.
13. Hoyert, D. L., Kochanek, K. D., and Murphy, S. L. (1999). Deaths: Final Data for 1997. *National Vital Statistics Reports* 47(19). Hyattsville, MD: National Center for Health Statistics.

CHAPTER TWO

Evolution of Epidemiology

Learning Objectives

▸ Describe the cause, source, nature, and historical impact of plague as it relates to public health.

▸ Discuss some of the major achievements of individuals who contributed to the early development of epidemiology.

▸ Differentiate among endemic, epidemic, and pandemic.

▸ Recognize the significance of Bills of Mortality and spot maps.

▸ Define multifactorial etiology; antecedent, immediate, and underlying cause of death; notifiable or reportable disease; vital event, record, and statistics; and vital statistics registration system.

Overview

Epidemiology gradually evolved as individuals sought to explain disease occurrence in a systematic way. The great epidemics and pandemics of history, such as plague, provided the incentives to understand and control human disease and suffering. Starting with Hippocrates, who was the first to explain disease on a rational basis, a long line of dedicated individuals, including John Graunt, William Farr, John Snow, Joseph Goldberger, and many others, shaped the development of epidemiology as a distinct discipline in public health.

Origins of Epidemiology

Between 1347 and 1351 over 30 percent of the population of Western Europe (some 25 million people) died of a highly contagious disease known as the Black Death, or **plague** as it is properly known.[1, 2] In 1348 alone, Venice lost 100,000 people, and at least 1,200 died daily in Vienna. Worldwide the number of deaths was over 60 million.[3] The desolation caused by plague (see table 2–1) can hardly be overestimated. According to John J. Hanlon and George E. Pickett, the authors of a classic public health text, "Probably nothing ever came so close to exterminating the human species."[3(p15)] So many dead bodies had to be disposed of that in some locations they were stacked in layers by the thousands and buried in large pits or discarded in the river.

Table 2–1 Some Basic Facts about Plague

Clinical Forms	Bubonic, Septicemic, and Pneumonic
Causative Agent	*Yersinia pestis,* a bacterium
Major Source	Bite of the infected Rat Flea, *Xenopsylla cheopis*
Description	*Bubonic plague*, which has an incubation period of 2–6 days, generally produces fever, chills, malaise, myalgia, nausea, sore throat, headache, and one or more painful, swollen lymph nodes, known as bubos, near the bite area. Bubonic plague may also be contracted by direct contact with infected tissues or body fluids. Untreated, bubonic plague has a case-fatality rate of 50–60%. *Septicemic plague* results from direct invasion of the circulatory system without node involvement or by secondary spread of bubonic plague. The prognosis is very poor. *Pneumonic plague*, like septicemic plague, can be primary or secondary. In secondary pneumonic plague either of the bubonic or septicemic forms can lead to lung involvement causing pneumonic plague. Primary pneumonic plague is spread person-to-person by infected respiratory droplets. It has an incubation period of 1–3 days. Pneumonic plague is characterized by a severe pneumonia with high fever, chills, cough, and bloody sputum.
Preventive and Control Measures	While relatively rare today (only about 1,000–2,000 cases per year worldwide), plague was the cause of millions of deaths in the Middle Ages. It is a disease with epidemic potential that needs to be taken very seriously when detected. Proper sanitation for rodent control is an important preventive measure. Use of appropriate insecticides and repellants may be recommended in areas where flea bites are possible. Isolation of active cases, antibiotic treatment (e.g., streptomycin), disinfection and proper disposal of discharges and contaminated clothing, and quarantine of contacts may be

References: Chin, J., ed. (2000). *Control of Communicable Diseases Manual*, 17th ed. Washington, DC: American Public Health Association; Centers for Disease Control and Prevention (1995). Plague Information: Health-care Worker Information. Available: http://www.cdc.gov/ncidod/diseases/plague/hlth-carw.htm (Access date: March 12, 2000.)

This, however, was not the first occurrence of plague as a **pandemic**, which is an epidemic on a grand scale, causing illness or death over very extensive areas and generally crossing international borders and afflicting large numbers of people.[6] Plague is estimated to have killed 100 million people in Europe and Asia between A.D. 500 and 650 and another 280,000 in Europe from 1098 to 1101. Altogether, epidemics and pandemics of plague may have accounted for as many as 138 million lives worldwide from A.D. 500 to 1923.[1] When we consider these and other historical pandemics of diseases, such as leprosy and syphilis,[3, 4] it is not difficult to see why these events were connected with the origins of epidemiology.[5] The great thinkers of the time sought to explain the devastation caused by plague and other diseases, while the more practical souls fought to control the carnage using whatever methods seemed to work. These efforts to understand and control disease in populations paralleled the early beginnings of epidemiology.

Early Pioneers of Epidemiology

The first "epidemiologists" were those who sought to explain the causes of disease and death in human populations in a systematic manner.[5] Epidemiology as a discipline evolved slowly as theories of disease causation were developed, refined, and tested. While many men and women contributed significantly to the early evolution of epidemiology (see table 2–2 on p. 16), the achievements of a few individuals stand out as milestones in the shaping of this dynamic field.

Hippocrates, a physician who lived about 460–377 B.C., is often credited as the *first true epidemiologist*. Although not always correct in his beliefs about disease causation, Hippocrates has an honored place in the history of epidemiology because he was one of the first to base his conclusions on observations.[5] Some of his important contributions to epidemiology are summarized below.

- He was the first individual who attempted to use rational versus supernatural means to explain disease occurrence.

- He recognized that disease not only affects individuals but populations as well.

- He wrote three books that dealt with epidemiologic concepts—*Epidemic I, Epidemic III*, and *Air, Water, and Places*.

- He differentiated between **endemic**, which refers to the constant presence or usual frequency of a specific disease in a given community,[6] and epidemic disease, which represents a clear increase in the number of cases of disease compared to what is normally expected for the particular time and place.

- He recognized associations between environmental and other factors (e.g., water conditions, housing, diet, climate, etc.) and certain diseases.[5]

Table 2–2 Selected Historical Contributions of Men and Women to Epidemiology

Individual	Life Span	Selected Contributions
Hippocrates	460–377 B.C.	The first to offer formally rational versus supernatural explanations for disease occurrence in terms of environmental and other factors
Girolamo Fracastoro	1478–1553	Believed to be the first to articulate formally a theory of disease transmission by contagion
John Graunt	1620–1674	Used the Bills of Mortality to describe disease occurrence in a systematic manner
Thomas Sydenham	1624–1689	Insisted that observation should guide the study of the natural history of disease rather than merely theoretical explanations
James Lind	1716–1794	Used the experimental approach to determine that dietary factors were influential in treating and preventing scurvy
Edward Jenner	1749–1823	Invented a vaccine against smallpox based on careful observation
William Farr	1807–1883	Used vital statistics and other statistical approaches to describe epidemiologic problems
John Snow	1813–1858	Demonstrated that cholera could be transmitted through contaminated water
Ignas Semmelweis	1818–1865	Used epidemiologic methods to identify the source of childbed (puerperal) fever and introduced handwashing with chlorinated lime to reduce its incidence
Peter Ludwig Panum	1820–1885	Demonstrated that acquired immunity results from infection with measles
Florence Nightingale	1820–1910	Used mortality statistics to justify improved hygienic standards at military hospitals
Louis Pasteur	1822–1895	Demonstrated that microorganisms cause disease and that vaccination could be employed as a sound approach to disease control
Robert Koch	1843–1910	Developed strict criteria for establishing bacterial causes of disease. Together with Pasteur, Koch is credited with firmly establishing the Germ Theory of Disease
Anna Wessels Williams	1863–1954	Isolated a strain of the diphtheria organism that was used to prepare an effective antitoxin against diphtheria
Joseph Goldberger	1874–1929	Used observational and experimental approaches to demonstrate that pellagra was caused by a protein-deficient diet

References: Fox, J. P., Hall, C. E., and Elveback, L. R. (1970). *Epidemiology: Man and Disease*. New York: Macmillan Company; Lilienfeld, D. E., and Stolley, P. D. (1994). *Foundations of Epidemiology*, 3rd ed. New York: Oxford University Press; Timmreck, T. C. (1998). *An Introduction to Epidemiology*, 2nd ed. Boston: Jones and Bartlett Publishers; Shearer, B. F., and Shearer, B. S., eds. (1996). *Notable Women in the Life Sciences: A Biographical Dictionary*. Westport, CT: Greenwood Press.

John Graunt (1620–1674) was a London tradesman who published a book in 1662 entitled *Natural and Political Observations Made Upon the Bills of Mortality*.[5] This landmark volume can be considered the forerunner of modern **vital statistics**,[3] which are introduced in exhibit 2–1. **Bills of Mortality** was the phrase used for the weekly and annual recording of births and deaths, which started in England as early as 1538.[6] Graunt is credited with quantifying disease patterns in London and associating births and deaths with age, sex, and other factors. He was one of the first to demonstrate statistically, for example, that there was a higher frequency of births and deaths among males than among females and that the infant mortality rate in London was unusually high in 1662. The impact of Graunt's work with the Bills of Mortality was clearly ahead of its time. In fact, it was over 175 years later that Graunt's early attempts to describe disease occurrence statistically came to fruition in the work of William Farr, another pioneer of epidemiology.

William Farr (1807–1883), described as the founder of modern epidemiology,[7] extended the work of Graunt by using vital statistics in a comprehensive and systematic manner to describe epidemiologic problems.[5] Working as a medical statistician for the General Register Office for England and Wales from 1839 to1879, Farr contributed to epidemiology in manifold ways. Some of his accomplishments include:

- Demonstrating the need for population studies to describe disease distribution and explain disease causation
- Promoting the concept of **multifactorial etiology** (i.e., the idea that some diseases, especially chronic diseases, have many interrelated causes)
- Recognizing the interrelationship between incidence (new cases of disease) and prevalence (existing cases of disease)
- Applying his understanding of the distribution and determinants of disease to prevention and control efforts
- Classifying diseases in a systematic fashion that eventually led to the International Classification of Diseases*
- Developing standardized statistical measures, such as the infant mortality rate, the standardized mortality rate, life tables, and mathematical models of epidemic curves[7]

Perhaps the most well known of the early pioneers of epidemiology is John Snow (1813–1858), a British anesthesiologist who administered chloroform to Queen Victoria during the birth of two of her children.[5] Snow was a founding member of the London Epidemiological Society, whose initial purpose was to determine the causes of cholera,[8] an acute enteric disease that was epidemic in London at the time and had been pandemic throughout most of the world during the nineteenth century.[9] Today, Snow's work is looked upon as an eminent example of *analytic epidemiology*.[10]

---

* The International Classification of Diseases (ICD) is an international system for categorizing health outcomes. The tenth version, for example, is known as the *International Statistical Classification of Diseases and Related Health Problems*, but is commonly referred to as *ICD-10* for short. It has 21 chapters and uses alphanumeric coding to classify virtually all known diseases.[6]

During an investigation of a cholera outbreak in London in 1849, Snow observed that deaths from cholera were highest in districts served by two water companies (the Lambeth Company and the Southwark and Vauxhall Company), both of which obtained their water supplies from sewage-contaminated areas of the Thames River. In 1852 the Lambeth Company relocated its source to a relatively uncontaminated area of the Thames. A subsequent cholera outbreak in 1853 provided Snow with an opportunity to compare cholera death rates in the districts served by each water company. Snow found that the death rate from cholera was over five times higher in districts served exclusively by the Southwark and Vauxhall Company when compared to those served only by the Lambeth Company.[11] There thus appeared to be an association between sewage-contaminated drinking water and cholera deaths. To test this hypothesis, Snow focused on those districts served by *both* water companies. In these districts, the death rate from cholera was intermediate between those served *only* by the Lambeth Company or by the Southwark and Vauxhall Company, respectively. Fortunately for Snow, in the districts served by both water companies, there was no discernible pattern in terms of which households obtained their water from one company or the other. For all intents and purposes, the households in these districts used one of the two water companies on a completely random basis. Through painstaking and careful data collection, Snow was able to verify that households receiving drinking water from the Southwark and Vauxhall Company had substantially higher death rates from cholera than those served by the Lambeth Company, thus lending support to his original hypothesis that sewage-contaminated water was associated with cholera deaths.[11] Snow's meticulous work demonstrates a *natural experiment* (a situation in nature that mimics a planned experiment) through which he was able to show confidently that cholera was associated with the ingestion of contaminated drinking water. The impact of Snow's findings was significant. Following publication of his report, legislation was passed requiring that all water companies in London provide filtered water by 1857.[8]

In another investigation, Snow examined patterns of an 1854 cholera outbreak in the Golden Square area of London. In this inquiry, known as "The Case of the Broad Street Pump," Snow carefully noted the location of all cholera deaths in the area by place of residence and place of work. He then noted the sites of the water well pumps in the area based on his hypothesis that cholera was transmitted through water. The distribution of deaths and the location of the well pumps were marked on what is commonly known today as a **spot map**.* Snow noticed that the cases clustered around the pump on Broad Street. After carefully eliminating other potential explanations and investigating the actual water sources of those who succumbed to cholera, Snow concluded that contaminated water at the Broad Street pump was the

---

* A spot map is a map showing the geographical location of each case of a disease or other attribute. It is frequently used in investigating localized disease outbreaks to discover place factors where cases cluster. Case clustering may suggest possible causes of the outbreak. Inferences from spot maps can be misleading, however, if the population at risk for the disease is not evenly distributed over the area.[6]

Exhibit 2–1 A Primer on Vital Statistics

Vital statistics refer to information derived from **vital events**, which are registered life events such as births, deaths, marriages, divorces, and certain diseases. In the United States, vital events must be reported by law. Typically, registration forms or certificates are completed and signed by authorized personnel. For example, birth and death certificates are normally completed and signed by the attending physician. **Vital records**, which are the completed registration forms or certificates of birth, death, marriage, etc., are generally filed with a local vital statistics registrar, who maintains the records in the county or parish where they occurred. Copies of the vital records are then forwarded to the state registrar for vital statistics, who forwards copies to the National Center for Health Statistics (NCHS) located in the Centers for Disease Control and Prevention within the U.S. Department of Health and Human Services. This system constitutes the **vital statistics registration system** of the United States. Vital statistics may be combined with census data to develop a variety of statistics that can be used to describe trends, make comparisons, and test hypotheses about the causes of morbidity and mortality. While the NCHS recommends standardized forms for the collection of vital statistics, states may adopt their own forms as long as the required information is collected.

Examples of Vital Records

Birth Certificates: Birth certificates contain demographic information about the child and parent(s), data relating to birth weight, complications of pregnancy and labor, previous births and terminations, visible birth defects, etc.

Death Certificates: Death certificates contain demographic and other information about the decedent and the causes of death. The causes of death recorded on death certificates include:

- **Immediate Cause of Death**: This is the disease or condition that directly led to death. It specifically excludes *modes* of dying, such as respiratory or heart failure. *Example:* pneumonia

- **Antecedent Cause of Death**: This is any disease or condition that gave rise to the immediate cause of death. *Example:* congestive heart failure

- **Underlying Cause of Death**: This is the cause or injury that *initiated* the chain of events that ultimately produced death. It is the *official cause of death* used in mortality statistics. *Example:* aortic valve disease

- *Other Significant Conditions:* These are important conditions that contributed to death but are not related to the other causes of death. *Examples:* coronary heart disease, diabetes

Reports of Notifiable Diseases: **Notifiable diseases** (also known as **reportable diseases**) are diseases or conditions that must be reported to the appropriate health authority whenever they are diagnosed. Reporting is usually by physicians, laboratories, or hospital personnel. The specific reporting methods and the specific diseases or conditions that must be reported vary from state to state. In general, notifiable diseases are those that require prompt public health action because of their severity, communicability, or because they may represent a failure of preventive measures already in place (e.g., immunizations, food safety inspections). Examples of notifiable diseases include salmonellosis, syphilis, measles, diphtheria, AIDS, tuberculosis, and lead poisoning. There are about 60 diseases that are legally reportable in all 50 states.

source of the epidemic.[11] As a final gesture, he had the pump handle removed, thereby curtailing the epidemic, which was almost over anyway.

Though John Snow was able to show conclusively that cholera could be transmitted through contaminated water by 1854, it took another 27 years for the etiologic agent, *Vibrio cholerae*, to be identified.[4] In his own work, entitled *On the Mode of Communication of Cholera*, Snow discussed common modes of person-to-person transmission and added that cholera could also be spread by "the mixture of the cholera evacuations with water used for drinking and culinary purposes, either by permeating the ground, and getting into wells, or by running along channels and sewers into the rivers from which entire towns are sometimes supplied with water."[12(p45)] What is so amazing is that the *germ theory of disease* (that microorganisms are responsible for most infectious diseases) had not been developed at the time of Snow's work. He was clearly ahead of his time.

Among the many other individuals who contributed to the development of epidemiology is Joseph Goldberger (1874–1929), an American physician who used experimentation to confirm his observations. In the early part of the twentieth century Goldberger studied pellagra, a condition that most believed to be an infectious disease at the time. Goldberger observed that pellagra was associated with rural areas and poverty and that it was prevalent in mental institutions but oddly absent among the nurses and attendants. This led him to hypothesize that the disease was caused by a nutritional deficiency. He was able to demonstrate both observationally and experimentally in selected populations that pellagra was caused by a protein-deficient diet. Today we know that pellagra is due specifically to a deficiency of nicotinic acid, a form of the B vitamin niacin, found in protein-rich foods such as red meat.[4, 13]

Today, a new set of pioneers is expanding the borders of epidemiology into new areas of clinical practice, environmental risk assessment, health care decision making, and health policy development. All of these applications, however, depend on a firm grasp of the basic principles and methods of epidemiology.

Summary

- Historical pandemics of devastating diseases like plague (Black Death) and leprosy were connected with the origins of epidemiology.

- As a discipline, epidemiology evolved slowly as theories of disease causation were developed, refined, and tested.

- Among the many noteworthy pioneers of epidemiology we can cite Hippocrates, who provided the first rational explanations for disease occurrence; John Graunt, who systematically evaluated the Bills of Mortality; William Farr, who brought the statistical analysis of epidemiologic problems to a new level; John Snow, who used epidemiologic methods to uncover the source and mode of transmission of cholera; and Joseph Goldberger, who used observation and experimentation to demonstrate the cause of pellagra.

New Terms

antecedent cause
   of death
bills of mortality
endemic
immediate cause
   of death

multifactorial etiology
notifiable disease
pandemic
plague
reportable disease
spot map

underlying cause of death
vital event
vital record
vital statistics
vital statistics
   registration system

Study Questions and Exercises

1. Match the historical contributions in Column B with the individuals in Column A.

    Column A

    ____ William Farr

    ____ Joseph Goldberger

    ____ John Graunt

    ____ Peter Ludwig Panum

    ____ Edward Jenner

    ____ Hippocrates

    ____ James Lind

    ____ Florence Nightingale

    ____ Louis Pasteur

    ____ John Snow

    ____ Girolamo Fracastoro

    Column B

    A. Probably first to express formally a theory of contagion

    B. The first to explain disease occurrence on a rational basis

    C. Used mortality data to get improvements at military hospitals

    D. Evaluated the Bills of Mortality

    E. Demonstrated cholera could be transmitted through water

    F. Demonstrated that immunity results from measles infection

    G. Promoted the concept of multifactorial etiology

    H. Showed that diet could prevent scurvy

    I. Invented a vaccine against smallpox

    J. Helped establish the Germ Theory of Disease

    K. Showed pellagra was caused by a protein-deficient diet

2. An 85-year-old woman with Type II diabetes, osteoporosis, and coronary heart disease tripped on a rug, fell, and fractured her right hip. She was admitted to the hospital within six hours by her daughter-in-law but died two days later at the hospital. Just four hours prior to her death she had extreme difficulty breathing and her skin became bluish in color. The attending physician said this was the result of a massive pulmonary embolism, a condition resulting from a large blood clot in the pulmonary artery. Using the definitions in exhibit 2–1, hypothesize as to the immediate, antecedent, and underlying causes of death.

3. Describe three diseases anywhere in the world that are currently endemic, epidemic, and pandemic, respectively. Explain why these diseases are classified as they are.

References

1. Major Plagues and Epidemics (no date). *Compton's Encyclopedia Online*. Available: http://www.optonline.com/Tables/90000f5_T.html (Access date: January 6, 2000.)
2. Janis, E. (1996). Bubonic Plague. Available: http://ponderosa-pine.uoregon.edu/students/Janis/menu.html (Access date: January 6, 2000.)
3. Hanlon, J. J., and Pickett, G. E. (1979). *Public Health Administration and Practice*. St. Louis: C. V. Mosby Company.
4. Goerke, L. S., and Stebbins, E. L. (1968). *Mustard's Introduction to Public Health*, 5th ed. London: Macmillan Company.
5. Fox, J. P., Hall, C. E., and Elveback, L. R. (1970). *Epidemiology: Man and Disease*. New York: Macmillan Company.
6. Last, J. M., ed. (1995). *A Dictionary of Epidemiology*. New York: Oxford University Press.
7. Susser, M., and Adelstein, A. (1987). The Work of William Farr. In *Epidemiology, Health, & Society: Selected Papers* (by M. Susser). New York: Oxford University Press, pp. 49–57.
8. Lilienfeld, D. E., and Stolley, P. D. (1994). *Foundations of Epidemiology*, 3rd ed. New York: Oxford University Press.
9. Chin, J., ed. (2000). *Control of Communicable Diseases Manual*, 17th ed. Washington, DC: American Public Health Association.
10. Susser, M. (1987). Epidemiologists in Society. In *Epidemiology, Health, & Society: Selected Papers* (by M. Susser). New York: Oxford University Press, p. 11.
11. Centers for Disease Control and Prevention (1992). *Principles of Epidemiology: An Introduction to Applied Epidemiology and Biostatistics*, 2nd ed. Atlanta: The Centers.
12. Snow, J. ([no date] 1988). On the Mode of Communication of Cholera. In *The Challenge of Epidemiology: Issues and Selected Readings*, C. Buck, A. Llopis, E. Najera, and M. Terris, eds. Washington, DC: Pan American Health Organization, pp. 42–45.
13. Goldberger, J. ([1914] 1988). Considerations on Pellagra. In *The Challenge of Epidemiology: Issues and Selected Readings*, C. Buck, A. Llopis, E. Najera, and M. Terris, eds. Washington, DC: Pan American Health Organization, pp. 99–102.

CHAPTER THREE

Selected Disease Concepts in Epidemiology

Learning Objectives

▸ Define and give examples of communicable and noncommunicable diseases.

▸ Apply the ecological model to a given disease.

▸ Differentiate between models of disease and models of health.

▸ Use the concepts of natural history of disease and levels of prevention to describe the development, progression, and control of a given disease.

▸ Give examples of primary, secondary, and tertiary prevention.

▸ Describe the differences among active, passive, and herd immunity.

▸ Define disease, health, incubation period, latency period, subclinical disease, carrier, antibody, and antigen.

Overview

Disease is an important concept in epidemiology, and many efforts have been made to explain its occurrence. All diseases undergo a familiar life cycle known as the natural history of disease, which for any given individual may involve one or more of four distinct stages—susceptibility, presymptomatic disease, clinical disease, and diminished capacity. At each stage there is a corresponding and appropriate level of prevention that may be applied to preclude, resolve, or limit the effects of the disease. Immunity to communicable diseases can be acquired by active or passive means. Protection can also be achieved indirectly by the phenomenon of herd immunity.

Concepts of Disease and Health

Disease, which refers to physiological or psychological dysfunction,[1] is an important concept in epidemiology since much of the field deals with communicable and noncommunicable disease distribution, etiology, prevention, and control. **Communicable diseases** are those that can be transmitted directly or indirectly to a susceptible person through contact, inhalation, or ingestion. They are commonly referred to as **infectious diseases**.[2] By contrast, **noncommunicable diseases** are those that cannot be transmitted to others, either directly or indirectly. These are **noninfectious diseases**, such as diabetes, skin cancer, or stroke.

Epidemiology also deals with other health-related problems and issues that are not technically diseases. For example, epidemiology may look at the distribution or causes of various risk behaviors, such as cigarette smoking, sedentary lifestyle, or high fat consumption. In addition, epidemiology may be concerned with understanding the antecedents of social problems, such as child abuse, violence, or crime. Attributes such as joy and wellness may also be studied epidemiologically. None of these, however, is appropriately classified as disease. Nevertheless, partly because of the historical concerns of epidemiology (discussed in chapter 2) and partly because of the toll disease still takes on the quality and longevity of human life, disease remains an important focus of epidemiology and needs to be studied and understood. Some of the concepts of disease may also apply to other health-related problems.

The **ecological model**, or epidemiologic triangle, represents an attempt to explain disease causation using a very simple paradigm. According to this model, disease is caused by an imbalance among *host*, *agent*, and *environmental factors* (see figure 3–1). *Host factors* represent intrinsic characteristics that influence an individual's susceptibility to disease. These include immune status, general health status, genetic makeup, lifestyle practices, age, sex, and socioeconomic status. *Agents* consist of biological, chemical, and physical hazards that can induce disease. Biological agents include pathogenic microorganisms, such as bacteria, viruses, and parasites. Chemical agents generally involve toxic substances, such as lead, mercury, and carbon monoxide. Physical agents include extreme temperatures, excessive noise, and ionizing radiation. *Environmental factors* are extrinsic characteristics that can affect exposure to the agent, effectiveness or virulence of the agent, or susceptibility of the host. Examples include weather conditions, adequacy of living conditions, general levels of sanitation, population density, and access to health care. According to the ecological model, disease results when the agent, host, and environment are no longer in balance. This can occur when environment (the fulcrum in figure 3–1) shifts or when either the agent or host are no longer aligned due to changes in agent effectiveness or host susceptibility.

Although the ecological model was originally conceived to explain the causes of communicable diseases, it has also been applied to noncommunicable diseases and other health-related problems, but with less success. One of the problems is that it can be difficult to differentiate some agents from environmental factors.[3] Noise, for example, could be classified as an agent because it

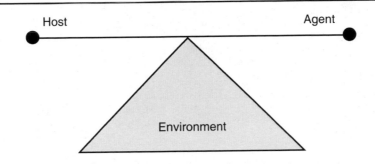

Host

Agent

Environment

Adapted from Centers for Disease Control and Prevention (1992). *Principles of Epidemiology: An Introduction to Applied Epidemiology and Biostatistics*, 2nd ed. Atlanta: The Centers, p. 36.

Figure 3–1 Ecological model of disease

induces hearing loss or as an environmental factor because it distracts attention, thereby increasing host susceptibility to injuries. In addition, G. E. Alan Dever argues that since the agent is traditionally considered essential for disease to occur, the ecological model represents a *single cause/single effect model* that is not applicable to noncommunicable diseases.[4] Indeed, he believes that a single cause/single effect model is not valid for most of the serious health problems facing contemporary society. When we consider chronic health problems and conditions, for example, *multiple cause/multiple effect models* appear to make more sense. According to these models, multiple factors like cigarette smoking, excessive alcohol consumption, stress, and poor diet can lead to multiple effects like heart disease, stroke, hypertension, and cancer.

    Holistic models of health go beyond the ecological model by looking at the factors that influence *health* versus disease. **Health** can be conceived as a state of well-being and positive functioning and not just the absence of disease.[5] Holistic models of health can serve as a basis for public health planning and policy making.[4] An example of an early holistic model is the *health field concept* developed by Marc Lalonde, former Canadian Minister of National Health and Welfare (see figure 3–2). Lalonde envisioned environment (e.g., food and water quality) lifestyle (e.g., drug and alcohol use), human biology (e.g., genetics and aging), and health care organization (e.g., accessibility, quality, and quantity of services) to be the key factors determining health.[6] The health field concept says that health exists when its four components are in balance. It is reasonable to conclude from this model that efforts to improve public health must include programs aimed at environmental protection and lifestyle management, as well as those directed toward optimizing human functioning and treating disease. Other models have gone beyond the relatively basic health field concept. One example is a model developed by R. G. Evans and G. L. Stoddart.[7] This model includes prosperity as a key element of community health (see figure 3–3).

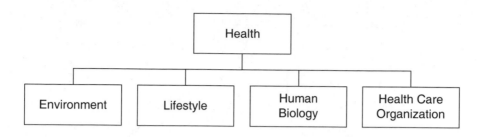

Reference: Lalonde, M. (1975). *A New Perspective on the Health of Canadians: A Working Document.* Ottawa: Information Canada.

Figure 3–2 Health field concept

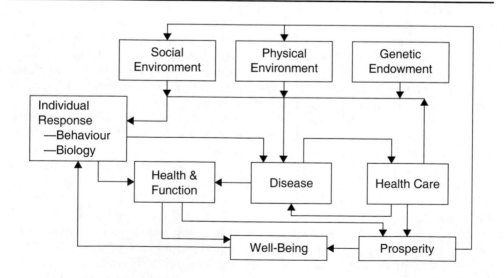

Source: Reprinted with permission from R. G. Evans, Morris L. Barer, and Theodore R. Marmor, eds. *Why Are Some People Healthy and Others Not? The Determinants of Health of Populations.* (New York: Aldine de Gruyter). Copyright ©1994 Walter de Gruyter Inc., New York.

Figure 3–3 Health model of Evans and Stoddart

Natural History of Disease

Every disease in a host follows a potentially predictable life cycle from onset to final outcome, which is known as its natural history. Understanding the **natural history of disease** is important to clinicians in establishing appropriate treatment and accurate prognosis, and it is vital to public health professionals in developing effective disease prevention and control strategies. Although the life cycle or natural history of a particular disease will vary somewhat from individual to individual, and different diseases will each have their own distinct natural histories, it is possible to identify four common stages that most diseases manifest:

- Stage of susceptibility
- Stage of presymptomatic disease
- Stage of clinical disease
- Stage of diminished capacity

The *stage of susceptibility* precedes the onset of disease. The disease has not yet developed, but the host is susceptible due to the presence of risk factors. Individuals with high serum cholesterol, hypertension, a sedentary lifestyle, and diabetes, for example, have an increased risk of developing coronary heart disease. Likewise, lack of sleep, excessive stress, and poor eating habits may predispose one to the common cold. Epidemiologists are continually seeking to identify and confirm risk factors for the major health problems that affect society. Ongoing research to determine if alcohol consumption is an important risk factor for breast cancer is one example.[8]

In the *stage of presymptomatic disease* the disease process has begun, but no overt signs or symptoms are evident to the host. For communicable diseases, this stage includes the **incubation period**, which is the time between the invasion of an infectious agent and the development of the first signs or symptoms of the disease. For noncommunicable diseases, it includes the **latency period** (or induction period), which is the time it takes for the disease to develop once the causes are in place. Cancer, for example, can be thought of as passing through three steps during the latency period. First, cancer is *initiated* by a carcinogen. Next, the cancer is *promoted* by the same or other agents, and third, the cancer *progresses* as cancerous cells divide and multiply. The latency period ends when cancer is manifested by signs or symptoms, or for practical purposes, when it is clinically detected and diagnosed.[1] The stage of presymptomatic disease also includes cases of **subclinical disease**, that is, disease that is fully developed but which produces no symptoms in the host (i.e., asymptomatic disease). A classic example concerns Typhoid Mary, the infamous cook and *carrier* of typhoid fever, who is believed to have infected as many as 53 people with typhoid fever over a period of 15 years.[9] The total number of infections that resulted from her presence could number in the thousands (see exhibit 3–1). A **carrier** of a communicable disease is an individual who has no symptoms of the disease but nevertheless harbors the causative agent, which can be transmitted to others.[1] Other examples of presymptomatic disease include atherosclerotic plaque buildup in the coronary arteries prior to the manifestation of any coronary heart disease symptoms and precancerous lesions of the cervix evident only from a Pap test.

Exhibit 3–1 A Brief Profile of Typhoid Mary

The infamous Typhoid Mary was really Mary Mallon, a New York cook who came to the United States from Ireland in 1883. In the summer of 1906 an outbreak of typhoid fever* occurred in the town of Oyster Bay on Long Island, New York. Though typhoid fever caused about 25,000 deaths in the United States in 1906, the outbreak in Oyster Bay surprised the three resident physicians, and local investigators were not able to find any obvious sources of contamination. Six of those living in the house where Mary was employed as a cook contracted typhoid fever, and one died. Concerned that they might not be able to rent the house, the owners commissioned George Soper, a sanitary engineer from the New York City Health Department, to investigate. After some initial dead ends, Soper began to focus his investigation on Mary Mallon, who had left unexpectedly about three weeks after the outbreak. Soper suspected she might be a healthy carrier of the disease. He later tracked her down in Manhattan where she was serving as a cook for another family. She reportedly threatened him when he asked her to be tested for the disease. Convinced she was a carrier, Soper looked into her work history and found that in the previous ten years she had worked for eight families, seven of whom came down with typhoid. A 1903 outbreak in Ithaca, New York, which claimed 1,300 lives, is believed to have originated with Mary Mallon. In March, 1907, Mary was taken, kicking and screaming, to a city hospital to be tested. Fecal samples showed high levels of *Salmonella typhi,* the bacillus that causes typhoid fever. Mary was offered to have her gall bladder removed, which would have ended her carrier state. She adamantly refused, claiming vociferously that she was not responsible for the outbreaks. Mary was therefore placed in an isolation cottage at Riverside Hospital on North Brother Island in New York. She remained there as a virtual prisoner and emerging celebrity until she was released three years later, ostensibly due to adverse public opinion. Conditions of her release stated that she would keep in touch with the health department and not work in food handling again. Several years later in 1915, she was found working as a cook in Sloane Maternity Hospital in Manhattan under the assumed name of Mrs. Brown. During her employment at the hospital she is believed to have infected at least 25 of the medical and support staff, two of whom died. She was handcuffed and taken back to a cottage on North Brother Island where she remained in relative isolation for the rest of her life. Mary died in 1938 around the age of 70 from complications of a stroke. According to one source, Mary Mallon still baked and sold cakes while on North Brother Island.

*Typhoid fever, which is characterized by sudden onset, causes sustained fever, severe headache, anorexia, malaise, splenomegaly, and sometimes rose-colored spots on the body. Although once prominent in the U.S., today less than 500 cases occur each year due to better sanitation measures aimed at water supplies, food, and milk. Untreated, typhoid fever has a case fatality rate of 10–20%.

References: Ochs, R. (no date). Dinner with Typhoid Mary. Available: http://www.lihistory.com/7/hs702a.htm (Access date: February 3, 2000.); Alcamo, I. E. (1997). *Fundamentals of Microbiology,* 5th ed. Menlo Park, CA: Benjamin/Cummings; Chin, J., ed. (2000). *Control of Communicable Diseases Manual,* 17th ed. Washington, DC: American Public Health Association.

In the *stage of clinical disease* the condition is clearly apparent, and the host experiences one or more overt signs or symptoms characteristic of the disease. This stage is where the disease is commonly diagnosed and treated by physicians. Clinical disease may range in degree of severity and advance slowly or rapidly depending upon a variety of host, agent, and environmental factors. As an example, influenza causes fever, headache, muscle aches, coughing, and fatigue in most adults for up to a week,[10] but in some, especially those with weak immune systems, symptoms may continue much longer. In addition, some individuals may appear only moderately upset by the symptoms, while others may find them quite oppressive. Some chronic diseases may be graded during this stage depending on their degree of progression. Cancer, for example, is classified by stages. *Stage one* cancers are localized and have not yet metastasized to other parts of the body. *Stage two* cancers have infiltrated underlying tissues more than stage one cancers, but they have still not metastasized to other parts of the body. *Stage three* cancers have metastasized to surrounding tissues, and *stage four* cancers have spread extensively throughout the body. This latter stage represents advanced cancer for which treatment is largely palliative.[2]

The final stage in the natural history of disease, the *stage of diminished capacity*, is characterized by a convalescent period or a residual disability. In the case of *convalescence*, there is a period following completion of clinical disease during which the individual has not yet returned to his or her former level of health. Though influenza has passed, for example, it may be several days or weeks before an individual feels enough strength to say he or she is well again. This represents the convalescent period. Many moderate to serious infectious diseases require some convalescence after the disease has run its course. *Residual disability* can result from diseases that produce temporary or protracted complications. Examples are poliomyelitis, which has left some of its victims with permanent physical disabilities, and influenza in the elderly, which can sometimes result in pneumonia. Also, heart attacks and strokes can leave individuals with limited functional capacity. The distinction between the convalescent period and residual disability is not always clear. In summary, the convalescent period represents the time it takes recovered (disease-free) individuals to get back on their feet, while residual disability refers to the development of complications or disability resulting directly from the clinical disease.

Ultimately, the natural history of a disease concludes in either full recovery or death. The number of stages a person passes through or the length of time one stays in a particular stage will vary depending on the particular disease, the overall health of the individual, and other factors. Individuals with chronic diseases, such as emphysema or a severe stroke, will remain in the clinical or diminished capacity stages for life.

Levels of Prevention

The definition of epidemiology encompasses preventing and controlling diseases in human populations. This is usually accomplished using three **levels of prevention**. *Primary prevention* seeks to reduce the frequency of new cases of disease occurring in a population and, thus, is most applicable to persons who are in the stage of susceptibility. *Secondary prevention* attempts to reduce the number of *existing* cases in a population and, therefore, is most appropriately aimed at those in the stage of presymptomatic disease or the early stage of clinical disease. *Tertiary prevention* tries to limit disability and improve functioning following disease or its complications, often through rehabilitation. Therefore, it is most applicable during the late clinical stage or the stage of diminished capacity.[11] The natural history of disease and the levels of prevention are closely linked. As illustrated in figure 3–4, appropriate levels of prevention may be applied at each stage of the natural history of disease.

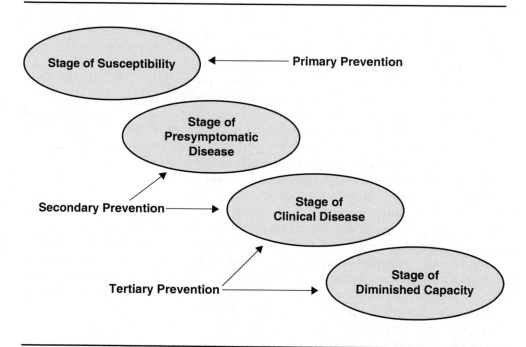

Figure 3–4 Stages in the natural history of disease and corresponding levels of prevention

Primary Prevention

Primary prevention strategies emphasize general health promotion, risk factor reduction, and other health protective measures. These strategies include health education and health promotion programs designed to foster healthier lifestyles and environmental health programs designed to improve environmental quality. Specific examples of primary prevention measures include immunization against communicable diseases; public health education about good nutrition, exercise, stress management, and individual responsibility for health; chlorination and filtration of public water supplies; and legislation requiring child restraints in motor vehicles.

Secondary Prevention

Secondary prevention focuses on early detection and swift treatment of disease. Its purpose is to cure disease, slow its progression, or reduce its impact on individuals or communities.[12] A common approach to secondary prevention is screening for disease, such as the noninvasive computerized test for the early detection of heart disease. This test uses computerized tomography scans to look for calcium deposition in the arteries, which can signal previously undetected heart disease. Other examples of screening include mammography for breast cancer detection; eye tests for glaucoma; blood tests for lead exposure; occult blood tests for colorectal cancer; the Pap test for cervical cancer; the breath test for *Helicobacter pylori*, the bacterium implicated in duodenal and gastric ulcers; and the Prostate-Specific Antigen (PSA) test for prostate cancer. In each case, screening is performed to detect disease early so prompt treatment can be initiated. Examples of other secondary prevention methods include treatment of hypertension to prevent complications and removal of skin cancer lesions as they occur.

Tertiary Prevention

Tertiary prevention strategies involve both therapeutic and rehabilitative measures once disease is firmly established.[5] Examples include treatment of diabetics to prevent complications of the disease and the ongoing management of chronic heart disease patients with medication, diet, exercise, and periodic examinations. Other examples include improving functioning of stroke patients through rehabilitation by occupational and physical therapy, nursing care, speech therapy, counseling, and so forth, and treating those suffering from complications of diseases such as meningitis, multiple sclerosis, or Parkinson's disease.

On a community level, providing high quality, appropriate, and accessible health care and public health resources is critical to assuring satisfactory primary, secondary, and tertiary prevention. Table 3–1 summarizes the three levels of prevention and provides examples of their applications at the community level.

Table 3–1 Examples of Levels of Prevention

Level of Prevention	Main Purpose	Examples at the Community Level
Primary	To prevent disease before it develops so as to maintain health	Smoking prevention programs, air pollution control enforcement, health education in the schools
Secondary	To diagnose and treat disease in its early stages so as to restore or improve health	Blood pressure screening for hypertension, vision screening in schools, case finding and referral for treatment of sexually transmitted diseases
Tertiary	To reduce complications of disease and improve functioning and quality of life where possible	Rehabilitation programs for heart attack victims, hospice programs for AIDS patients, group counseling for those with chronic fatigue syndrome

Immunity to Disease

Antibodies are involved in producing immunity to disease. When certain foreign substances, such as those introduced by pathogenic bacteria or viruses, enter the body, antibodies are formed as a defensive response. Antibodies are protein substances or globulins derived from B and T lymphocytes, which originate in the bone marrow. They are *specific* to the particular invading substance, known as an **antigen**, and thus provide highly selective protection.[2] Because antigens stimulate antibody production, we often speak of antigen-antibody reactions. Antibody production is important to epidemiology because *titers* (concentrations) of specific antibodies can be measured in individuals and used to indicate the relative immunity of different populations to specific diseases, as well as to identify asymptomatic cases of disease.[1]

Disease immunity can be classified as active or passive. **Active immunity** occurs when the body produces antibodies in reaction to an infection or a vaccine.[2] Vaccines typically use attenuated, modified, or killed pathogenic organisms, or their inactive toxins, to achieve active immunity in the host without producing disease.[1] **Passive immunity** can be acquired in three ways:

- By injection of a serum (a refined suspension containing antibodies already produced by another host, e.g., immune globulin)
- By placental transfer (i.e., transfer of a mother's antibodies to her developing fetus during pregnancy)
- By breast-feeding (i.e., transfer of a mother's antibodies to her child through breast milk)

The major differences between active and passive immunity have to do with how rapidly protection against a given disease is conferred and how long the protection lasts. In general, active immunity takes about two to three weeks to confer immunity, while passive immunity is immediate. On the other hand, active immunity often lasts a lifetime, while passive immunity persists about two weeks if received from a serum and up to six months if received by placental transfer or breast-feeding.[2]

Another concept related to disease immunity is **herd immunity**, which refers to the resistance of a group or population to the spread of a specific disease through the group. This resistance is due to the fact that a high proportion of the group members is immune to the particular disease. Herd immunity can be thought of as simply group immunity. It is important to epidemiology because it renders populations less susceptible to epidemics from particular diseases. The reason for this becomes clearer when one realizes that:

> *The probability of a communicable disease spreading in a population depends on the number of susceptible people in that population and the likelihood that a susceptible person will come into contact with someone who is infected with the disease.*

Thus, the higher the proportion of immune individuals in a population, the less chance there is that a susceptible person will come into contact with an infected person. Herd immunity is most often achieved by prior immunity resulting from previous immunization or recovery from an active case of the disease. Theoretically, when at least 85–90% of a population are immune to a given disease, herd immunity should be expected to protect most of the other 10–15%.[9, 13] Therefore, it would seem that the ideal goal of 100% immunization touted for many vaccine-preventable diseases is not always necessary to prevent disease outbreaks. One problem with this thinking, however, is that the remaining susceptible people frequently represent a demographic subgroup where the members live in close proximity to each other. If the disease is introduced into the subgroup, a localized outbreak could occur.[13] Therefore, it is important to realize that the concept of herd immunity assumes a relatively well distributed population of immune persons.

Many vaccines are available for use in the United States to prevent potentially serious communicable diseases. General recommendations for adult immunizations may be modified depending on the history of childhood vaccinations and prior diseases. However, a list of the more common vaccines that are currently available for adult immunization is presented in table 3–2 on page 34. Routine childhood vaccines include the following:

- Hepatitis B (Hep B) vaccine
- Diphtheria, tetanus, pertussis (DTaP) vaccine
- *Haemophilus influenzae* type b (Hib) vaccine
- Polio (IPV) vaccine
- Measles, mumps, rubella (MMR) vaccine
- Varicella (Var) vaccine
- Hepatitis A (Hep A) vaccine

With the exception of the Hep A vaccine, which is recommended only in selected states or regions where hepatitis A is a concern,[14] all childhood vaccines are recommended for general administration to children before the age of two.

Summary

- Disease is an important concept in epidemiology because much of the field deals with its distribution, etiology, prevention, and control. In recent years, epidemiology has expanded to encompass all types of health-related problems and issues.

- The ecological model is a relatively simple paradigm for explaining disease causation in terms of host, agent, and environmental factors. According to this model, disease occurs when these three factors are not in balance. While useful in explaining infectious diseases, the model seems less applicable to many contemporary health issues and, therefore, has often been replaced by more complex models, including holis-

Table 3–2 Commonly Available Vaccines for Adults in the United States*

Vaccine	Purpose	General Applicability
Tetanus and Diphtheria Toxoids (Td) Vaccine	To prevent tetanus (lockjaw) and diphtheria	All adults every 10 years
Influenza Vaccine	To prevent influenza	Adults at high risk (e.g., over age 65, chronically ill, pregnant), or at risk of transmitting influenza to high-risk individuals, each year during the fall
Pneumococcal Pneumonia (PPV) Vaccine	To prevent pneumococcal pneumonia	Adults at high risk (e.g., over age 65, presence of certain chronic illnesses or other conditions, Alaskan natives, certain Native Americans)
Measles and Mumps Vaccines	To prevent measles and mumps	Adults born prior to 1956 without written documentation of immunization on or before age one
Rubella Vaccine	To prevent rubella (German measles)	Adults, especially women, without written documentation of immunization on or before age one or those whose blood tests show no previous rubella infection
Polio Vaccine	To prevent polio	Adults at increased risk (e.g., certain travelers, lab workers, unvaccinated adults whose children will receive the live vaccine)
Varicella Vaccine	To prevent varicella (chickenpox)	Adults uncertain if they have had chickenpox, health care workers who have not had chickenpox, and certain other high-risk groups
Hepatitis A Vaccine	To prevent hepatitis A	Adults at high risk (e.g., travelers to areas where hepatitis A is endemic, sexually active homosexual men, illegal drug users, and certain other high-risk groups)
Hepatitis B Vaccine	To prevent hepatitis B	Adults at high risk (e.g., health care workers, hemophiliacs, sexually active homosexual men, illegal drug users, and certain other high-risk groups)

*The guidelines presented in this table are for summary purposes only. Individuals should seek a qualified health professional for specific medical advice, including vaccine applicability, contraindications, and possible side effects.

Reference: Zanca, J. A. (November, 1998). Adult Vaccines: Who Should Get What, and When? In *Closing the Gap* (Office of Minority Health). Washington, DC: U.S. Public Health Service.

tic models of health, such as the Health Field Concept and the model of Evans and Stoddart. Health is usually conceived of as a state of well-being and positive functioning and not just the absence of disease.

- Understanding the natural history of disease, its four stages (susceptibility, presymptomatic disease, clinical disease, and diminished capacity), and the three levels of prevention (primary, secondary, and tertiary) are helpful in developing effective public health interventions.

- Immunity to disease may be due to active immunity, which occurs when the body produces its own antibodies in reaction to an infection or vaccine, or to passive immunity, which occurs when one receives antibodies produced by another host. Herd immunity is group immunity due to a high proportion of immune individuals in a population and tends to reduce the epidemic potential of a given disease when the immune population is well distributed.

- There are many vaccines available in the United States that can be used to prevent potentially serious communicable diseases in children and adults.

New Terms

active immunity	ecological model	levels of prevention
antibody	health	natural history of disease
antigen	herd immunity	noncommunicable disease
carrier	incubation period	noninfectious disease
communicable disease	infectious disease	passive immunity
disease	latency period	subclinical disease

Study Questions and Exercises

1. Use the ecological model to explain the occurrence of plague in medieval Europe. (Note that chapter 2 discusses plague.)

2. Describe in detail the natural history of coronary heart disease and provide specific examples of prevention strategies that can be applied at the individual and community levels at each stage of the natural history of the disease. Identify the prevention strategies by level of prevention.

3. In school immunization programs, it is usually impossible to achieve a 100% immunization rate due to legitimate objections by parents on the grounds of religion, medical contraindications, or other reasons. Explain why and under what circumstances 100% immunization for a given disease may not be required to protect the students and their families from an outbreak of the disease.

4. Use the health field concept to explain the low prevalence of childhood malnutrition in the United States.

References

1. Last, J. M., ed. (1995). *A Dictionary of Epidemiology*. New York: Oxford University Press.
2. Hurster, M. M. (1997). *Communicable and Non-Communicable Disease Basics: A Primer*. Westport, CT: Bergin and Garvey.
3. Page, R. M., Cole, G. E., and Timmreck, T. C. (1995). *Basic Epidemiological Methods and Biostatistics: A Practical Guidebook*. Boston: Jones and Bartlett Publishers.
4. Dever, G. E. A. (1980). *Community Health Analysis: A Holistic Approach*. Germantown, MD: Aspen.
5. Beaglehole, R., Bonita, R., and Kjellström, T. (1993). *Basic Epidemiology*. Geneva: World Health Organization.
6. Lalonde, M. (1975). *A New Perspective on the Health of Canadians: A Working Document*. Ottawa: Information Canada.
7. Evans, R. G., and Stoddart, G. L. (1994). Producing Health, Consuming Health Care. In *Why Are Some People Healthy and Others Not? The Determinants of Health of Populations*, R. G. Evans, M. L. Barer, and T. R. Marmor, eds. New York: Aldine de Gruyter, pp. 27–64.
8. Swanson, C. A., Coates, R. J., Malone, K. E., Gammon, M. D., Schoenberg, J. B., Brogan, D. J., McAdams, M., Potischman, N., Hoover, R. N., and Brinton, L. A. (1997). Alcohol Consumption and Breast Cancer Risk Among Women Under Age 45 Years. *Epidemiology*: 8(3): 231–237.
9. Timmreck, T. C. (1998). *An Introduction to Epidemiology*, 2nd ed. Boston: Jones and Bartlett Publishers.
10. Chin, J., ed. (2000). *Control of Communicable Diseases Manual*, 17th ed. Washington, DC: American Public Health Association.
11. Duncan, D. F. (1988). *Epidemiology: Basis for Disease Prevention and Health Promotion*. New York: Macmillan.
12. Mausner, J. S., and Kramer, S. (1985). *Mausner & Bahn Epidemiology—An Introductory Text*. Philadelphia: W. B. Saunders Company.
13. Centers for Disease Control and Prevention (1992). *Principles of Epidemiology: An Introduction to Applied Epidemiology and Biostatistics*, 2nd ed. Atlanta: The Centers.
14. American Academy of Pediatrics (2000). Immunization Protects Children 2000 Immunization Schedule. Available: http://www.aap.org/family/parents/immunize.htm (Access date: February 3, 2000.)

CHAPTER FOUR

An Overview of Epidemiologic Study Designs

Learning Objectives

▸ Explain the differences between observational and experimental epidemiology.

▸ Summarize the differences among descriptive, analytic, and experimental studies.

▸ Identify the four types of ecological studies.

▸ Distinguish among preventive, intervention, and therapeutic trials, respectively.

▸ Correctly classify descriptions of epidemiologic studies as to their specific study designs.

▸ Define unit of analysis, ecological unit, ecological fallacy, primary and secondary sources, and quasi-experimental study.

▸ Compare and contrast reference population, experimental population, and study sample; and exposure and outcome, respectively.

Overview

Epidemiologic studies can be broadly categorized as observational or experimental. Observational studies, which include descriptive and analytic studies, do not involve direct intervention and control by the investigators. Descriptive studies include ecological and cross-sectional studies, as well as case reports and case series, which are common in clinical applications. Analytic studies also include ecological and cross-sectional studies, in addition to case-control, cohort, and hybrid studies. Experimental studies, which involve direct intervention and control by the investigators, consist of randomized controlled trials and community trials. Unlike descriptive studies, both analytic and experimental studies test predetermined hypotheses about the associations between exposures and outcomes.

Introduction

This chapter introduces the more commonly used study designs in epidemiology. Since some of these designs are referred to in subsequent chapters, it is important that you have a working knowledge of them before proceeding further. Chapters 10–13 provide additional details on specific types of studies, including a discussion of potential sources of error and basic methods of analysis.

Before we begin discussing epidemiologic study designs some terms related to *exposure* and *outcome* need to be explained. In epidemiology, when the term **exposure** is used, such as in the statement, "the exposure is associated with heart disease," it refers to a potential risk factor, whether that factor represents an actual exposure (e.g., environmental tobacco smoke), a behavior (e.g., sedentary lifestyle), or an individual attribute (e.g., age). **Exposure status** is a term for classifying individuals or groups according to their level of exposure, as defined above. **Outcome** is the disease or other health-related problem that is being studied (e.g., heart disease), and **outcome status** is the classification on the outcome. Both exposure status and outcome status can be dichotomous (e.g., exposed or unexposed; diseased or not diseased) or have several levels (e.g., high, moderate, low, or no exposure; severe, moderate, mild, or no disease). Unless otherwise indicated, we will describe studies where both exposure and outcome are dichotomous.

The application of the above terms can be illustrated by a study designed to assess the risk of lung cancer (the *outcome*) from cigarette smoking (the *exposure*). This study might compare the risk of developing lung cancer among smokers (the *exposed group*) to the risk of developing lung cancer among nonsmokers (the *unexposed group*). In this example, exposure status refers to whether or not one smokes cigarettes. Outcome status refers to whether or not one develops lung cancer.

Categories of Epidemiologic Studies

There are two broad categories into which epidemiologic studies can be classified. These categories are:

- Observational studies
- Experimental studies

Observational studies are epidemiologic studies where the investigators collect, record, and analyze data on subjects as they naturally divide themselves by potentially significant variables.[1] By contrast, **experimental studies** involve some type of intervention and control by the investigators. Most important, the investigators control the exposure status of the subjects. In observational studies, the exposure status of the subjects is not under the control of the investigators. To illustrate this difference, consider two possible ways of studying the effect of vitamin C supplementation on the prevention of the common cold. In an *observational study*, investigators might select a sample of individuals, query them about their use of vitamin C, and then follow up to see if those who routinely take a certain amount of vitamin C develop fewer colds than those who do not. In an *experimental study*, the investigators may randomly assign volunteers to take a prescribed amount of vitamin C or to take an inactive substance (i.e., a placebo), and then follow up to see if the exposed group develops fewer colds than the unexposed group. In the first example, there was no intervention or control by the investigators (i.e., the subjects were not asked to change their exposure status). The investigators simply observed what occurred in the exposed and unexposed groups. In the second example, the investigators intervened by altering the subjects' exposure (i.e., the investigators controlled the exposure by determining that some subjects would take the vitamin and some would not). Thus, the investigators intervened into the lives of the subjects.

Observational studies encompass *descriptive* and *analytic epidemiology* (see chapter 1). Descriptive epidemiology involves **descriptive studies**, and analytic epidemiology involves **analytic studies**, both of which are discussed below. *Experimental studies* encompass a third dimension of epidemiology, **experimental epidemiology**, which focuses on experimental approaches to identifying the determinants of morbidity or mortality in human populations. To recapitulate briefly, epidemiologic studies may be observational or experimental. Observational studies include both descriptive studies and analytic studies, while experimental studies exist in a class by themselves. This is illustrated in figure 4–1.

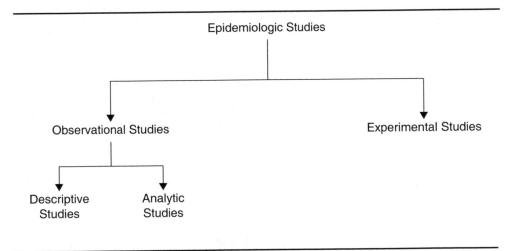

Figure 4–1 Classification of epidemiologic studies

Descriptive Studies

Descriptive studies are a class of epidemiologic studies that focus on characterizing morbidity or mortality in populations by person, place, or time variables and that have no *a priori* hypotheses. That is, they are not designed to test preconceived suppositions about the relationships between exposures and outcomes. Instead, their focus is on describing what exists. For example, an investigator may study the frequency and quantity of alcohol consumption among college students by various demographic factors, such as age, sex, race/ethnicity, socioeconomic background, and academic level. In this example, the investigator is simply observing *what exists* in a population in order to discover patterns that may later turn out to have some predictive value.

Descriptive studies can be very useful and do not always require original data collection. In fact, quite often epidemiologists use data previously collected from other sources (e.g., federal or state agencies, private health insurers, school systems) to summarize specific health problems. Descriptive studies are helpful in generating hypotheses about disease causation. This is why descriptive studies often precede more advanced epidemiologic investigations. Descriptive studies are also useful in demonstrating trends, such as the secular trend in the U.S. infant mortality rate for all races, which has been characterized by a marked, sustained decline of over 70% since 1965.[2] In addition, descriptive studies may be valuable to health professionals by providing a profile of susceptible populations that can aid diagnosis and assist in planning and allocating scarce health care resources in communities.[3]

There are four common types of descriptive studies: *case reports, case series, ecological studies,* and *cross-sectional studies.* A **case report** is a detailed description of an individual patient. Published case reports provide a valuable educational service by bringing unusual or rare conditions to the attention of other clinicians. This in turn can lead to speculation about possible risk factors or causes of the problem and, at the same time, stimulate further investigation. Birth defects from thalidomide, a sedative widely used in Europe during the 1960s, and fetal alcohol syndrome were first described in case reports.[4] Though common in clinical epidemiology, case reports are not in the strictest sense epidemiologic studies since they are not population based, a hallmark of epidemiologic studies.

A **case series** is an extension of the case report that describes the characteristics of a group or cluster of individuals with the same disease or symptoms. Case series attempt to quantify various aspects of the group so as to present a relatively complete profile of the illness. It was a case series, for example, that first identified toxic shock syndrome, which was later determined by analytic epidemiologic studies to be strongly associated with the use of Rely brand tampons.[5] Today, we know that this rare but severe condition is associated with strains of *Staphylococcus aureus*, a toxin-producing bacterium.[6] Like case reports, case series are not strictly epidemiologic studies. Nevertheless, as was the case with toxic shock syndrome, they can stimulate the initiation of epidemiologic investigations.

While clinical epidemiology frequently employs case reports or case series to describe health-related problems, classical epidemiology often employs **ecological studies** and **cross-sectional studies**. Ecological and cross-sectional studies can be descriptive or analytic, depending on whether or not there are hypotheses to be tested. Case reports and case series are exclusively descriptive designs. Descriptive ecological and cross-sectional studies are discussed in the next section along with their analytic counterparts because of similarities in the descriptive and analytic designs. Descriptive ecological and cross-sectional studies differ from their analytic counterparts primarily due to the fact that they have not been designed to test specific relationships between exposure and outcome and, therefore, may not have valid comparison groups. Without a valid comparison group it is impossible to say confidently whether any particular outcome is really due to a given exposure.[7]

Analytic Studies

Unlike descriptive studies, *analytic studies* are designed to test hypotheses about the association between an *exposure* of interest and a particular *outcome*. This can be illustrated graphically as follows:

$$\text{Exposure} \xrightarrow{?} \text{Outcome}$$

As mentioned previously, analytic studies, like descriptive studies, are *observational* and not experimental (see figure 4–1). There are five common types of analytic studies in epidemiology, in addition to hybrid studies, which represent combinations of two or more of the other study designs. They are:

- Ecological studies
- Cross-sectional studies
- Case-control studies
- Prospective cohort studies
- Retrospective cohort studies
- Hybrid studies

Ecological studies and *cross-sectional studies* can also be classified as descriptive studies as discussed in the previous section. In fact, some epidemiologists disagree as to how these two designs are best classified. The reason for the disagreement has to do with limitations on the inferences that can be drawn from associations identified in these study types. One solution is to consider the *intent* of the study. If the intent in a particular application is simply to *describe* a given health problem, then the study should be classified as descriptive. On the other hand, if the intent is to *test* a predetermined hypothesis, even in a preliminary way, then the study can be regarded as an analytic study. Therefore, both ecological and cross-sectional studies can be descriptive when their intent is to describe morbidity or mortality by person, place, or time variables and analytic when their intent is to test predetermined hypotheses about the associations between specific exposures and specific outcomes. This will become clearer once these study designs have been explained.

Ecological Studies

In order to understand ecological studies, it is important to grasp what is meant by **unit of analysis**. Unit of analysis refers to that which is being studied.[8] In most epidemiologic studies the unit of analysis is the individual. In other words, epidemiologists typically study individuals in order to draw conclusions about groups. To say, for example, that smokers are at a significantly higher risk of lung cancer than nonsmokers is to draw a conclusion about a group of people (smokers) presumably based on a study of individuals, some of whom smoke and some of whom do not. The unit of analysis in the ecological study, however, is the *group* versus the individual. The group, or **ecological unit**, as it has been traditionally referred to, represents an aggregate of individuals, such as countries, states, counties, cities, census tracts, hospitals, or schools. As discussed in chapter 10, ecological units can also represent time periods, such as groups in 2000 and 2002.

Because in ecological studies the unit of analysis is the group, investigators have a *summary* measure of exposure and a *summary* measure of outcome for each group being compared.[9] Data on exposure and outcome for individuals have not been collected. For example, an analytic ecological study conducted in Taiwan examined the association between chlorinated drinking water (the exposure) and cancer mortality (the outcome) among 28 municipalities (the groups or ecological units).[10] The investigators found a positive correlation between the use of chlorinated drinking water and mortality from rectal, lung, bladder, and kidney cancer. It is critical to understand that only municipalities as a whole were studied, and the investigators had no comparable data for the individuals in these communities. Therefore, the only association identified by the investigators was at the *group level*. It is not known what the association is at the individual level due to the study design. In other words, it was the municipalities chlorinating their drinking water that had the higher rates of cancer compared to the municipalities not chlorinating their water. The association between drinking chlorinated water and cancer among individuals was not examined. If we assume that individuals who drink chlorinated water are at a higher risk of certain cancers based on the study findings, we commit an **ecological fallacy**, which is an "error of reasoning" that one commits when group associations are used to draw conclusions about associations at the individual level that may not necessarily exist.[8] The problem with drawing conclusions at the individual level based on group associations can be further understood if one considers that in the example it is possible that those who tended to die from cancer were more likely to be individuals who drank water from unchlorinated alternate sources, such as bottled water or private wells (possibly contaminated), instead of the chlorinated municipal drinking water supply. If the proportion of this group was higher in the municipalities with chlorinated water than in those without chlorinated water, then this could explain the group association even though no similar association exists with chlorine on the individual level. Ecological fallacies are problematic because we usually cannot tell whether an association that exists on a group level also exists on an individual level based on an ecological study alone.

Despite their limitations, ecological studies are valuable to epidemiologists because ecological studies are relatively quick and inexpensive to perform and they provide clues to possible associations between exposures and outcomes of interest. In this light, they may be a good choice for the initial investigation of preliminary hypotheses that have not yet been widely examined. In some instances, group associations may be just as important or more important than individual associations in understanding multifactorial etiology.[11] For example, one may want to know if countries with nationalized health care have lower rates of infant mortality than countries without nationalized health care. In this case, the variables, nationalized health care and country-specific infant mortality, are group phenomena that are most appropriately studied at the group level. More is said about this in chapter 10.

Hal Morgenstern has identified four types of ecological study designs: [12]

- *Exploratory studies.* These are *descriptive* ecological studies that look at variations in outcomes across ecological units, such as countries, states, etc. Exposure is not assessed in these studies, and the purpose is to search for spatial patterns that might suggest etiologic hypotheses. An example of results from an exploratory study appears in figure 4–2. In this illustration, average annual injury death rates for each of 11 different countries were compared. England and Wales had the lowest rate of 31 injury deaths per 100,000 population, while France had the highest rate of 75 injury deaths per 100,000. Scotland was in the middle with an injury death rate of about 50 per 100,000. The data in this example do not appear to suggest any obvious explanations for the pattern. Further analysis, however, may reveal important differences between countries that could serve as a basis for additional study. Differences in death registration and reporting practices among the countries are possible explanations that are being investigated.[13]

- *Multiple-group comparison studies.* These are ecological studies that look for or test associations between average exposure levels (e.g., per capita consumption of dietary fat) and overall outcome rates (e.g., mortality rates from coronary heart disease) among several groups (e.g., countries). A typical research question might be, "Do countries with high levels of dietary fat intake have higher rates of coronary heart disease than those with low levels of fat intake?" To answer this question, one could obtain published information on average dietary fat intake for each of the countries in the sample and information on country-specific mortality rates from coronary heart disease. These data would represent **secondary sources*** and most likely would come from different agencies (e.g., the Food and Agricultural Organization and the World Health Organization, respectively). Typically, these data would have been collected for other purposes, and data linking fat intake and heart disease on the individual level would not be available.

---

* Secondary sources are sources of data that have not been collected firsthand. Therefore, they represent non-original sources. When investigators use other people's data in their research instead of data they have collected themselves, they are relying on secondary sources. **Primary sources** represent original data collected firsthand.[8]

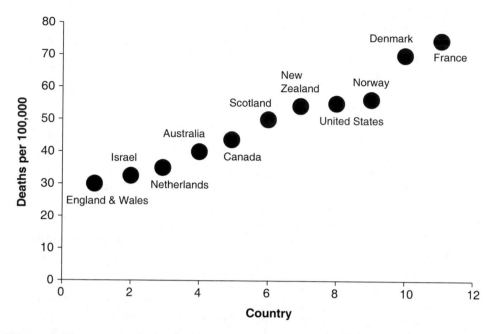

Reference: Fingerhut, L. A., Cox, C. S., Warner, M., et al. (1998). International Comparative Analysis of Injury Mortality: Findings from the ICE on Injury Statistics. *Advance Data from Vital and Health Statistics*, No. 303. Hyattsville, MD: National Center for Health Statistics.

Figure 4–2 Average annual injury death rates

- *Time-trend studies*. These ecological studies are also known as time-series studies. Their purpose is to detect changes in the average exposure level and outcome rates for a single population over time.
- *Mixed studies*. These studies examine the changes in average exposure level and outcome rates for several populations over time. They can be thought of as a combination of multiple-group comparison and time-trend studies.

The major difference between descriptive and analytic ecological studies is that the former are not designed to test predetermined hypotheses, although they may be useful in generating hypotheses for further study. Analytic ecological studies are conducted to test hypotheses, even if only in a preliminary way. Therefore, these studies always evaluate the relationship between one or more exposures and one or more outcomes. Hypotheses should be evident either explicitly or implicitly in published analytic studies. Keep in mind that having a hypothesis means that the investigator intended to test a *specific* association between an exposure and an outcome *before* the study began. Chapter 10 discusses other issues related to ecological studies.

Cross-Sectional Studies

Analytic cross-sectional studies assess both exposure and outcome status at the same point in time or during a brief period of time, where the individual is the unit of analysis. Thus, data on exposure and outcome can be said to be collected simultaneously. These studies generally survey, interview, examine, or observe a representative sample of individuals from a population. Figure 4–3 illustrates the basic format of an analytic cross-sectional study. Note that once the sample is selected, both exposure and outcome status are determined. Being analytic, there is one or more a priori hypotheses about the relationships between specific exposures and outcomes that the study seeks to verify. An example is a study conducted by J. A. Metz and colleagues that sought to determine if blood pressure and dietary intake of calcium (the exposures) were associated with bone mass (the outcome).[14] After selecting a sample of men, the investigators measured the subjects' blood pressure, assessed their dietary intake, and tested their bone mass all in the same time frame. They found that blood pressure levels showed an inverse association, and calcium intake a positive association, with regional measures of bone mass, a factor important in osteoporosis. Because the temporal sequence in which exposure and outcome occurred was not clear, the authors were careful not to suggest that the associations were causal. In order for an exposure to be classified as a risk factor or a cause of an outcome it must, among other things, *precede* the outcome. This, by the way, is one of the limitations of most cross-sectional studies. It is often difficult to establish a clear time separation between exposure and outcome because these attributes are assessed at the same time. One cannot always be sure whether exposure preceded outcome or outcome preceded exposure.

In a *descriptive* cross-sectional study, there is no hypothesis; the study is designed to uncover patterns of distribution by person, place, or time variables that may suggest hypotheses for further study. In some descriptive cross-sectional studies, only exposure or only outcome is assessed. A study

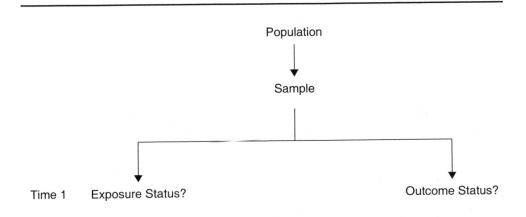

Figure 4–3 Cross-sectional study design

designed simply to determine HIV prevalence,* that is, the number of those infected with HIV in a specific community at a particular time, is an example of a descriptive cross-sectional study where exposure factors are of no current interest. Cross-sectional studies need to be well designed if the results are to be meaningful. Additional details regarding the cross-sectional design, its limitations, interpretation, and analysis can be found in chapter 10.

Case-Control Studies

Case-control studies begin by classifying subjects according to their outcome status. Cases of the disease being investigated are selected along with a comparable group of controls who do not have the outcome in question. The cases and controls are then queried or examined for exposures of interest (see figure 4–4). Ideally, only *new* cases of disease are included in the

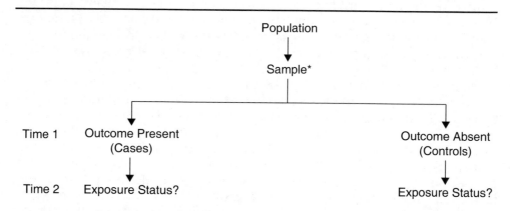

*Frequently in case-control studies cases and controls are selected separately

Figure 4–4 Case-control study design

study, and only *past* exposures are assessed. This is done to maintain an appropriate temporal sequence between exposure and outcome, which is necessary to make statements about risk or causation. A positive association between exposure and outcome resulting from a case-control study is said to exist when the proportion of cases with the exposure is significantly greater than the proportion of controls with the exposure, all other factors being equal. The case-control method is illustrated in a study of the relationship between environmental tobacco smoke (ETS) and lung cancer. In this study, the researchers interviewed 292 nonsmoking subjects with lung cancer (the cases) and 1,338 nonsmoking controls about prior exposure to ETS. Among the findings was a 164% increase in the risk of lung cancer among those who

* Prevalence, which is discussed in chapter 5, is the usual measure of disease frequency in cross-sectional studies. Generally, when studies employ prevalence, one may suspect that they are descriptive or analytic versions of cross-sectional studies. In fact, some epidemiologists refer to cross-sectional studies as prevalence studies.

were exposed to the highest levels of ETS in their transportation vehicles.[15] Case-control studies are discussed further in chapter 11.

Prospective Cohort Studies

Unlike case-control studies, **prospective cohort studies** (PCSs) begin by classifying subjects without the outcome of interest on the basis of exposure status. The subjects, known as the cohort, are then followed longitudinally into the future to determine if the rate of development of the study outcome is significantly higher in the exposed group compared to the unexposed group (see figure 4–5). A finding that the incidence (see chapter 5) of the outcome is higher in the exposed versus the unexposed group implies that the exposure is associated with the outcome, all other factors being equal. If this is the case, the exposure can be said to increase the risk of the outcome. In one sense, PCSs are the opposite design of case-control studies. Case-control studies start with the outcome and end with the exposure, while PCSs start with the exposure and end with the outcome. One other major difference is that PCSs, especially those investigating chronic diseases, generally take a long time to complete. The investigators must provide sufficient time for the study disease to develop, which may take many years. The longer the latency period, the longer the follow-up period needs to be. The fact that the disease has already occurred in case-control studies removes the need for a follow-up period.

The Framingham Heart Study, which was referred to in chapter 1, and a study conducted by E. J. Jacobs, M. J. Thun, and L. F. Apicella[16] are examples of PCSs. The latter is a U.S.-based study, which ran from 1982 to 1991 and examined the relationship between cigar smoking (the exposure) and death from coronary heart disease (the outcome) in 121,278 men 30 years of age and older. The subjects completed a baseline questionnaire in 1982 designed to assess smoking history and determine the presence of other risk factors. Only subjects who were free of heart disease at baseline were included in the study. The results showed that males less than 75 years old who smoked cigars at the beginning of the study had a 30% higher risk of dying from cor-

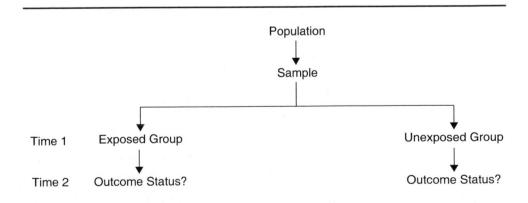

Figure 4–5 Basic cohort study design

onary heart disease compared to those who did not smoke cigars. It is important to note that this investigation excluded subjects who already had heart disease at the beginning of the study. This is critical if the findings are to be attributed to the observed exposure. It is also important in PCSs to reassess the exposure at regular intervals if it can change over time. In this way, subject exposure can be reclassified where necessary and the change accounted for in the analysis. This and other pertinent design issues concerning prospective cohort studies are examined in chapter 12.

Retrospective Cohort Studies

Retrospective cohort studies (RCSs) are a variation of the basic cohort study design. In these studies a *historical* cohort is reconstructed from existing data sources at the beginning of the study. The cohort is considered historical because it represents a group of people as they once were in the past. For example, researchers conducting an RCS on the effects of pesticide exposure on cancer mortality might reconstruct a cohort of factory workers who were employed by a particular pesticide manufacturer from 1960 to 1965 using personnel records supplied by the company. Because of the time element, we would expect few of the members of this cohort to be working for the company today. In fact, some may even be deceased. Nevertheless, the attempt is to assemble *on paper* a cohort that would have existed between 1960 and 1965. Once the cohort has been identified, the next step is to classify the subjects by exposure status. This can be difficult unless good records are available to identify exposed and unexposed groups. One might classify the exposed group, for instance, as those who worked with pesticides on a routine basis and the unexposed group as those who did not. This information might be available from company records indicating job classifications. Other records (e.g., company medical records) would need to be reviewed to identify factors that could confound the association or otherwise invalidate the study. Assuming this information was available, the final step would be to see what happened to each of the cohort members. This would involve follow-up of cohort members from 1960 to the present, perhaps by contacting the subjects themselves, their families or relatives, or by consulting cancer registries, death certificates, and other data sources. Similar to the PCS, we would want to know whether the exposed group had a higher mortality rate from cancer than the unexposed group. In other words, does pesticide exposure increase the risk of cancer?

Both RCSs and PCSs assess exposure *first* and outcome *second*; however, this is done in different time frames. Prospective cohort studies assess exposure status in the *present* (defined as exposure status at the beginning of the study) and outcome status in the *future* (defined as disease status by the end of the study). By contrast, RCSs assess exposure in the *past* (defined as exposure status at the time the cohort actually existed) and outcome status in the *present* (defined as the disease status at the time of the study). Thus, RCSs follow the cohort from the past to the present, and PCSs follow the cohort from the present to the future. This difference in time frame is illustrated in figure 4–6.

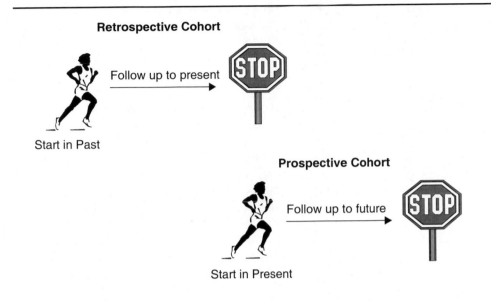

Figure 4–6 Retrospective versus prospective cohort study designs

Hybrid Studies

Not all analytic epidemiologic studies fit neatly into the above categories. Some studies combine features of two or more designs. These studies can be referred to as **hybrid studies**.[17] While a detailed discussion of these designs is beyond the scope of this book, it should be helpful to outline briefly a few of the more common types.

- **Nested case-control study.** This increasingly popular study design involves a case-control study within a prospective cohort study. Cases are selected from those who develop the study disease during the follow-up period in a cohort study. Controls are selected from cohort members who have not developed the disease during the same time period. One reason these studies are appealing is because of the increasing number of large, well-established cohort studies that can serve as data sources.[11] Another reason is because the cases and controls are more likely to be comparable than in traditional case-control designs since they both come from the same well-defined population. This has the effect of minimizing potential selection bias (see chapter 8) that is problematic in many case-control studies.[11, 17] A variation of the nested case-control study is the **nested case-cohort study**. Instead of selecting controls from cohort members who do not develop the disease, a sample is selected randomly from all members of the cohort at the beginning of the study. Those subjects who later become cases can be sorted out during the analysis phase. The *nested* *case-cohort study* provides a simple way of identifying controls for subsequent case-control studies and can provide data on the prevalence of various risk factors.[11, 18] The term "nested" in these two hybrid studies refers to the fact that the studies are embedded or "nested" within larger cohort studies.

- **Panel study.** This type of study combines features of the cross-sectional and prospective cohort designs. It can be viewed as a series of cross-sectional studies conducted on the same subjects (the panel) at successive time intervals, sometimes referred to as *waves*. This design allows investigators to relate changes in one variable to changes in other variables over time.[1, 9] For example, a California study identified the employment and depression status of a group at the first wave of a two-wave panel study.[19] At the second wave, the investigators found that those who were not depressed at the first wave but who subsequently lost their jobs were over twice as likely to suffer depressive symptoms as those who did not lose their jobs. In other words, the investigators were able to link changes in employment status to changes in depression status.

- **Repeated surveys.** In this design successive cross-sectional studies are performed over time on the same *study population*, but each sample is selected independently. Therefore, the actual subjects can be expected to differ from one survey to the next, although the samples will be representative of the study population. Repeated surveys differ from panel studies in that panel studies follow the same *individuals* from survey to survey, which allows investigators to link individual exposures to individual outcomes over time. Repeated surveys are useful in identifying overall trends in health status and factors that may help to explain them.[17] Several large repeated surveys are conducted by the National Center for Health Statistics, which is a part of the Centers for Disease Control and Prevention in the U.S. Department of Health and Human Services. An example is the Health and Nutrition Examination Survey (see appendix C).

Experimental Studies

Like analytic studies, experimental studies are designed to test hypotheses between specific exposures and outcomes. The major difference is that in experimental studies the investigator has direct control over the study conditions.[1] Of particular significance, the investigator controls the exposure status. Though very important to epidemiology, these studies are employed less frequently than observational studies due in part to ethical limitations. Many experimental studies on people are only feasible under conditions of uncertainty about the intervention. This is especially true if serious side effects are possible. In general, the investigators must show that the intervention has enough promise to justify exposing some individuals to the intervention but not so much as to justify denying others of the potential benefits.[7]

There are two major types of experimental studies in epidemiology—**randomized controlled trials** and **community trials**. Randomized controlled trials are often known as **clinical trials** because of their frequent use in clinical environments. This design, however, has applications in epidemiology that go beyond the clinical setting, and, hence, the term randomized controlled trials better reflects this broader use. Community trials differ from randomized controlled trials in two important ways. First, they are not always randomized. Nonrandomized community trials are technically **quasi-experimental studies** because they do not involve random assignment to the experimental and control groups. Quasi-experimental studies are studies where the investigator does not have full control over the assignment or timing of the intervention but where the study is still conducted as if it were an experiment.[1] Second, they employ a different unit of analysis. The unit of analysis in randomized controlled trials is the individual, while in community trials it is the group. A brief description of experimental study designs is presented below and additional details are discussed in chapter 13.

Randomized Controlled Trials

Randomized controlled trials (RCTs) involve three fundamental steps, which are illustrated in figure 4–7. These steps are:

1. Selection of an appropriate study sample
2. Random allocation of subjects into experimental and control groups
3. Follow-up and outcome assessment

The selection of the **study sample** is normally a three-step process in itself. First, the **reference population** is selected. This represents the population to which the investigator hopes to generalize the study findings (e.g., adult females with Type II diabetes). Next, the **experimental population** is defined. This is a practical representation of the reference population (e.g., a sample of adult females with Type II diabetes served by 10 large medical clinics in central Michigan). Finally, *volunteers* from the experimental population who meet the eligibility criteria for the study are selected for inclusion in the study sample.[7]

One of the most important aspects of RCTs is **random allocation**, which helps to assure that all subjects have the same probability of being assigned to an experimental group or to the control group.[20] This can virtually eliminate selection bias and confounding (see chapter 8) that could result from differences among the study groups and, therefore, increases study validity, making this design the most powerful research method in epidemiology.

There are three basic types of RCTs:[21]

- **Preventive trials.** These studies, also known as *prophylactic trials*, focus on *individuals without the study disease* (i.e., those in the stage of susceptibility). Their purpose is to determine if a particular intervention reduces the risk of some adverse outcome. For example, a preventive trial was conducted at the Stanford University School of Medicine to see if reducing the use of television, videotape, and video games among a sample of elementary school students reduced obesity.[22] The experimental group received a six-month educational program designed to reduce television, videotape, and video game use, while a control group did not receive any intervention. Results at the end of the intervention period revealed statistically significant reductions in body mass index, triceps skinfold thickness, waist circumference, and waist-to-hip ratio among the experimental subjects compared to the controls. This study also illustrates a *nonclinical* application of an RCT.

- **Intervention trials.** These RCTs focus on *high risk individuals* (i.e., those in the stage of presymptomatic disease). Their purpose is to test interventions to see if they can forestall disease development. A trial to determine the efficacy of treating hypertensive individuals with ascorbic acid to lower blood pressure might be considered an intervention trial to forestall the development of heart disease and stroke.[23] The line between intervention and therapeutic trials, however, is not always clear, and it could make sense to classify this study as a therapeutic trial (see below).

- **Therapeutic trials.** These trials focus on *patients with existing disease or disability* (i.e., those in the stages of clinical disease or diminished capacity). Their objective is to test interventions that might cure disease or improve a patient's quality of life. Therapeutic trials are commonly used in testing new drugs and medical procedures. The titles of the following published studies illustrate this study design: "A Randomized, Controlled Trial of the Effects of Remote, Intercessory Prayer on Outcomes in Patients Admitted to the Coronary Care Unit";[24] "Effectiveness of Manual Physical Therapy and Exercise in Osteoarthritis of the Knee. A Randomized, Controlled Trial."[25]

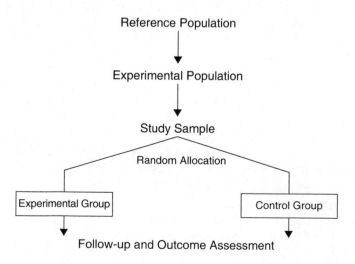

Figure 4–7 Randomized controlled trial

Community Trials

Instead of randomly assigning *individuals* to experimental or control groups as in the RCT, community trials assign interventions to *entire communities* or other groupings of people (e.g., schools). In the most basic scenario, one community receives the intervention, and another serves as a control. Community trials involve at least four important steps:

1. Selection of the participating communities
2. Collection of baseline data on the study outcome
3. Assignment and application of the community intervention
4. Follow-up, outcome assessment, and evaluation

A classic example of a community trial is the Newburgh-Kingston Caries-Fluoride Study that began about 1944.[26] Two cities in New York, Newburgh and Kingston, agreed to participate in the experiment. Both cities had populations of about 30,000 and were approximately 35 miles from each other on the West Bank of the Hudson River. Both cities were also using fluoride-deficient water. After collecting baseline data on the number of decayed, missing, and filled tooth surfaces (DMFS) in the two cities, Newburgh's water supply was subjected to continuous fluoridation beginning in 1945. The fluoride content of Kingston's water was not altered. After ten years of follow-up, child and adolescent rates of DMFS were substantially lower in Newburgh than in Kingston. In the youngest age group reported, the rate of DMFS after 10 years was 58% lower in the experimental versus the control group. In a published article on their findings the authors stated that "[the analysis] demonstrates conclusively two important facts—fluoridation is effective in reducing dental caries and it is a safe public health practice."[26(p235)]

Randomization was not used in assigning the intervention in the Newburgh-Kingston study, but it has been used in recent community trials, especially those involving a large number of communities. Sometimes practical matters dictate whether or not random assignment of the intervention is feasible or even desirable. For example, maybe only one community will agree to an intervention, or a community may have resources that make the intervention easier to implement, such as a local television station for broadcasting educational messages. Where possible, random assignment of the intervention is a good idea since it guards against unconscious or conscious preferences on the part of the investigator that could bias study results.[21] Whether or not randomization is used in community trials, the ideal is to have communities that are truly comparable except for the intervention.

A relatively recent community trial using randomization was Communities Mobilizing for Change on Alcohol (CMCA).[27] This experimental study involved 15 communities and randomly assigned a community organizing intervention designed to reduce the accessibility of alcohol to adolescents under the legal drinking age. The results showed that the CMCA intervention had some significant and beneficial effects on the personal behaviors of 18–20 year olds and on the practices of some of the alcohol establishments, based on data collected before and after the intervention.

Identifying Epidemiologic Study Designs

By now you should have a good idea of the basic epidemiologic study designs and should be able to identify them in the public health and biomedical literature. To assist you in this task, exhibit 4–1 presents an algorithm for identifying the major designs, and table 4–1 presents a summary of the sequence in which exposure and outcome are assessed in the most common analytic and experimental designs, as well as key characteristics.

Table 4–1 also presents alternate names for each study type. It is important to note that some of the names that have been applied to epidemiologic studies are too general to be very useful. The terms prospective study, longitudinal study, and follow-up study, for example, have all been applied to prospective cohort studies, but they could also apply to panel studies and repeated surveys, as well as to some case-control studies, randomized controlled trials, and community trials. Likewise, case-control studies have been referred to as retrospective studies because exposure status is usually assessed retrospectively. This same term, however, has been applied to retrospective cohort studies, which also look at exposure status retrospectively. Some ecological and cross-sectional studies may also involve retrospective assessment. It is, therefore, important not to rely on these general terms as a sole method for determining study designs. The titles used for epidemiologic studies in this chapter have had wide acceptance and use and are unlikely to be a source of confusion.

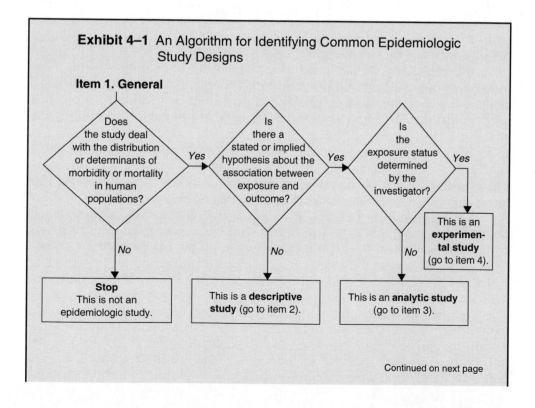

Exhibit 4–1 An Algorithm for Identifying Common Epidemiologic Study Designs

Item 1. General

Does the study deal with the distribution or determinants of morbidity or mortality in human populations? — Yes → Is there a stated or implied hypothesis about the association between exposure and outcome? — Yes → Is the exposure status determined by the investigator? — Yes → This is an **experimental study** (go to item 4).

No ↓ **Stop** This is not an epidemiologic study.

No ↓ This is a **descriptive study** (go to item 2).

No ↓ This is an **analytic study** (go to item 3).

Continued on next page

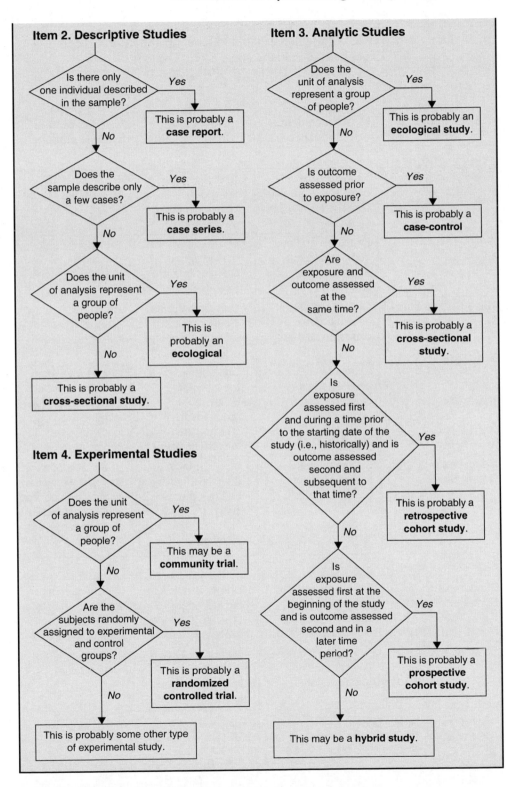

Item 2. Descriptive Studies

Is there only one individual described in the sample?

Yes → This is probably a **case report**.

No ↓

Does the sample describe only a few cases?

Yes → This is probably a **case series**.

No ↓

Does the unit of analysis represent a group of people?

Yes → This is probably an **ecological**

No ↓

This is probably a **cross-sectional study**.

Item 4. Experimental Studies

Does the unit of analysis represent a group of people?

Yes → This may be a **community trial**.

No ↓

Are the subjects randomly assigned to experimental and control groups?

Yes → This is probably a **randomized controlled trial**.

No ↓

This is probably some other type of experimental study.

Item 3. Analytic Studies

Does the unit of analysis represent a group of people?

Yes → This is probably an **ecological study**.

No ↓

Is outcome assessed prior to exposure?

Yes → This is probably a **case-control**

No ↓

Are exposure and outcome assessed at the same time?

Yes → This is probably a **cross-sectional study**.

No ↓

Is exposure assessed first and during a time prior to the starting date of the study (i.e., historically) and is outcome assessed second and subsequent to that time?

Yes → This is probably a **retrospective cohort study**.

No ↓

Is exposure assessed first at the beginning of the study and is outcome assessed second and in a later time period?

Yes → This is probably a **prospective cohort study**.

No ↓

This may be a **hybrid study**.

Table 4–1 Typical Characteristics of the Most Common Analytic and Experimental Epidemiologic Study Designs

Type of Epidemiologic Study	Exposure–Outcome Assessment Sequence	Key Identifying Characteristics	Some Alternative Designations*
Analytic Designs			
Ecological Study	Exposure and outcome status are often assessed during the same time period	• Unit of analysis is the group • Conclusions are about groups	Ecologic study, correlational study
Cross-Sectional Study	Exposure and outcome status are assessed during the same time period	• Unit of analysis is the individual • Conclusions are tentative	Prevalence study, prevalence survey
Case-Control Study	Outcome status is assessed before exposure status	• Unit of analysis is the individual • Ideally, exposure precedes outcome	Retrospective study, case-referent study, case-comparison study
Prospective Cohort Study	Exposure status is assessed before outcome status	• Unit of analysis is the individual • Follow-up proceeds from study initiation forward in time	Prospective study, concurrent cohort study, cohort study, longitudinal study, follow-up study, incidence study
Retrospective Cohort Study	Exposure status is assessed before outcome status	• Unit of analysis is the individual • Follow-up proceeds from the past to the time of study initiation	Historical cohort study, nonconcurrent cohort study, nonconcurrent prospective study, historical prospective study
Experimental Designs			
Randomized Controlled Trial	Exposure status is assessed before outcome status	• Unit of analysis is the individual • Investigator controls exposure status	Clinical trial, randomized clinical trial, randomized controlled clinical trial
Community Trial	Exposure status is assessed before outcome status	• Unit of analysis is the group • Investigator controls exposure status	Community intervention trial

*The list of alternative designations is not exhaustive. Many of these names are too general to be very useful (e.g., retrospective study, prospective study, prevalence study, etc.), since the terms may be applied to more than one design under different circumstances.

Summary

- Epidemiologic studies can be broadly classified as observational or experimental. In observational studies, exposure status refers to what exists among the subjects as they naturally divide themselves with regard to potentially significant inherent or acquired characteristics. These studies include both descriptive and analytic designs. In experimental studies, the investigators determine the exposure status of the subjects by selecting and employing one or more interventions.

- Descriptive studies do not test hypotheses. Instead, they focus on describing what exists in a population by person, place, or time variables. Descriptive studies are often helpful in generating hypotheses for further study or providing health professionals with a clearer picture of community health problems that can be useful in the health planning process.

- The major types of descriptive studies are ecological and cross-sectional studies, which are also classified as analytic studies when the intent is to test a hypothesis, and case reports and case series, which are frequently used in clinical epidemiology.

- Analytic studies are designed to test hypotheses. These studies include analytic ecological studies, analytic cross-sectional studies, case-control studies, cohort studies (prospective and retrospective), and various hybrid designs, including nested case-control and case-cohort studies, panel studies, and repeated surveys.

- Experimental studies are also designed to test hypotheses. The two major types of experimental studies in epidemiology are randomized controlled trials and community trials. A major difference between the two is the unit of analysis. In randomized controlled trials the unit of analysis is the individual; in community trials it is the group. Randomized controlled trials include three types—preventive, intervention, and therapeutic trials.

New Terms

analytic study	experimental population	preventive trial
case-control study	experimental study	primary source
case report	exposure	prospective cohort study
case series	exposure status	quasi-experimental study
clinical trial	hybrid study	randomized controlled trial
community trial	intervention trial	reference population
cross-sectional study	nested case-cohort study	repeated surveys
descriptive study	nested case-control study	retrospective cohort study
ecological fallacy	observational study	secondary source
ecological study	outcome	study sample
ecological unit	outcome status	therapeutic trial
experimental epidemiology	panel study	unit of analysis

Study Questions and Exercises

Using the key below, classify each of the following descriptions of epidemiologic studies according to study type. Also give reasons for your selections.

A. Descriptive Study

B. Analytic Ecological Study

C. Analytic Cross-Sectional Study

D. Case-Control Study

E. Retrospective Cohort Study

F. Prospective Cohort Study

G. Randomized Controlled Trial

H. Community Trial

_____ 1. A total of 825 insulation workers employed between 1941 and 1944 was identified from the personnel records of three large insulation manufacturing plants in the southeastern U.S. in 1975. During the period 1941–1975, 26 deaths from lung cancer were discovered among the workers. Only six lung cancer deaths, however, were reported among a comparable group of 700 coworkers who did not work with insulation during the same time period. The investigators had postulated that exposure to the insulation material increases the risk of lung cancer.

_____ 2. To see if hypnosis could reduce chronic pain, investigators randomly assigned 120 volunteers with osteoarthritis to either hypnosis therapy or a control group. Pain levels were checked among the subjects every three months during the 12-month study using validated pain measures. Those assigned to the hypnosis group reported reduced pain compared to those in the control group after three and six months, but not after nine and 12 months, of follow-up.

_____ 3. The prevalence of Type II diabetes was determined from a randomly selected sample of 3,000 adults over 50 years of age in a large city in the Southwest. Based on clinical examinations and testing, the prevalence of diabetes was 7.5% in men and 6.2% in women. The prevalence of diabetes increased with age more among the women than the men. Also, the rates in both men and women were higher than they had been in past years.

_____ 4. A study was undertaken to test the hypothesis that chewing tobacco increases the risk of stomach cancer. Detailed historical data on chewing tobacco use were collected from 400 subjects with newly diagnosed stomach cancer and 400 subjects without stomach cancer. The results revealed that chewing tobacco was not a significant risk factor for stomach cancer.

_____ 5. Two hundred babies were followed from birth to age five to determine if those whose mothers smoked during pregnancy were more likely to have respiratory infections in the first five years of life than those whose mothers did not smoke during pregnancy. The findings supported the investigators' assumption that smoking during pregnancy increases the frequency of respiratory infections in young children.

_____ 6. To study a presumed inverse relationship between black tea consumption and cardiovascular disease, investigators randomly selected a sample of 13,500 subjects, 50–64 years of age, and queried them about tea consumption and current treatment for cardiovascular disease. No significant association was found between drinking black tea and having cardiovascular disease.

___ 7. To find out if planting grass on the top of buildings would be effective in reducing air pollution levels in polluted cities, investigators selected two adjacent cities with similar demographic profiles and air pollution levels. The officials of one city agreed to plant grass on all its public buildings in the downtown area and on all private buildings where consent could be obtained. The other city did not plant any grass on the top of any of its buildings. After two years of follow-up, the city that planted grass on the buildings had lower air pollution levels than the city that did not plant any grass, although the difference was not statistically significant.

___ 8. A sample of residents of Grover County (population 43,000) was invited to participate in a survey to determine the prevalence of *Helicobacter pylori*, a bacterium that causes ulcers. Five thousand residents participated and were given diagnostic blood tests. The results revealed that *H. pylori* was about two times more common among men than women in the county. The overall proportion of positive tests was a surprising 58%.

___ 9. Fifty patients recently diagnosed with hepatitis A were selected along with another group of 50 subjects without hepatitis A. The groups were then interviewed to determine if they had had any body piercing within the last two months. To assure the groups were comparable, they were matched for age, sex, and race. The findings revealed that the body piercing was more likely among the group with hepatitis A than those without the disease after controlling for other factors.

___ 10. In order to determine if vitamin D (the "sunshine" vitamin) is associated with reduced levels of ovarian cancer, an epidemiologist identified 10 geographic regions in Sweden and obtained data on annual days of sunlight and ovarian cancer rates for each region. The findings indicated that those regions with the most days of sunlight per year had significantly lower rates of ovarian cancer than those areas with the fewest days of sunlight per year. The epidemiologist reported her findings at the Scandinavian Conference on Cancer.

References

1. Last, J. M., ed. (1995). *A Dictionary of Epidemiology*. New York: Oxford University Press.
2. Hoyert, D. L., Kochanek, K. D., and Murphy, S. L. (1999). Deaths: Final Data for 1997. *National Vital Statistics Reports* 47(19). Hyattsville, MD: National Center for Health Statistics.
3. Friedman, G. D. (1980). *Primer of Epidemiology*, 2nd ed. New York: McGraw-Hill Book Company.
4. Fletcher, R. H., Fletcher, S. W., and Wagner, E. H. (1988). *Clinical Epidemiology: The Essentials*, 2nd ed. Baltimore: Williams and Wilkins.
5. Centers for Disease Control (1992). *Tampons and Toxic Shock Syndrome*. 1992 EIS Course (available from the Association of Teachers of Preventive Medicine, Washington, DC). Atlanta: The Centers.

6. Chin, J., ed. (2000). *Control of Communicable Diseases Manual*, 17th ed. Washington, DC: American Public Health Association.

7. Hennekens, C. H., and Buring, J. E. (1987). *Epidemiology in Medicine*. Boston: Little, Brown and Company.

8. Vogt, W. P. (1993). *Dictionary of Statistics and Methodology*. Newbury Park, CA: Sage.

9. Kelsey, J. L., Thompson, W. D., and Evans, A. S. (1986). *Methods in Observational Epidemiology*. New York: Oxford University Press.

10. Yang, C. Y., Chiu, H. F., Cheng, M. F., and Tsai, S. S. (1998). Chlorination of drinking water and cancer in Taiwan. *Environmental Research* 78(1): 1–6.

11. Szklo, M., and Nieto, F. J. (2000). *Epidemiology: Beyond the Basics*. Gaithersburg, MD: Aspen.

12. Morgenstern, H. (1982). Uses of Ecologic Analysis in Epidemiologic Research. *American Journal of Public Health* 72(12): 1336–1344.

13. Fingerhut, L. A., Cox, C. S., Warner, M., et al. (1998). International Comparative Analysis of Injury Mortality: Findings from the ICE on Injury Statistics. *Advance Data from Vital and Health Statistics*, No. 303. Hyattsville, MD: National Center for Health Statistics.

14. Metz, J. A., Morris, C. D., Roberts, L. A., McClung, M. R., and McCarron, D. A. (1999). Blood Pressure and Calcium Intake Are Related to Bone Density in Adult Males. *British Journal of Nutrition* 81(5): 383–388.

15. Kreuzer, M., Krauss, M., Kreienbrock, L., Jockel, K. H., and Wichmann, H. E. (2000). Environmental Tobacco Smoke and Lung Cancer: A Case-control Study in Germany. *American Journal of Epidemiology* 151(3): 241–250.

16. Jacobs, E. J., Thun, M. J., and Apicella, L. F. (1999). Cigar Smoking and Death from Coronary Heart Disease in a Prospective Study of U.S. Men. *Archives of Internal Medicine* 159(20): 2413–2418.

17. Kleinbaum, D. G., Kupper, L. L., and Morgenstern, H. (1982). *Epidemiologic Research: Principles and Quantitative Methods*. Belmont, CA: Lifetime Learning Publications.

18. Hulley, S. B., Cummings, S. R., Browner, W. S., Grady, D., Hearst, N., and Newman, T. B. (2001). *Designing Clinical Research: An Epidemiologic Approach*, 2nd ed. Philadelphia: Lippincott Williams & Wilkins.

19. Dooley, D., Catalano, R., and Wilson, G. (1994). Depression and Unemployment: Panel Findings from the Epidemiologic Catchment Area Study. *American Journal of Community Psychology* 22(6): 745–765.

20. Streiner, D. L., Norman, G. R., and Blum, H. M. (1989). *PDQ Epidemiology*. Toronto: B.C. Decker.

21. Lilienfeld, D. E., and Stolley, P. D. (1994). *Foundations of Epidemiology*, 3rd ed. New York: Oxford University Press.

22. Robinson, T. N. (1999). Reducing Children's Television Viewing to Prevent Obesity: A Randomized Controlled Trial. *Journal of the American Medical Association* 282(16): 1561–1567.

23. Duffy, S. J., Gokee, N., Holbrook, M., Huang, A., Frei, B., Keaney, J. F., Jr., and Vita, J. A. (1999). Treatment of Hypertension with Ascorbic Acid. *Lancet* 354(9195): 2048–2049.

24. Harris, W. S., Gowda, M., Kolb, J. W., Strychaez, C. P., Vacek, J. L., Jones, P. G., Forker, A., O'Keefe, J. H., and McCallister, B. D. (1999). A Randomized, Controlled Trial of the Effects of Remote, Intercessory Prayer on Outcomes in Patients Admitted to the Coronary Care Unit. *Archives of Internal Medicine* 159(19): 2273–2278.

25. Deyle, G. D., Henderson, N. E., Matckel, R. I., Ryder, M. G., Garber, M. B., and Allison, S. C. (2000). Effectiveness of Manual Physical Therapy and Exercise in Osteoarthritis of the Knee. A Randomized, Controlled Trial. *Annals of Internal Medicine* 132(3): 173–181.

26. Ast, D. B., and Schlesinger, E. R. (1956). The Conclusion of a Ten-year Study of Water Fluoridation. *American Journal of Public Health* 46(3): 265–271.

27. Wagenaar, A. C., Murray, D. M., Gehan, J. P., Wolfson, M., Forster, J. L., Toomey, T. L., Perry, C. L., and Jones-Webb, R. (2000). Communities Mobilizing for Change on Alcohol: Outcomes from a Randomized Community Trial. *Journal of Studies on Alcohol*: 61(1): 85–94.

CHAPTER FIVE

Common Measures of Morbidity and Mortality

Learning Objectives

▸ Compare and contrast incidence and prevalence.

▸ Calculate and interpret the cumulative incidence rate, the person-time incidence rate, the point prevalence rate, and the period prevalence rate.

▸ Calculate and interpret the crude death rate, cause-specific mortality rate, proportionate mortality ratio, infant mortality rate, neonatal mortality rate, maternal mortality rate, perinatal mortality rate, fetal death rate, case fatality rate, survival rate, years of potential life lost rate, crude birth rate, and the fertility rate.

▸ Explain the rationale, use, and interpretation of confidence intervals.

▸ Define population at risk, person-time units, rate base, risk, steady-state conditions, target population, and point estimate.

Overview

Incidence measures how many new cases of a disease or other event occur in a population. There are two types of incidence rates—the cumulative incidence rate and the person-time incidence rate. Prevalence measures how many cases exist in a population at a specified time. Prevalence rates include the point prevalence rate and the period prevalence rate. Other common frequency measures in epidemiology include the crude death rate, cause-specific mortality rate, proportionate mortality ratio, infant mortality rate, and others. These are frequently used as indices of population health status. Because most rates in epidemiology are based on samples of a defined population, confidence intervals are used to indicate their precision as population estimates.

Measures of Incidence

Incidence deals with what is new. Specifically, incidence is the number of *new* events (e.g., new cases of a disease) occurring in a defined population during a specified time period. It is also sometimes called the *incidence number* or *incident number*. Thus, when we say that 12 new cases of HIV infection occurred in a community during 2001 we are talking about incidence. Incidence can refer to conditions of morbidity, mortality, or other occurrences, such as the incidence of smoking among teenagers. When combined with an appropriate denominator incidence becomes an **incidence rate**.* The incidence rate is one of the most useful and versatile statistical measures in epidemiology. There are two basic types of incidence rates, which are described in the following sections.

Cumulative Incidence Rate

The **cumulative incidence rate** is fairly easy to conceptualize and is calculated as follows:

(5.1)

$$IR_C = \frac{\text{Number of new events occurring during a specified time period}}{\text{Population at risk}} \times 10^n$$

The notation IR_C refers to the cumulative incidence rate, and 10^n is the **rate base**. The rate base is 10 raised to a power of two or more. Since the exponent n is a whole number, the rate base will have a value of 100, 1,000, 10,000, 100,000, etc. The purpose of the rate base is to assure that the reported rate is always expressed as a number equal to or greater than one for a given population size. The reason for using a rate base will become clear shortly when an example of a cumulative incidence rate is presented. First, however, we need to define the **population at risk**. The population at risk (PAR) refers to those in a defined population who are *at risk* of the event but are event-free at the beginning of the specified time period. Sometimes the PAR is estimated using the average or mid-interval population during the specified time period (e.g., July 1 for a calendar year). The estimate is generally used: (a) when information on the risk status of the population is either unknown or known for only a small fraction of the defined population, or (b) when the defined population is undergoing significant change during the specified time period so that the beginning population is no longer representative of the PAR. To differentiate between the actual PAR and estimates based on the average population, the actual PAR is sometimes referred to as the **initial population at risk**. Inevitably, when students begin calculating the cumulative incidence rate for the first time, some questions arise about who to include or exclude from the numerator and denominator. Exhibit 5–1 addresses these issues.

---

* The term incidence is not always distinguished from incidence rate. Sometimes when incidence is used, one really means incidence rate. It is important to look at the context in which the terms are used to avoid any confusion.

Exhibit 5–1 Determining the Correct Numerator and Denominator in the Cumulative Incidence Rate

One issue that frequently arises when students begin calculating cumulative incidence rates is who to include or exclude from the numerator and the denominator. Before addressing this issue, it is important to note that *all those who are included in the numerator of a cumulative incidence rate are also included in the denominator.* In fact, the cases that go in the numerator come from the denominator, the population at risk. It is not possible, therefore, to have individuals in the numerator who do not also belong to the denominator. Part of the confusion comes from the fact that the numerator and denominator are determined in different time periods. The denominator is determined first, and then as new cases develop they are included in the numerator. In most cases, students find it easier to determine the correct numerator than the correct denominator.

Who should be included in the numerator?

Some students wonder whether or not recurrent events during a specified time period should be included in the numerator of a cumulative incidence rate. If, for example, one person in a population at risk has two strokes during the follow-up period, should both strokes be counted in the numerator? The general answer to this question is no, since the numerator is a count of people who develop the disease and not a count of diseases. Cases refer to *people* with the disease. If all strokes are counted, it would be theoretically possible to have an incidence rate that exceeds 100%. Nevertheless, there may be some instances where it makes sense to include all events that occur during a specified time period. However, this is not the usual definition of a cumulative incidence rate.

Who is included in the denominator?

Determining who to include or exclude from the denominator in a cumulative incidence rate is not as easy as it may first seem. By definition, the population at risk (PAR) includes only those in the defined population who are *at risk* of developing a given event (e.g., disease) at the beginning of a specified time period. In practice, this usually means excluding those who have the disease at the start of the specified time period on the assumption that they are no longer at risk of developing the disease or of becoming *new* cases. This works fairly well for those who have diseases that confer lifetime immunity, such as measles, mumps, or chickenpox. It also works well for lifelong chronic diseases, such as diabetes, multiple sclerosis, or Parkinson's disease. But, what about events like injuries, strokes, or the common cold that can reoccur? Should individuals with these and similar conditions be excluded from the PAR? The answer lies in what is being investigated. If one is concerned with *entirely new* (first-time) events, then anyone who *has or has had* the disease should be excluded from the PAR. On the other hand, if one is only concerned with events that are new *for the specified time period*, then previous cases who are still susceptible to the event should be included. For example, if one wanted to know the incidence of first-time strokes in Chicago during the year 2000, one should exclude from the PAR anyone who had had a stroke any time prior to 2000. However, if one wanted to know how many total strokes occurred in Chicago for the first time during 2000, then it would be necessary to include survivors with a history of stroke prior to 2000 in the PAR. Usually, for chronic diseases, new cases mean first-time cases only. For acute diseases where recovery is possible, the PAR usually includes all those who were not in a disease state at the beginning of the specified time period and who were not immune to the disease, whether or not they have had the disease in the past.

The cumulative incidence rate, which is often calculated in longitudinal-type studies, is important in epidemiology because it measures **risk** (probability). Specifically, the cumulative incidence rate measures the risk that a person will develop a given disease (or other event) in a specified time period. For any given population, the cumulative incidence rate represents a population member's *average* risk of developing the disease during the period of observation. Technically, this assumes that the person does not die from a cause other than the disease during the study interval.[1, 2] A variant of the cumulative incidence rate is the *attack rate*, which is discussed in chapter 14. Example 5–1 illustrates how a cumulative incidence rate is calculated.

Example 5–1: Cumulative Incidence Rate

Imagine that, in January 1996, a team of epidemiologists identified a sample of 4,500 men, 65–74 years of age, in Cedar Rapids, Iowa, for a study of prostate cancer. Tests indicated that 7% of the men already had prostate cancer and, therefore, were not at risk. The rest of the men were followed prospectively for five years to determine the cumulative incidence rate of prostate cancer in the sample. By the end of the five years of follow-up 156 of the men had developed prostate cancer. What was the five-year cumulative incidence rate of prostate cancer in this group?

Solution:

Formula 5.1 is used to calculate the cumulative incidence rate.

$$IR_C = \frac{\text{Number of new events occurring during a specified time period}}{\text{Population at risk}} \times 10^n$$

For convenience, let's represent the formula as $IR_C = (X / Y) \times 10^n$, where X = the number of new events occurring during a specified time period, Y = the PAR, and 10^n = the rate base.

Step 1: Determine the numerator or X. The 156 men who developed the disease were new cases that developed during the five-year follow-up period. Therefore,

X = 156 new cases of prostate cancer

Step 2: Determine the denominator or Y.

Y = 4,500 − (4,500 × 0.07) = 4,500 − 315 = 4,185 men, 65–74 years of age

Because 7% of the men were not at initially at risk, they were not included in the study (i.e., they were not followed up). Therefore, they have been subtracted from the original sample of 4,500. It is important to realize, however, that the remaining 4,185 men include the 156 who subsequently became prostate cancer cases. This is because in cumulative incidence rates the new cases (the numerator) always arise from the PAR (the denominator).

Step 3: Complete the calculation of the cumulative incidence rate (IR_C) using a rate base that will produce a rate that is at least one for the selected rate base. In this example, 100 is the smallest rate base that will produce a rate of at least one per 100.

$IR_C = (X / Y) \times 10^n = (156 / 4,185) \times 10^n = 0.037 \times 10^2 = 3.7$ cases per 100 men

Answer: The five-year cumulative incidence rate of prostate cancer was 3.7 cases per 100 men, 65–74 years of age, in Cedar Rapids, Iowa during the period 1996 through 2000.

Comments:

1. The rate base is a convention in epidemiology that is used for the convenience of not having to report decimal fractions. In actuality, 0.037 is the same as 3.7 per 100, 37 per 1,000, 370 per 10,000, etc. Usually, we select the smallest rate base to achieve its purpose, since larger rate bases appear less precise. Exceptions are made when we want to maintain a common rate base when comparing several different rates or when we select a larger rate base because that is the way a particular rate is commonly reported in the literature. A convenient way to determine the appropriate rate base is to divide X by Y and then determine what rate base is needed to produce a rate that is at least one per the selected rate base.

2. It is important to note that the solution to this problem represents results during a particular time period, among a particular group, and at a particular place. Unless this information is clear from the context, it is important to specify the relevant time, person, and place factors. *Since the cumulative incidence rate can normally be expected to increase with the time of observation,* it is especially important to indicate the period the cumulative incidence rate encompasses. For example, the five-year cumulative incidence rate of prostate cancer would be expected to be greater than the one-year rate.

3. The study alluded to in this problem is a descriptive study. There is no a priori hypothesis, and only outcome is being assessed. The study begins with a cross-sectional study and then involves longitudinal follow-up. This reiterates a point made in the last chapter. Terms like "longitudinal study" or "follow-up study" are too general for one to assume that they imply a cohort study.

Person-Time Incidence Rate

A second type of incidence rate is the **person-time incidence rate**, also known as **incidence density**, **force of morbidity**, or simply, incidence rate. This rate may seem a little less straightforward than the cumulative incidence rate, but it has several advantages, which will be noted shortly. Like the cumulative incidence rate, the person-time incidence rate is also commonly used in longitudinal-type studies, especially cohort studies. The person-time incidence rate can be calculated as follows:

(5.2)

$$IR_{P-T} = \frac{\text{Number of new events occurring during a specified time period}}{\text{Total person-time units at risk}} \times 10^n$$

While the numerator and the rate base in the person-time incidence rate are exactly the same as those in the cumulative incidence rate, the denominator differs. **Person-time units** represent a single, combined measure of the number of persons at risk of a specified outcome and the time they were at risk. The most common person-time unit is *person-years*. A person-year represents one person at risk for one year, two persons at risk for half a year, or any other combination of persons and time whose product is one. Similarly, four person-years can mean one person at risk for four years, two persons at risk for two years, four persons at risk for one year, etc. The *total person-time units at risk*, the denominator in the person-time incidence rate, is the sum of the person-time units at risk for all individuals in the sample. This can be expressed mathematically as follows:

(5.3)

$$T = \Sigma t_i$$

where T = the total person-time units at risk, and Σt_i = the sum of each individual's person-time units at risk. Before we discuss the person-time incidence rate further, it should be helpful to work through an example.

Example 5–2: Person-Time Incidence Rate

Assume another study of prostate cancer was initiated in Des Moines, Iowa, in January of 1997. This time 1,000 men, 55–64 years of age, with no prior evidence of prostate cancer were enrolled in the study. The men were then followed by the investigators for four years until the end of the year 2000. Each year during the study, the men were examined and tested for the presence of prostate cancer. The results of the annual examinations revealed the following:

    10 cases were confirmed after 1 year

    15 additional cases were confirmed after 2 years

    20 additional cases were confirmed after 3 years

    25 additional cases were confirmed after 4 years

What was the person-time incidence rate of prostate cancer in this group?

Solution:

Formula 5.2 is used to calculate the person-time incidence rate.

$$IR_{P\text{-}T} = \frac{\text{Number of new events occurring during a specified time period}}{\text{Total person-time units at risk}} \times 10^n$$

For convenience, let's represent the formula for the person-time incidence rate as:

$IR_{P\text{-}T} = (X / T) \times 10^n$, where X = the number of new events occurring during a specified time period, T = the total person-time units at risk, and 10^n = the rate base.

Step 1: Determine the number of new cases, or X, which in this example is the number of those who developed prostate cancer during the four-year follow-up period. Note that all subjects were initially free of prostate cancer. Therefore,

$$X = 10 + 15 + 20 + 25 = 70 \text{ new cases of prostate cancer}$$

Step 2: Determine the total person-time units at risk, or T, the denominator in the person-time incidence rate, which is equivalent to the sum of each individual's person-time units at risk (i.e., Σt_i). The person-time units at risk must be calculated for every subject in the group, both those who developed the disease and those who did not, and then added together to get the appropriate denominator. For those who developed prostate cancer we can calculate their portion of T as follows:

    10 cases were confirmed after 1 year: 10 persons $\times$ 1 year = 10 person-years

    15 cases were confirmed after 2 years: 15 persons $\times$ 2 years = 30 person-years

    20 cases were confirmed after 3 years: 20 persons $\times$ 3 years = 60 person-years

    25 cases were confirmed after 4 years: 25 persons $\times$ 4 years = 100 person-years

The total person-time units at risk contributed by the 70 cases is:

$$10 + 30 + 60 + 100 = 200 \text{ person-years}$$

After we have accounted for the person-time units contributed by the 70 cases, we must also account for the person-time units contributed by the remaining sample, which in this example are those who did *not* develop prostate cancer. Even though these subjects did not develop the study disease, they were at risk during the entire four years of study and, therefore, must be included in the denominator of the person-time incidence rate. Since 70 subjects developed prostate cancer, there were 930 (i.e., 1,000 − 70 = 930) who did not. These individuals were observed for four years. Therefore, the total person-time units contributed by those who did not develop prostate cancer is:

$$930 \text{ persons} \times 4 \text{ years} = 3,720 \text{ person-years}$$

As a final step, we add the person-time units at risk contributed by both those who did and those who did not develop the study disease. The calculation of the total person-time units at risk is:

$$T = 200 \text{ person-years} + 3,720 \text{ person-years} = 3,920 \text{ person-years}$$

The entire calculation of T can be represented as follows:

$$T = (10 \times 1) + (15 \times 2) + (20 \times 3) + (25 \times 4) + [(1,000 - 70) \times 4] = 3,920 \text{ person-years}$$

Step 3: Calculate the IR_{P-T} using a rate base that will produce a rate that is at least one for the selected rate base.

$$IR_{P-T} = (X / T) \times 10^n = (70 / 3,920) \times 10^n = 0.018 \times 10^2 = 1.8 \text{ cases per 100 person-years}$$

Answer: The person-time incidence rate of prostate cancer is 1.8 cases per 100 person-years among men 55–64 years of age in Des Moines, Iowa during the period 1997 through 2000.

Comments:

1. When calculating a person-time incidence rate note that once the subjects develop the study disease, they are no longer at risk and, therefore, no longer contribute person-time units to the denominator. Similarly, *subjects who are lost to follow-up, die from causes other than the study disease, or withdraw from the study are only counted for the time they were in the study.* In this example, the only reason some individuals did not complete the study was because they contracted the study disease.

2. The rate base is selected in the same manner as for the cumulative incidence rate. Since the rate is 0.018 cases per person-year, a rate base of 100 allows us to express this as 1.8 cases per 100 person-years.

3. Since time is already represented in the person-time incidence rate, it would be inappropriate to indicate that this is a four-year incidence rate. It is proper, however, to indicate the observation period along with person and place information if these are not clear from the context.

4. As in the previous example, this is a descriptive study with a follow-up period (i.e., a type of panel study).

Person-Time Versus Cumulative Incidence Rates

The person-time incidence rate has some practical advantages over the cumulative incidence rate when used in follow-up (e.g., cohort) studies. First, it allows investigators to account for subject losses due to withdrawals, deaths, or other reasons during the follow-up period, and, second, it can accommodate subjects entering a study at different times. These advantages are due to the fact that the denominator of the person-time incidence rate only includes the time the subjects are actually observed. Those who are observed for longer time periods contribute more to the denominator than those who are observed for shorter time periods. For example, if a subject completes only one year of a five-year study, the subject contributes only one person-year to the denominator. If another subject completes the entire five years, this subject contributes five person-years to the denominator.

In contrast to the person-time incidence rate, the cumulative incidence rate assumes that the entire population at risk is observed (i.e., at risk) for the entire study period and that the subjects all enter the study at the same time. The denominator does not take into consideration that subjects may be at risk for varying lengths of time. For example, in a five-year study if one subject gets the disease after one year, and hence is no longer at risk, and another subject completes the entire five years disease free, both subjects contribute the same amount to the denominator. In other words, the length of time at risk makes no difference in the size of the denominator of the cumulative incidence rate. Thus, the cumulative incidence rate is less flexible than the person-time incidence rate because it requires that all subjects enter the study at the same time and assumes that each subject is at risk for the same time period.

Another difference between the two types of incidence rates has to do with what they attempt to assess. The cumulative incidence rate measures the *risk* of disease development, while the person-time incidence rate measures the *rate* of disease development. Technically, the cumulative incidence rate is a proportion. It is the proportion of the population at risk that develops the disease in a given time frame. It estimates an individual's risk of developing a given disease. The person-time incidence rate, on the other hand, is a measure of the rate at which new cases of a disease are occurring in a population. It attempts to evaluate the rate of disease flow into a population. *Incidence density* and *force of morbidity* are descriptive terms that seem to capture the essence of the person-time incidence rate.*

Although they measure different things, under certain conditions the person-time incidence rate can be used to approximate the cumulative incidence rate and vice versa. This is illustrated in example 5–3 using the following formulas:

(5.4 a and b)

$$\text{(a)} \quad IR_C \cong IR_{P\text{-}T} \times Y$$

$$\text{(b)} \quad IR_{P\text{-}T} \cong IR_C / Y$$

---

* The preceding discussion concerning the differences between cumulative and person-time incidence rates has been somewhat oversimplified for the sake of brevity. For those who want a more complete explanation see Kleinbaum, Kupper, and Morgenstern.[2] The term "rate" is loosely applied to various statistical measures in epidemiology, including the cumulative incidence rate. Many so-called rates are really ratios or proportions (ratios where the numerator is included in the denominator). This usage is long-standing in epidemiology and is not discussed further in this text except where it helps to clarify a particular concept.

where Y = the length of the study period in years. In order to apply this formula, the following conditions must be met: (a) the incidence should be relatively constant, and (b) the incidence rates must be relatively low (i.e., less than 0.10), or the length of the study period (Y) must be relatively short (i.e., equal or less than 5 years).[3]

Example 5–3: Relationship Between Cumulative Incidence and Person-Time Incidence Rates

Between January 1, 2000 and December 31, 2001, 5,000 men working in highly stressful jobs in Los Angeles County, California, were enrolled in a study of the relationship between stress and gastric ulcers. Clinical examinations revealed that all subjects were free of gastric ulcers at the beginning of the study. The authors reported the following statistics at the conclusion of the study:

10 men developed gastric ulcers after 6 months

15 additional men developed gastric ulcers after 1 year

20 additional men developed gastric ulcers after 18 months

100 men who had not developed gastric ulcers dropped out of the study after 1 year

Based on this information, calculate the person-time incidence rate (in person-years), the cumulative incidence rate, and compare the two measures. Also, calculate and compare the rates using the estimate methods in formulas 5.4a and b.

Solution:

Step 1: Calculate the person-time incidence rate of gastric ulcers in the group.

$$IR_{P-T} = \frac{\text{Number of new events occurring during a specified time period}}{\text{Total person-time units at risk}} \times 10^n$$

The number of new cases of gastric ulcers during the two-year study period is:

10 + 15 + 20 = 45 cases of gastric ulcers

Next we need to calculate the total person-time units at risk, which is the sum of each individual's person-time units at risk. Based on the information provided, this can be calculated as follows:

10 cases after 6 months:	10 persons × 0.5 year = 5 person-years
15 cases after 1 year:	15 persons × 1 year = 15 person-years
20 cases after 18 months:	20 persons × 1.5 years = 30 person-years
100 non-case dropouts after 1 year:	100 persons × 1 year = 100 person-years

In addition, we must account for the remaining subjects in the study. These were individuals who did not develop the disease and who did not drop out of the study.

5,000 subjects − (45 cases + 100 dropouts) = 5,000 − 145 = 4,855 subjects

Since these subjects were followed for two years, their total contribution in person-time units is:

4,855 persons × 2 years = 9,710 person-years

Therefore, the total number of person-years is:

$$5 + 15 + 30 + 100 + 9{,}710 = 9{,}860 \text{ person-years}$$

The person-time incidence rate ($IR_{P\text{-}T}$), therefore, is:

$$IR_{P\text{-}T} = (45 \, / \, 9{,}860) \times 10^n = 0.0046 \times 10^3 = 4.6 \text{ cases per 1,000 person-years}$$

Step 2: Calculate the cumulative incidence rate.

$$IR_C = \frac{\text{Number of new events occurring during a specified time period}}{\text{Population at risk}} \times 10^n$$

Because all individuals were free of the study disease at the beginning of the study, the initial population at risk was 5,000. Also, as shown in step one, there were 45 cases. So,

$$IR_C = (45 \, / \, 5{,}000) \times 10^n = 0.0090 \times 10^3 = 9.0 \text{ cases per 1,000 population}$$

Step 3: Compare the two rates.

Although the cumulative incidence rate appears to be nearly twice the person-time incidence rate, it is necessary to remember that the cumulative incidence is based on a two-year period. In reality, the two rates in this example are very similar. Assuming the incidence rates are relatively constant, and since they are relatively small and over a short time period, we can estimate one rate from the other using formulas 5.4 a and b:

$$IR_C \cong IR_{P\text{-}T} \times \text{length of the study period in years}$$
$$IR_C \cong (4.6 \text{ per 1,000 person-years}) \times 2 \text{ years} = 9.2 \text{ cases per 1,000 persons}$$
$$\text{(or per 9.2 per 1,000 population or 4.6 per 1,000 population per year)}$$

$$IR_{P\text{-}T} \cong IR_C \, / \, \text{length of the study period in years}$$
$$IR_{P\text{-}T} \cong (9.0 \text{ per 1,000 persons}) \, / \, 2 \text{ years} = 4.5 \text{ per 1,000 persons per year}$$
$$\text{(or 4.5 per 1,000 person-years)}$$

Answer: The person-time incidence rate of gastric ulcers was 4.6 per 1,000 person-years, and the two-year cumulative incidence rate of gastric ulcers was 9.0 per 1,000 population. In this example, the cumulative incidence rate could be estimated from the person-time incidence rate and vice versa. The estimated cumulative incidence rate was 9.2 per 1,000 population compared to the calculated rate of 9.0 per 1,000 population. Similarly, the estimated person-time incidence rate was 4.5 per 1,000 person-years compared to the calculated rate of 4.6 per 1,000 person-years. In both cases, the estimates were nearly identical to the calculated rates. Also, the person-time and cumulative incidence rates are similar if the cumulative incidence rate is expressed on an average annual basis (i.e., as 4.5 per 1,000 population per year).

Measures of Prevalence

Whereas incidence deals with what is *new*, **prevalence** deals with what *exists*. By definition, prevalence is the number of cases of a given disease or other attribute (e.g., drug use, obesity) that exists in a defined population at a specified time. It is also sometimes referred to as the *prevalence number*. Unlike incidence, prevalence does not include mortality, which always represents a first-time or new event. To say that there are 21 cases of leukemia in a particular community at a given time is to make a statement about prevalence. **Prevalence rate*** refers to the *proportion* of a defined population that has a specific disease or attribute at a specified time. It is expressed in a manner similar to the cumulative incidence rate, although, unlike the cumulative incidence rate, it does not measure risk. More will be said about this later in the chapter.

There are two basic types of prevalence rates reported in the epidemiologic literature: the point prevalence rate and the period prevalence rate. The **point prevalence rate** is like a *snapshot* of the proportion of a disease that exists in a defined population, which is generally considered to be the entire population being investigated. Theoretically, the point of time is instantaneous, although in practice it usually represents a particular day or specific date. It can also be an event in time, such as the prevalence rate of cleft palate at birth. Point prevalence is the most commonly reported prevalence rate. Generally, unless otherwise indicated or implied, when a prevalence rate is cited it is most likely a point prevalence rate. The point prevalence rate is calculated as follows:

(5.5)

$$\text{Point PR} = \frac{\text{Number of persons with a specific disease or attribute at a specific point in time}}{\text{Total defined population at the same time}} \times 10^n$$

While the point prevalence rate can be viewed as a snapshot of the prevalence rate, the **period prevalence rate** can be thought of as involving time-lapse photography. It shows what has existed over a period of time. Conceptually, the period prevalence rate is the sum of the point prevalence rate at the beginning of a specified time period plus the cumulative incidence rate for the remainder of the specified time period. It differs from the point prevalence rate as the following formula indicates:

(5.6)

$$\text{Period PR} \quad \frac{\text{Number of persons with a specific disease or attribute anytime during a specified time period}}{\text{Total defined population during the specified time period}} \times 10^n$$

In the period prevalence rate all cases that existed anytime during the specified time period are included in the numerator regardless of outcome. Hence, even if a case dies during the specified time period, that case is still included in the numerator. The denominator for a period prevalence rate is generally the average or mid-interval population for the specified time period.

A variant of the period prevalence rate is the **lifetime prevalence rate**. This refers to the proportion of individuals in a defined population who have had a given disease or attribute at any time in their lives. Thus, the time

---

* As with incidence measures, the term prevalence is sometimes used when prevalence rate is meant. It is important to look at the context in which the terms are used to avoid any confusion.

period for the lifetime prevalence rate represents the lifetimes of the individuals in the population. We can expect the lifetime prevalence rate for a given health-related problem to be greater than the point or the "less than lifetime" period prevalence rates in the same population. In fact, since period or lifetime prevalence rates may give the impression that the magnitude of a particular problem is greater than other problems that may be represented by point prevalence rates, it is important to know what type of prevalence rate is being reported in epidemiologic studies. Many common conditions (e.g., the common cold, heartburn, injuries) have lifetime prevalence rates in adults at or near 100%.

Prevalence is most commonly measured in cross-sectional studies and repeated surveys. It is a useful measure in health planning because it represents the *disease burden* of a community. Alexander Walker[4] refers to prevalence as a status report. The relationship between incidence and prevalence rates is discussed in the following section. Examples of prevalence rate calculations are presented below.

Example 5–4: Point Prevalence Rate

Assume 3,465 women, 60–74 years of age, were screened for the presence of osteoporosis at a major women's health fair held January 3–10, 2002, in Phoenix, Arizona. A total of 974 cases were identified. What was the prevalence rate of osteoporosis in this group?

Solution:

$$\text{Point PR} = \frac{\text{Number of persons with a specific disease or attribute at a specific point in time}}{\text{Total defined population at the same time}} \times 10^n$$

For convenience, let's represent this formula as: Point PR = $(X / Y) \times 10^n$, where X = the number of persons with the disease at a specific point in time, Y = the defined population at the same time, and 10^n = the rate base. Therefore,

$$X = 974 \text{ cases of osteoporosis}$$
$$Y = 3,465 \text{ women, 60–74 years of age}$$
$$\text{Point PR} = (974 / 3,465) \times 10^n = 0.281 \times 10^2 = 28.1 \text{ cases per 100 women}$$

Answer: The point prevalence rate of osteoporosis was 28.1 cases per 100 women, 60–74 years of age, based on the findings at the women's health fair in Phoenix, Arizona, held January 3–10, 2002.

Comments:

1. Although not specifically indicated in the problem, it is implied that the prevalence rate to be calculated is the point prevalence rate. The cases of osteoporosis were those that existed at a point in time (i.e., at the time of the health fair). That the health fair ran for eight days does not alter this fact. Only cases that existed at the time of examination are reported.

2. The defined population includes all women who were screened. As with the cumulative incidence rate, the numerator of a prevalence rate arises from the denominator, which is the reference group. The reference group for the osteoporosis cases are those who were screened.

3. The rate base is selected in the same manner as that for incidence rates. A rate base of 100 is the smallest rate base that will make the prevalence rate at least one per the selected rate base.

4. As with incidence rates, it is important to note that the result is indicative of particular persons at a particular time and place. Unless this information is clear from the context, it is important to specify the relevant person, time, and place factors.

5. The screening referred to in this problem does not really represent an epidemiologic study per se, but it is descriptive and cross-sectional in design.

Example 5–5: Period Prevalence Rate

From January 1 to March 14, 2001, 112 cases of salmonellosis were reported to health officials in Shelby County, a county with a population of 210,000. An additional 10 cases were reported March 15–30. On March 31, six new cases of salmonellosis were reported. Routine surveillance in the county indicated that four of the above reported cases in Shelby County died due to complications. Based on this information, what was the prevalence rate of salmonellosis in Shelby County during the first quarter of 2001?

Solution:

$$\text{Period PR} \quad \frac{\text{Number of persons with a specific disease or attribute anytime during a specified time period}}{\text{Total defined population during the specified time period}} \times 10^n$$

For convenience, let's represent the formula for the period prevalence rate as: Period PR = $(X / Y) \times 10^n$, where X = the number of persons with the disease anytime during a specified time period, Y = the defined population during the specified time period, and 10^n = the rate base. Since, by definition, period prevalence includes all cases that existed anytime during the specified time period, the four cases that died from salmonellosis must not be excluded. They were cases at some time during the first quarter, and therefore they must be counted in the numerator. Therefore,

$$X = 112 + 10 + 6 = 128 \text{ cases of salmonellosis}$$

The defined population includes everyone in Shelby County, since no restrictions are placed on the population by demographic or other factors. Thus,

$$Y = 210,000 \text{ people}$$

$$\text{Period PR} = (128 / 210,000) \times 10^n = 0.00061 \times 10^4 = 6.1 \text{ cases per 10,000 population}$$

Answer: The period prevalence rate of salmonellosis was 6.1 cases per 10,000 population in Shelby County during the first quarter of 2001.

Comments:

1. Period prevalence is the appropriate measure to use in solving this problem. The problem requests the prevalence rate over a period of time (i.e., the first quarter of 2001), which is what the period prevalence rate measures.

2. The rate base is selected as in the previous examples. In this case, a rate base of 10,000 is the smallest rate base that will produce a prevalence rate of at least one per the selected rate base.

3. As in the other examples, it is important to indicate the relevant person, place, and time factors unless this information is clear from the context.

4. This is not an epidemiologic study, but it is a part of descriptive epidemiology.

Relationship between Incidence and Prevalence

Intuitively, it makes sense that incidence and prevalence are related. If there is an increase in the incidence of a nonfatal chronic disease in a community, it would be expected that the prevalence of that disease would also increase. In other words, if many new cases of the disease are developing in the community, and these cases continue to live with the disease, then, unless there is significant migration into or out of the community, we would expect the prevalence of the disease in the community to rise. This relationship is illustrated in figure 5–1 where incidence is depicted by water flowing from a faucet into a basin, and prevalence is represented by the water level in the basin. When the inflow is heavy, the basin readily fills. The process, however, is mediated by another factor, which is represented by the basin drain. This factor is disease resolution. If the disease resolves quickly by recovery or death, this will have the effect of reducing the prevalence unless the inflow is heavy enough to sustain the water level in the basin. However, even if the disease readily resolves itself, a large inflow will not be able to increase the prevalence materially.

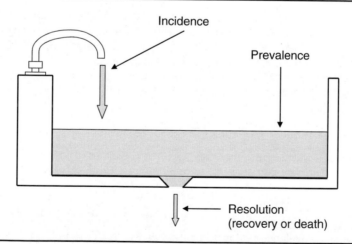

Figure 5–1 Relationship between incidence and prevalence

Person-Time Incidence and Point Prevalence Rates

When a population is stable and the incidence and prevalence rates are unchanging, we have what are known as **steady-state conditions**. Under these conditions we can easily predict the person-time incidence rate if we know the point prevalence rate. This can be very useful because the prevalence rate is usually much easier to obtain than the incidence rate. While the prevalence rate is normally attained in a one-time survey or cross-sectional study, the incidence rate usually requires both an initial assessment of outcome status and a follow-up assessment. Therefore, incidence studies are usually more costly and time consuming than prevalence studies.

Assuming steady-state conditions, the person-time incidence rate can be estimated from the point prevalence rate using the following formula:

(5.7)

$$IR_{P\text{-}T} = \frac{\text{Point PR}}{D\,(1 - \text{Point PR})}$$

where $IR_{P\text{-}T}$ = the person-time incidence rate, Point PR = the point prevalence rate, and D = the average duration of the disease from diagnosis until recovery or death.[2] If in addition to meeting the requirement for steady-state conditions, the disease prevalence is low (say, less than 10 per 100), formula 5.7 can be simplified to $IR_{P\text{-}T} \cong$ Point PR / D. For ease of calculation, the rates should be expressed as *decimal fractions* and the average duration in years if person-years are to be reported. For example, say a given disease has a point prevalence rate of 20 cases per 1,000 population and an average duration of three years from diagnosis to resolution. The person-time incidence rate for this example could be estimated as follows: 0.02 / [3 (1 – 0.02)] = 0.02 / [3 (0.98)] = 0.02 / 2.94 = 0.0068. Therefore, the estimated person-time incidence rate is 6.8 per 1,000 person-years, using a rate base of 1,000 and assuming steady-state conditions. Note that 0.02, a decimal fraction, is equivalent to 20 per 1,000. Using decimal fractions avoids the problem of what to do with the rate bases during the arithmetic procedures. Since the prevalence rate is also low (i.e., less than 10 per 100), we could have estimated the person-time incidence rate using the formula $IR_{P\text{-}T} \cong$ Point PR / D. In this case the estimate would be 0.02 / 3 = 0.0067, which is 6.7 per 1,000 person-years, and very close to what was calculated using formula 5.7.

Cumulative Incidence and Point Prevalence Rates

While the cumulative incidence rate is a good estimate of disease risk, the point prevalence rate is not. This is due to the fact that the magnitude of the point prevalence rate is influenced by the duration of the disease (i.e., by recovery or death). The cumulative incidence rate, on the other hand, is not affected by duration. That is, whether cases recover or die has no influence on the number of new cases developing in a defined population. Therefore, the cumulative incidence rate reflects the risk of disease development, while the point prevalence rate reflects risk and duration, which can be difficult to untangle. For this reason prevalence rates should not be used to estimate risk. In the Framingham Heart Study initial examinations of males and females in the 30–44-year age group revealed identical prevalence rates of coronary heart disease of five per 1,000. Eight years of follow-up, however, showed something else. The cumulative incidence rate for the males was 24 per 1,000 versus only one per 1,000 for the females. Had the prevalence rates been used to estimate the risk of heart disease, one would have concluded incorrectly that there was no difference in risk between the males and females. The reason for the similarity in prevalence rates and the difference in cumulative incidence rates between the sexes has to do with duration of the disease. The males tended to die from more fatal myocardial infarctions than the females, while the females tended to develop more nonfatal cases of angina pectoris than the males.[5] Thus, the disease in the males tended to be of shorter duration, resulting in a low prevalence rate compared to the cumulative incidence rate, and the disease in the females tended to be of longer duration, resulting in a high prevalence rate compared to the cumulative incidence rate. The prevalence rates were affected by the duration of the disease, but the cumulative incidence rates were not. Table 5–1 compares some of the more common characteristics of cumulative incidence and point prevalence rates.

Table 5–1 General Characteristics of Incidence and Prevalence

Cumulative Incidence Rate	Point Prevalence Rate
• Dynamic concept indicating change in disease status over time	• Static concept indicating existing disease status at a particular time
• A good estimate of the risk of disease	• An unreliable estimate of the risk of disease
• Unaffected by recovery or death	• Affected by recovery or death

General Health and Population Indices

There are a number of frequency measures used in epidemiology as general indicators or indices of the health status of a population. Many of these measures relate to mortality since these data are more readily available on chronic diseases than are data on morbidity. In addition, there are several indicators of population dynamics (e.g., the **crude birth rate** and the **fertility rate**), which indicate changes in population growth. Figure 5–2 on page 77 lists some of the more common indices used in epidemiology. The rate bases shown are those most frequently reported. As should be clear from the preceding discussion, other rate bases may be used in specific circumstances.

The **crude death rate** (CDR) is actually a type of cumulative incidence rate. The event being measured is death and, since everyone is at risk of dying, the population at risk is the entire population. The CDR in the United States was reported in the late 1990s to be 864.7 deaths per 100,000 population.[6] Another common index is the **cause-specific mortality rate**, which measures the risk of death due to a specific cause. When leading causes of death are reported in the literature, cause-specific mortality rates are being used. In the same report citing the crude death rate, the leading cause of death in the United States was heart disease with a cause-specific mortality rate of 271.6 per 100,000.[6] This was over 4.5 times greater than that for cere-

1. Crude Birth Rate	$\dfrac{\text{Number of live births during a specified time period}}{\text{Mid-interval population}} \times 1{,}000$
2. Fertility Rate	$\dfrac{\text{Number of live births during a specified time period}}{\text{Mid-interval population of women aged 15–44 years}} \times 1{,}000$
3. Crude Death Rate (CDR)	$\dfrac{\text{Number of deaths during a specified time period}}{\text{Mid-interval population}} \times 1{,}000$ (or 100,000)
4. Cause-Specific Mortality Rate	$\dfrac{\text{Number of deaths from a specific cause during a specified time period}}{\text{Mid-interval population}} \times 100{,}000$
5. Proportionate Mortality Ratio (PMR)	$\dfrac{\text{Number of deaths from a specific cause during a specified time period}}{\text{Total number of deaths in the same time period}} \times 100$
6. Infant Mortality Rate	$\dfrac{\text{Number of deaths in infants aged 0–1 year during a specified time period}}{\text{Number of live births in the same time period}} \times 1{,}000$
7. Neonatal Mortality Rate	$\dfrac{\text{Number of deaths in infants aged less than 28 days during a specified time period}}{\text{Number of live births in the same time period}} \times 1{,}000$
8. Perinatal Mortality Rate	$\dfrac{\text{Number of fetal deaths after 28 weeks or more of gestation + Number of infant deaths within 7 days of birth during a specified time period}}{\text{Number of live births + Number of fetal deaths after 28 weeks or more of gestation}} \times 1{,}000$
9. Fetal Death Rate	$\dfrac{\text{Number of fetal deaths after 20 weeks or more of gestation during a specified time period}}{\text{Number of live births + Number of fetal deaths after 20 weeks or more of gestation}} \times 1{,}000$
10. Maternal Mortality Rate	$\dfrac{\text{Number of deaths due to childbirth during a specified time period}}{\text{Number of live births in the same time period}} \times 100{,}000$

Most of these indices are routinely reported on a calendar basis. The rate bases are those in most common use.

Figure 5–2 Common health and population indices used in epidemiology

brovascular diseases, the third leading cause of death. It was also 30% higher than the second leading cause of death, malignant neoplasms.

The **proportionate mortality ratio** (PMR) appears similar to the cause-specific mortality rate, but is actually quite different. Instead of measuring the *risk* of dying from a specific cause of death, it measures how important a particular cause of death is in relation to all deaths occurring in a given population. A high PMR means that a certain cause of death contributes substantially to all deaths in a particular group, but it tells us nothing about the risk of dying from that cause. The PMR, which is a ratio, depends not only on how many deaths occur from a specific cause but also on how many total deaths occur. For example, in a recent report, the cause-specific mortality rate for diabetes was 38.4 per 100,000 among 55–64 year olds, but only 1.6 per 100,000 among 25–34 year olds,[6] implying that the risk of dying from diabetes was 24 times higher in the 55–64-year-old group than the 25–34-year-old group. The PMR, however, was somewhat lower in the older versus the younger age group (3.1 per 1,000 vs. 4.1 per 1,000). The explanation for this difference is that the total number of deaths (i.e., the denominator of the PMR) was significantly smaller in the 25–34 year olds than in the 55–64 year olds.

Other common health status indices include the **infant mortality rate**, the **neonatal mortality rate**, the **maternal mortality rate**, the **perinatal mortality rate**, and the **fetal death rate** (see figure 5–2). Note that the first three of these rates have the number of live births in the denominator. This is not the exact population at risk, but it is a convenient estimate, and one that is reliably reported and readily available. The population at risk for the maternal mortality rate, for example, should be the number of pregnancies during the specific time interval, but as this is virtually impossible to obtain, the number of live births provides a convenient estimate. The denominators for the perinatal mortality rate and the fetal death rate are also denominators of convenience. With regard to the infant and neonatal mortality rates, which are usually reported on a calendar year basis, some of the infant deaths in one year may be from births that occurred in the previous year. For example, some deaths that occurred in January of a particular calendar year may represent births that occurred in December of the previous year. Nevertheless, these routinely reported rates are good indices of the health status of a population and are valuable in identifying potential public health problems, establishing trends, and making comparisons to other populations or periods of time. We would be very concerned, for example, about the quality of health care and public health services in a population if the infant mortality rate was increasing or high compared to similar populations.

Other Measures of Morbidity and Mortality

Case Fatality Rate

One mortality rate that deserves special mention is the **case fatality rate** (CFR). This is not an index of community health status but, instead, is a measure of prognosis for those with a given disease. It represents the rate at which cases die from a disease; hence, it is an indicator of a disease's deadliness. The CFR for untreated bubonic plague is estimated to be about 55%. That for meningococcal meningitis, a serious acute bacterial infection affecting primarily children and young adults, is 5–15% with early diagnosis, therapy, and supportive measures.[7] The CFR can be calculated using the following formula:

(5.8)

$$CFR = \frac{\text{Number of deaths from a specific disease during a specified time period}}{\text{Number of cases of the disease during the same time period}} \times 10^n$$

The 10^n is the rate base, which is usually 10^2 (or 100). As the previous examples illustrate, the CFR is usually expressed as a percentage. Like some of the previous mortality rates, the CFR is not really a rate. It is the proportion of cases who die during a given time period. It should be expected, however, that some of the cases will have developed in time periods prior to that of the deaths, so the cases and deaths are not necessarily linked. As an example of the calculation of a CFR, assume that, in 2001, 40 cases of a given disease were diagnosed in a certain community and that 12 persons diagnosed with the disease died. The CFR would be calculated as: $(12 / 40) \times 10^n = 0.30 \times 10^2 = 30\%$.

Survival Rate

Another measure related to the CFR is the **survival rate** (SR), which is also a measure of prognosis and useful in applications in clinical epidemiology. It measures the probability of surviving a specified period of time.[8] The SR is usually expressed as a percent and is calculated as:

(5.9)

$$SR = \frac{\begin{array}{c}\text{Number of newly diagnosed patients with a given disease} - \text{Number} \\ \text{of deaths observed among the patients in a specified time period}\end{array}}{\begin{array}{c}\text{Number of newly diagnosed patients with} \\ \text{the disease in the same time period}\end{array}} \times 10^n$$

For example, say one wanted to calculate the five-year survival rate for breast cancer. Suppose there were 150 newly diagnosed breast cancer cases in a sample, and the investigators followed the patients to determine the five-year survival rate. During five years of follow-up, 45 of the cases died from breast cancer. The survival rate would be calculated in the following manner: SR = $[(150 - 45) / 150] = (105 / 150) \times 10^n = 0.70 \times 10^2 = 70\%$. Thus, 70% of the patients survived five years after diagnosis. The SR assumes that death is the only reason that patients do not complete the prescribed follow-up period. It does not account for losses to follow-up or attrition (i.e., patients discontinuing their participation). Life table analysis and similar survival analysis techniques have been developed to handle these situations, and are discussed by Moyses Szklo and F. Javier Nieto[9] and others. Another limitation of the SR (and the CFR) is that deaths may not always be related to the disease, so the SR may be influenced by unrelated events, such as injuries, accidental poisonings, and so forth. However, if the sample size is large, the influence of these factors is likely to be minimal.

Years of Potential Life Lost

Years of potential life lost (YPLL) and its variants (e.g., years of productive life lost) measure the relative impact of premature death on society and can be used to establish public health priorities. In contrast to other mortality measures, they are weighted toward deaths at younger ages. Hence, a death of a 10 year old contributes substantially more to the YPLL than the death of a 60 year old.[10] This weighting has a definite economic overtone, but it does dramatize the societal impact of some diseases. The YPLL can be calculated for all premature deaths or only those from specific causes (see figure 5–3).

   To calculate YPLL, one must first decide upon a suitable *endpoint*. The endpoint represents an age that is considered *not* to constitute premature or untimely death. Typical endpoints are 65, 70, or 75 years or average life expectancy. Once the endpoint has been determined, every death in a popu-

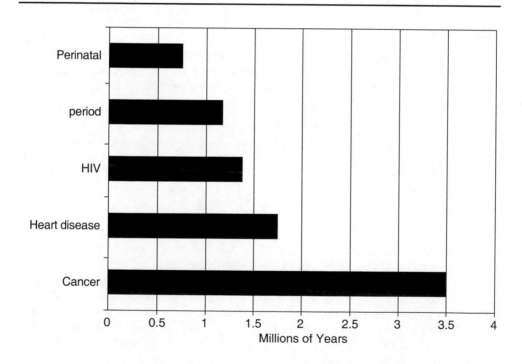

Source: National Center for Prevention and Control (1997). Years of Potential Life Lost Before Age 65 Due to Injury. Available: http://www.cdc.gov/ncipc/images/yp1995.gif (Access date: March 3, 2000.)

Figure 5–3 Years of potential life lost before age 65 by causes of death, U. S., 1995

lation that occurs *before* the endpoint is subtracted from the endpoint to obtain the number of years of potential life lost. This can be represented mathematically as:

(5.10)

$$YPLL = \Sigma \, (E - a_i)$$

where Σ = sum of, E = the chosen endpoint (e.g., 65 years), and a_i = the age of an individual who dies prior to the endpoint. Thus, this formula represents the sum of the differences between the endpoint and age at premature death for all individuals in the population who have not yet reached the endpoint. When YPLL is calculated from a distribution of deaths by age categories, the *midpoints* of the age categories are used.

   The YPLL rate is a measure of the number of years of potential life lost in relation to the population younger than the selected endpoint in a specified time period. It is calculated as follows:

(5.11)

$$YPLL \ Rate = \frac{YPLL}{Number \ in \ the \ population \ below \ the \ selected \ endpoint} \times 10^n$$

where YPLL is calculated as shown in formula 5.10, the denominator is the population younger than the chosen endpoint (e.g., those under 65 years of age), and 10^n is usually 10^3 or 1,000. The following examples are illustrative:

Example 5–6: Years of Potential Life Lost before 65 Years

Health officials reported five deaths in Spring Valley in 2001. Three of these deaths were of persons under the age of 65. One death occurred in a 19-year-old male due to a motorcycle injury. The other two deaths occurred from drowning when a brother and sister went swimming in an unsupervised quarry. The boy was 11 and his sister was nine. The estimated population of Spring Valley was 5,400, and 65% of the population was under the age of 65. What are the YPLL before 65 years overall and for each cause of death, respectively? Also, what is the overall YPLL rate for Spring Valley in 2001?

Solution:

Step 1: Calculate the overall YPLL.

$$YPLL = \Sigma \, (E - a_i)$$

where Σ = sum of, E = the endpoint of interest, and a_i = the age of an individual who dies prior to the endpoint. Therefore,

$\Sigma \, (E - a_i) = (65 - 19) + (65 - 11) + (65 - 9) = 46 + 54 + 56 = 156$ years of potential life lost

Step 2: Calculate the YPLL specific for each cause of death.

The YPLL due to motorcycle injury is:

$$65 - 19 = 46 \text{ years of potential life lost}$$

and the YPLL due to drowning is:

$$(65 - 11) + (65 - 9) = 54 + 56 = 110 \text{ years of potential life lost}$$

Step 3: Calculate the overall YPLL rate.

$$\text{YPLL Rate} = \frac{\text{YPLL}}{\text{Number in the population below the selected endpoint}} \times 10^n$$

For convenience, let's represent the formula as: YPLL rate = $(X / Y) \times 10^n$, where X = YPLL, Y = the population under age 65, and 10^n = the rate base. Therefore,

$$X = 156 \text{ years}$$
$$Y = 5,400 \times 0.65 = 3,510 \text{ people under age 65}$$
$$X / Y = 156 / 3,510 = 0.0444$$

YPLL rate = $0.0444 \times 1,000 = 44.4$ years of potential life lost per 1,000 population under age 65

Answer: In Spring Valley, 2001, 156 years of potential life were lost before age 65, 46 due to motorcycle injury and 110 due to drowning. The YPLL rate was 44.4 per 1,000 population under age 65.

Comments:

1. Since the age of 65 is chosen as the endpoint, the two deaths that occurred in those 65 years or older are not considered in calculating the YPLL, and the population 65 years or older is not included in the denominator of the YPLL rate.

2. The overall YPLL before age 65 in Spring Valley in 2001 was 156. This implies that 156 years of potential life could have been saved if the deaths could have been prevented.

3. Drowning was the most important cause of death in Spring Valley in terms of YPLL before age 65. Over twice as many years of potential life were lost before age 65 due to drowning compared to motorcycle injury.

4. The sum of the YPLL due to motorcycle injury and drowning is equal to the total YPLL before age 65 because these were the only causes of death in the population among those less than 65 years of age. Had there been other causes of death before age 65, the sum of the YPLL due to motorcycle injury (46 years) and drowning (110 years) in this population would have been less than the total YPLL before age 65.

5. The YPLL rate is the number of years of potential life that were lost for every 1,000 persons in Spring Valley who were not yet 65 years of age. A rate base of 1,000 is common, but any suitable rate base may be chosen.

6. Unless it is clear from the context, it is a good idea to indicate the population, place, and time observed when reporting the YPLL or the YPLL rate. In this case it was the population of Spring Valley in the year 2001.

Example 5–7: Years of Potential Life Lost before 70 Years

The following statistics were reported for Humboldt County in 2001:

Age Group	Population	Deaths
0–9	3,610	3
10–19	2,500	2
20–39	5,125	3
40–59	4,950	8
60–69	3,945	12
70 and over	2,900	13

Based on these data, calculate the total YPLL before age 70 and the YPLL rate.

Solution:

Step 1: Calculate the YPLL.

$$YPLL = \Sigma \, (E - a_i)$$

where Σ = sum of, E = the endpoint of interest, and a_i = the midpoint of an individual age category where a death occurred prior to the endpoint. *The midpoint is determined by summing the initial and ending age for each age category, adding one, and dividing the sum by two.* Since all deaths in each age category are assumed to have occurred at the midpoint, the number of deaths in a category is multiplied by the difference between age 70 and the midpoint (i.e., $E - a_i$). Based on the data in the above table, the YPLL is thus calculated as follows:

$$\Sigma \, (E - a_i) = [3 \, (70 - 5)] + [2 \, (70 - 15)] + [3 \, (70 - 30)] + [8 \, (70 - 50)] + [12 \, (70 - 65)] =$$
$$195 + 110 + 120 + 160 + 60 = 645 \text{ years of potential life lost}$$

Step 2: Calculate the YPLL rate.

$$YPLL \text{ Rate} = \frac{YPLL}{\text{Number in the population below the selected endpoint}} \times 10^n$$

For convenience, let's represent the formula as: YPLL rate = $(X / Y) \times 10^n$, where X = YPLL, Y = the population under age 70, and 10^n = the rate base. Therefore,

$$X = 645 \text{ years}$$
$$Y = 3{,}610 + 2{,}500 + 5{,}125 + 4{,}950 + 3{,}945 = 20{,}130 \text{ people under age 70}$$
$$X / Y = 645 / 20{,}130 = 0.0320$$

YPLL rate = $0.0320 \times 1{,}000 = 32.0$ years of potential life lost per 1,000 population under age 70

Answer: In Humboldt County in 2001, 645 years of potential life were lost before age 70, and the YPLL rate was 32.0 per 1,000 population under age 70.

Comments:

1. Since the age of 70 is chosen as the endpoint, the deaths that occurred in those 70 years and over are *not* considered in calculating the YPLL. Also, the population 70 years and over is not included in the denominator of the YPLL rate.

2. To calculate the YPLL, it was necessary first to determine the midpoint for each age category. This is accomplished by summing the beginning and ending age of an age category, adding one, and dividing the result by two (e.g., for the 0–9-year age group, the midpoint = $[0 + 9 + 1] / 2 = 5$). The one is added because the ending age (e.g., nine) is virtually a year long since it actually extends to within a day of the next year (i.e., 10). The midpoint is then subtracted from the endpoint (i.e., 70 years) and multiplied by the number of deaths in that category. In example 5–6 we had each individual's age at death, which we subtracted from the endpoint. We do not have this information in this example; therefore, we have assumed that all deaths in a particular age category were on average at the midpoint of the interval. For example, multiplying the difference between the endpoint and the midpoint in the first age category by three is the same as adding 70 – 5 three times, since all deaths in the category were presumed to have occurred at age five, which is the midpoint of the 0–9 age group as defined above.

3. The overall YPLL before age 70 in Humboldt County in 2001 was estimated to be 645. This means that based on the chosen endpoint of 70 years, approximately 645 years of potential life could have been saved if the deaths could have been prevented. The reason this number is approximate is because exact ages at death are not available and

were therefore estimated using the midpoints of the age categories. Exact ages may not always be available when secondary data sources are being used.

4. The YPLL rate is the estimated number of years of potential life that were lost for every 1,000 persons in Humboldt County who were not yet 70 years of age. A rate base of 1,000 is common, but any suitable rate base may be used.

5. Unless it is clear from the context, it is important to indicate the population, place, and time observed when reporting the YPLL or the YPLL rate. In this case it was the population of Humboldt County in the year 2001.

Confidence Intervals for Rates

Because it is often impossible or impractical to measure an entire population of interest, epidemiologic rates are typically based on samples of populations. Samples, however, characterize only a fraction of the **target population**, that is, the population to which we would like to generalize the findings.[11] Therefore, the sample rate is only an estimate of the population rate, and one that will vary depending on the characteristics of the sample chosen. In statistics, the sample rate is considered a **point estimate** of the population rate, that is, a sample statistic used to estimate a population parameter.[12] The precision of the point estimate is a function of how representative the sample is of the target population, and the representativeness of the sample depends on the *sampling technique* and *chance variation*. Random sampling techniques tend to increase the probability, but not guarantee, that a sample will be representative of a target population because chance variation can still occur. The role of chance can be estimated, however, though not controlled. Therefore, rates calculated from samples will vary in how well they represent the rate in the target population.

One way of estimating the precision of a sample rate is to calculate a **confidence interval**, which is the range of values in which the population parameter is likely to fall based on statistical probability. The most commonly reported confidence interval for rates in epidemiology is the *95% confidence interval*. It is defined as follows:

> *The 95% confidence interval is the range of sample estimates in which we are 95% confident that the population rate lies.*

Figure 5–4 provides an example of a 95% confidence interval for a rate. The 95% represents the **confidence level**, the range represents the *confidence interval*, and the start and end of the range represent the **confidence limits**. The lower rate is known as the **lower confidence limit** (LCL), and the upper rate is known as the **upper confidence limit** (UCL). With regard to the example in figure 5–4, we can state that we are 95% confident that the population rate lies between 4.2 per 1,000 and 5.4 per 1,000. This implies, of course, that we cannot be 100% certain because for every 100 samples drawn ran-

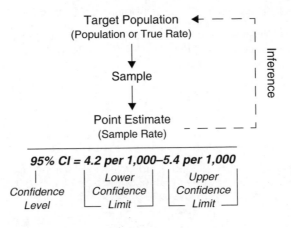

Figure 5–4 Anatomy of a 95% confidence interval (CI)

domly from the population, we would expect that 5% would produce point estimates outside these boundaries because of chance variation. Nevertheless, we have a high degree of confidence about the relative magnitude of the population rate.

A confidence interval is affected by sample size, sample variance, and the confidence level chosen. Narrow confidence intervals indicate more precision than wide confidence intervals. In general, for a given confidence level, the greater the sample size, or the less the sample variance, the more precise the point estimate, and thus the narrower the confidence interval. On a relative basis it is easier to be 50% confident about the probable range of a population rate than to be 99% confident. Therefore, the greater the confidence level for a particular sample, the wider the confidence interval.

Because of their extensive use and importance in epidemiology, you will be reading more about specific types of confidence intervals in subsequent chapters. For now it is important that you understand their usefulness with sample measures of morbidity and mortality and that you know how to interpret them properly. Methods for estimating 95% confidence intervals for incidence and prevalence rates are presented in exhibit 5–2. There are also a number of statistical computer programs available and Internet sites that will calculate various confidence intervals.

Exhibit 5–2 Estimating Confidence Intervals for Rates

If we assume that the number of cases is distributed normally, we can calculate approximate 95% confidence intervals for the following measures using methods derived from Ahlbom.*

95% Confidence Interval (CI) for the Cumulative Incidence or Prevalence Rate

$$95\% \ CI = r \pm 1.96 \ \sqrt{r \ (I - r) / n}$$

where r = the cumulative incidence rate or prevalence rate stated as a decimal fraction and n = the appropriate denominator (i.e., population at risk or total population).

Example: On September 14, 2000, a cross-sectional survey of 24,000 residents of a western state revealed that there were 145 cases of tuberculosis. What is the prevalence rate and 95% confidence interval?

Solution: r = the prevalence rate = 145 / 24,000 = 0.006 (stated as a decimal fraction); n = 24,000

$$95\% \ CI = 0.006 \pm 1.96 \ \sqrt{0.006 \ (1 - 0.006) / 24,000} =$$

0.006 − [1.96 (0.0004)] = 0.005 (this is the lower confidence limit)

0.006 + [1.96 (0.0004)] = 0.007 (this is the upper confidence limit)

95% CI = 0.005–0.007 = 5.0 per 1,000 − 7.0 per 1,000 (using a rate base of 1,000)

95% Confidence Interval (CI) for the Person-Time Incidence Rate

$$95\% \ CI = r \pm 1.96 \ \sqrt{e / T^2}$$

where r = the person-time incidence rate stated as a decimal fraction, e = the number of new events, and T = the total person-time units at risk.

Example: A prospective cohort study revealed that 65 new cases of stroke developed over 1,300 person-years of observation. What is the person-time incidence rate and 95% confidence interval?

Solution: r = the person-time incidence rate = 65 / 1,300 = 0.05 (stated as a decimal fraction); e = 65 and T = 1,300

$$95\% \ CI = 0.05 \pm 1.96 \ \sqrt{65 / 1,300^2} =$$

0.05 − [1.96 (0.006)] = 0.04 (this is the lower confidence limit)

0.05 + [1.96 (0.006)] = 0.06 (this is the upper confidence limit)

95% CI = 0.04–0.06 = 4.0 per 100 person-years − 6.0 per 100 person-years (using a rate base of 100)

*Ahlbom, A. (1993). *Biostatistics for Epidemiologists*. Boca Raton, FL: Lewis Publishers.

Summary

- Incidence refers to the number of new cases of a disease. When combined with the appropriate denominator and rate base, two types of incidence rates can be calculated—the cumulative incidence rate, which is incidence divided by the population at risk, and the person-time incidence rate, which is incidence divided by the total person-time units at risk. Technically, the cumulative incidence rate is a measure of the risk of disease development, and the person-time incidence rate is a measure of the rate of disease development. Under certain circumstances one rate can be used to estimate the other.

- Prevalence is the number of existing cases of disease in a population. The prevalence rate is the proportion of the total defined population with the disease. There are two major types of prevalence rates—the point prevalence rate, which is the prevalence rate at a specific point in time, and the period prevalence rate, which is the prevalence rate over a period of time. Under steady-state conditions, if one knows the point prevalence rate and the average duration of a disease, it is possible to calculate the person-time incidence rate.

- Other common frequency measures in epidemiology are used to indicate health status of a population. These measures include the crude death rate, the cause-specific mortality rate, the proportionate mortality ratio, the infant mortality rate, and years of potential life lost. In addition, the crude birth rate and the fertility rate can be used as indicators of population growth. The case fatality rate and the survival rate are measures of disease prognosis.

- Since most rates are based on samples of a population, confidence intervals are commonly used to estimate the probable range in which the population rate lies. The 95% level is the most common confidence level reported in epidemiology. Sample size, sample variance, and the chosen confidence level affect the range of confidence intervals. In general, the narrower the range of the confidence interval, the more precise the point estimate and vice versa.

New Terms

case fatality rate
cause-specific
  mortality rate
confidence interval
confidence level
confidence limits
crude birth rate
crude death rate
cumulative incidence rate

fertility rate
fetal death rate
force of morbidity
incidence
incidence density
incidence rate
infant mortality rate
initial population
  at risk

lifetime prevalence rate
lower confidence limit
maternal mortality rate
neonatal mortality rate
perinatal mortality rate
period prevalence rate
person-time incidence
  rate
person-time units

point estimate	proportionate mortality ratio	target population
point prevalence rate	rate base	upper confidence limit
population at risk	risk	years of potential
prevalence	steady-state conditions	life lost
prevalence rate	survival rate	YPLL rate

Study Questions and Exercises

1. San Carlos County Health Department reported 17 new cases of tuberculosis in the first half of 2001 and 18 additional cases during the second half of the year. The population of the county was 204,500 at the beginning of the year and 215,000 at the end of the year. What was the incidence rate of tuberculosis in San Carlos County in 2001? Also, what type of incidence rate does this represent?

2. During the period July 1 to December 31, 2000, 76 cases of measles were reported among 12–19 year olds in a Russian community of 32,000. Ten percent (3,200) of the residents were 12–19 years old on April 1, and the size and age distribution of the population has remained constant. An investigation of the cases in the 12–19-year age group revealed that 22 of the reported cases were contracted prior to July 1. In addition, another 18 cases developed in April and May but were clinically resolved before July 1. What was the cumulative incidence rate of measles in 12–19 year olds in this Russian community during the period July 1–December 31, 2000?

3. An epidemiologic study of breast cancer among elderly women followed 1,400 women, 65–79 years of age, without evidence of breast cancer over several years. Every two years the investigators examined the women for breast cancer. The results were as follows: 12 new cases at the first evaluation, 11 new cases at the second evaluation, 23 new cases at the third evaluation, and 28 new cases at the fourth (final) evaluation. The investigators also noted that 35 of the women had withdrawn from the study at the third evaluation. Based on this information, calculate and interpret the person-time incidence rate of breast cancer in this group and the associated 95% confidence interval.

4. Health authorities in Egypt reported that 22 injuries requiring hospitalization occurred in a community of 65,000 during a recent national holiday. Eight additional cases occurred during the following month, and two of these died from their injuries. What was the prevalence rate of injuries requiring hospitalization on the holiday and for the period as a whole?

5. In Ferguson Junction last year four deaths occurred in males aged 3, 12, 24, and 75 years, and two deaths occurred in females aged 14 and 85 years. The population of Ferguson Junction last year was 24,000, of which 10% were 70 years or older. Based on these data, calculate the total years of potential life lost (YPLL) before age 70 and the YPLL rate. Interpret your findings.

6. Each of the following statements suggests a common epidemiologic measure that could be calculated if the all the data had been supplied in the statement. For example, the first statement suggests the crude death rate. The numerator for this rate (82 deaths from all causes) is provided, and the denominator is the population of Randall County, which could be obtained from census data. For each of the other statements indicate what epidemiologic measure is being suggested and indicate the reasons for your answer.

   a. In Randall County there were 82 deaths from all causes last year.

   b. Twelve cases of rabies were reported for the first time in Asheville this year.

   c. Of 10 new cases of ovarian cancer diagnosed in Darrington County, only four were living after five years.

   d. Ten percent of all deaths are caused by suffocation in Summit County.

   e. Of the 130 babies born in Shannon County last year, 14 died within four weeks.

   f. Last year 21 deaths occurred in Culver City from accidental drowning.

   g. Sixty percent of the population of Orion has had the flu in the last two years.

   h. Of the 45 cases of hemorrhagic stroke admitted to Community Memorial Hospital last year, 12 died within two days of admission.

References

1. Ahlbom, A., and Norell, S. (1990). *Introduction to Modern Epidemiology*, 2nd ed. Chestnut Hill, MA: Epidemiology Resources, Inc.
2. Kleinbaum, D. G., Kupper, L. L., and Morgenstern, H. (1982). *Epidemiologic Research: Principles and Quantitative Methods*. Belmont, CA: Lifetime Learning Publications.
3. Hennekens, C. H., and Buring, J. E. (1987). *Epidemiology in Medicine*. Boston: Little, Brown and Company.
4. Walker, A. M. (1991). *Observation and Inference: An Introduction to the Methods of Epidemiology*. Chestnut Hill, MA: Epidemiology Resources, Inc.
5. Mausner, J. S., and Kramer, S. (1985). *Mausner & Bahn Epidemiology—An Introductory Text*. Philadelphia: W. B. Saunders Company.
6. Hoyert, D. L., Kochanek, K. D., and Murphy, S. L. (1999). Deaths: Final Data for 1997. *National Vital Statistics Reports* 47(19). Hyattsville, MD: National Center for Health Statistics.
7. Chin, J., ed. (2000). *Control of Communicable Diseases Manual*, 17th ed. Washington, DC: American Public Health Association.
8. Greenberg, R. S., Daniels, S. R., Flanders, W. D., Eley, J. W., and Boring, J. R. (1996). *Medical Epidemiology*, 2nd ed. Norwalk, CT: Appleton and Lange.
9. Szklo, M., and Nieto, F. J. (2000). *Epidemiology: Beyond the Basics*. Gaithersburg, MD: Aspen.
10. Centers for Disease Control and Prevention (1986). Premature Mortality in the United States: Public Health Issues in the Use of Years of Potential Life Lost. *Morbidity and Mortality Weekly Reports* 35(2S): 1s–11s.
11. Last, J. M., ed. (1995). *A Dictionary of Epidemiology*. New York: Oxford University Press.
12. Vogt, W. P. (1993). *Dictionary of Statistics and Methodology*. Newbury Park, CA: Sage.

CHAPTER SIX

Comparing Rates in Epidemiology

Learning Objectives

▸ Distinguish among crude, specific, and adjusted rates.

▸ Explain the rationale for rate adjustment/standardization.

▸ Perform and interpret the results of age adjustment using both the direct and indirect methods.

▸ Calculate and interpret relative risk, percent relative effect, rate ratio, odds ratio, risk and rate differences, attributable risk, attributable risk percent, population attributable risk, and population attributable risk percent and their rate counterparts.

▸ Perform and interpret the results of significance testing for dependent rates.

▸ Define absolute risk, confounding, odds, p-value, sampling error, and z-score.

Overview

Because comparisons of crude rates are often distorted by differences in the underlying population distributions, direct or indirect rate adjustment is frequently performed to remove the distortion and permit fair comparisons between the rates. Measures of association, such as the relative risk, rate ratio, and odds ratio, tell us about the strength of the relationship between a given exposure and outcome, while measures such as risk and rate differences, including attributable and population attributable risks and their percents, tell us about the public health impact of eliminating harmful exposures from either the exposed groups or the population as a whole. Tests of statistical significance tell us the probability that observed differences between rates are due to sampling error. A statistically significant difference is considered an unlikely result of sampling error; hence, it probably represents a real difference between the rates.

Crude and Specific Rates

Most of the epidemiologic measures referred to in chapter 5 were crude or specific rates. **Crude rates** are *overall* or *summary rates* for a defined population and are determined by dividing the total number of events of interest in a given time period by the defined population and multiplying the result by a selected rate base. **Specific rates** are rates for *distinct subgroups* within a defined population. For example, in a recent year, the overall infant mortality rate in the U.S. was 7.2 deaths per 1,000 live births. Among males, however, the rate was 7.9 per 1,000, and for females it was 6.5 per 1,000.[1] The overall rate in this example is the *crude* infant mortality rate. The rates for males and females are the *sex-specific* infant mortality rates.

Specific rates can be calculated for any subgroup of a defined population, although the most commonly reported specific rates are those based on age, sex, or race/ethnicity. In determining specific rates, it is essential to know the *defined population*. If the defined population only includes women, for example, then sex-specific rates cannot be calculated. In regard to the infant mortality rate, age-specific rates could be calculated, but each age-specific category would have to represent less than one year in length.

Crude rates are useful because with *just one rate* we get an overall summary of the actual experience of a defined population. The crude rate is actually a *weighted average* of the specific rates. Thus, if a defined population is 60% male and 40% female, and if the rate is 12 per 100 for males and 16 per 100 for females, then the crude rate is: (12 per 100 × 0.60) + (16 per 100 × 0.40) = 13.6 per 100. Crude rates make comparisons relatively simple. For example, in a recent year, the crude death rate in Florida was almost 2.5 times higher than that in Alaska (1,054.3 deaths per 100,000 population in Florida compared to 422.6 deaths per 100,000 population in Alaska).[2]

While crude rates are relatively easy to calculate and compare, they can be mine fields when it comes to interpreting the results of the comparisons. Before we can conclude that Florida is a much riskier place to live than Alaska, we have to be sure that the populations are similar in other important respects. If they differ significantly with regard to other factors that are related to the risk of death, then we cannot be sure whether or not any observed difference in the crude death rates is due to living in one of the states or to one or more of these factors. Some common factors that can distort comparisons of crude morbidity or mortality rates include differences in population distributions by age, sex, race/ethnicity, certain lifestyle behaviors, and the presence of certain diseases. For example, since age is closely related to the risk of death, if two populations have very different age distributions,* then it is possible that the age differences themselves might explain partially or fully any observed difference in the crude death rates. As you are probably aware, Florida has a large proportion of retired individuals, which skews the age distribu-

---

* Age distribution refers to the proportions or percentages of a population in different age groups. For example, a given population may have 1.5% of its population in the less than one year age category, 6.5% in the 1–4-year age category, 17.0% in the 5–14 age category, etc. The sum of the percentages for all age groups in the population will equal 100%.

tion of the population toward the older age groups. In fact, according to U.S. Census estimates, 18.4% of the population of Florida was 65 years or older in the example referred to earlier. Alaska, on the other hand, has a relatively young population. Only 5.3% of its residents were 65 or older.[3] Therefore, we would expect Florida to have a higher crude death rate than Alaska simply because of its older population and not necessarily due to any increased risk of living among the palm trees compared to the scenic panorama of Alaska.

Unlike crude rates, specific rates (e.g., rates in specific age, sex, or racial/ethnic subgroups) normally can be compared between populations *without* fear of distortion due to **confounding*** by the factor(s) used to categorize the subgroups (e.g., age, sex, or race/ethnicity). This is because specific rates, unlike crude rates, represent subgroups that are similar with regard to the categorizing factor. For example, we can compare the death rate among 30–34 year olds in Florida with that among 30–34 year olds in Alaska without worrying about the effects of differing age distributions between the populations, since the age groups are same. When age-specific rates are compared, however, they should represent relatively narrow age ranges (i.e., 10 or fewer years); otherwise, there may still be significant differences in how the ages are distributed within the age categories among the populations being compared. The problem with comparing specific rates among populations is the number of comparisons that may be necessary. When there are numerous specific rates to be compared, the task can become unwieldy. To overcome this problem we can use adjusted rates.

Adjusted Rates

Adjusted rates are summary rates that have been modified statistically to remove the confounding effect of one or more factors, such as differences in the age, sex, or racial/ethnic distributions of the populations being compared. Adjusted rates are statistically derived using a procedure known as **rate adjustment** or **rate standardization**. The rate adjustment procedure controls for, or adjusts, any distortion in the magnitude of the crude rates due to the confounding factor(s). Hence, it allows us to compare summary rates without the confounding effect of differences in underlying population distributions, which are incidental to the intended comparisons. It should be illuminating to note that after adjusting for age differences in the comparison of crude death rates in Florida and Alaska, the *age-adjusted* death rates were remarkably similar (462.7 per 100,000 for Florida and 461.0 per 100,000 for Alaska),[2] implying that differences in age distributions between the states were responsible for the large difference between the crude death rates. Rate adjustment allows us to calculate adjusted rates that permit fair comparisons of summary rates without the unwanted effects of confounding factors.

In the above example, different age distributions distorted (i.e., confounded) the apparent association between state of residence and the risk of

---

* Confounding is a distortion in the degree of association between a study factor and outcome due to a mixing of effects between the exposure and an incidental factor (known as a confounding factor or confounder). Chapter 8 discusses confounding in greater detail.

death, making Florida appear to be a much riskier place to live than Alaska, based on a comparison of crude death rates. This distortion was removed by rate adjustment, which produced adjusted rates that could be fairly compared, and which appeared to show virtually no difference in the risk of death between the states. Nevertheless, it is important to note that adjusted rates are artificial rates; they do not reflect the actual rates in the populations. In addition, their magnitude may depend on the **standard population*** used in the rate adjustment procedure. Although it is difficult to interpret an adjusted rate on its own, it is very meaningful when compared to other rates that have been adjusted using the same standard population. Table 6–1 provides a summary of the advantages and disadvantages of crude, adjusted, and specific rates.

Table 6–1 Advantages and Disadvantages of Crude, Adjusted, and Specific Rates*

Type of Rate	Advantages	Disadvantages
Crude	• True summary rate • Easy to calculate	• Difficult to interpret comparisons when populations differ by relevant variables (e.g., age, sex, or race)
Adjusted	• Summary rate • Permits unbiased comparisons	• Hypothetical rate • Magnitude may depend on standard population selected
Specific	• Permits unbiased comparisons • Allows detailed comparisons among various subgroups	• Unwieldy to compare many specific rates between populations

*Adapted from Mausner, J. S., and Kramer, S. (1985). *Mausner & Bahn Epidemiology—An Introductory Text.* Philadelphia: W. B. Saunders Company. (Reprinted with permission from W. B. Saunders. Copyright © W. B. Saunders, Philadelphia, PA).

Age Adjustment

Although rates may be adjusted for any factors that may distort a comparison of crude rates, the factor most commonly adjusted is age. Therefore, for the remainder of this section we will focus on **age adjustment** (also known as **age standardization**). Age adjustment is just one type of rate adjustment, as is adjustment for sex, race, smoking status, and so on. The basic methods of rate adjustment are the same no matter what factors serve as the basis for the adjustment. It will simplify the discussion, however, to focus on just one type of rate adjustment.

---

* The standard population is the population that forms the basis for the comparisons in rate adjustment. It has a known distribution with regard to the factors being adjusted.

The basic reason for age adjustment is to control for age differences in the populations being compared that might otherwise distort or confound a comparison of crude rates. Age adjustment allows us to calculate summary rates that would exist if each population being compared had the same age distribution.

Methods of Age Adjustment

There are two common methods of age adjustment—the **direct method** and the **indirect method**. The type and quality of data available determines the method to be used. The *direct method* is the method of choice when the age-specific rates for the populations being compared are available (or can be calculated) and when they are also stable. The *indirect method* is an alternative method when one or more of the age-specific rates of the populations being compared is unavailable (due to missing data) or unstable. Age-specific rates may be unstable due to a small number of events (e.g., less than 10) in one or more of the age-specific subgroups or due to unreliable reporting procedures.

Both methods of rate adjustment permit fair comparisons of summary rates; however, the procedures are somewhat different. In the *direct method* we determine an adjusted rate for each population being compared after applying the specific rates of each population to the standard population. In the *indirect method* we determine how the summary rate changes in the population with unavailable or unstable specific rates, after applying the specific rates of the standard population. This usually results in the calculation of a standardized ratio, which will be described shortly.

To illustrate age adjustment I will use a simple, though imperfect, analogy where two crude rates are different only because of confounding by different age distributions in the two populations being compared. Identical twin brothers each looked into a different trick mirror at an amusement park. One looked tall and thin, and the other looked short and fat. When they both looked into a regular mirror, however, there were no differences in their appearance. In this example, the images in the trick mirrors represent the crude rates. If they were to be compared, they would appear quite different. The trick mirrors represent the different age distributions, which distort the images (i.e., the crude rates). The regular mirror represents the standard population, and the images in the regular mirror exemplify the adjusted rates. Here it is clear that the rates are really the same. By controlling the distortion of the trick mirrors (the different age distributions) we can make a fair comparison of the brothers. This analogy represents the *direct method* of rate adjustment where the two populations with different age distributions were adjusted using a standard population so they could be fairly compared without the distortion caused by different age distributions.

Now imagine that one of the twins (Edward) moves over to the other trick mirror in which his twin (Denison) is looking. Here, though their images are distorted, they both look the same. This analogy exemplifies the *indirect method* of age adjustment. The first trick mirror Edward looked in represents the population with unavailable or unstable specific rates, and the second trick mirror represents the standard population. The images in the second mirror represent the results of the rate adjustment. Though not representative of their true selves, the twins appear the same. Now that you have a general conceptual idea of these two methods, we will discuss how to conduct rate adjustment in detail using the direct and indirect methods, respectively.

Use of the Direct Method

The direct method of age adjustment is the preferred method. It requires, however, that we have or can calculate age-specific rates in the populations being compared and that the specific rates are stable. The first step in the direct method is to select a standard population. The standard population is generally an existing population that is understood to be stable, or a derived population. Exhibit 6–1 provides two examples of derived standard populations. The first is based on the 1940 U.S. population distribution. The second is an artificially produced standard population that is derived from the two adult populations being compared.

The choice of a standard population in the direct method is arbitrary, but the specific population chosen will affect the magnitude of the adjusted rates. However, the choice of the standard population does not affect the comparison of rates adjusted using the same standard population. For example, if one adjusted rate is twice that of another adjusted rate, using the same standard population, then it will remain twice that rate even if the adjustment is performed again using a different standard population. This is important because adjusted rates are meant to be compared, as long as they are derived from the same standard population. Alone, they have little use.

Adjusted rates do not represent actual rates in a population, and they cannot be verified unless one knows the standard population. It could be misleading to compare one adjusted rate using one standard population to another adjusted rate using a very different standard population. For this reason it is important to indicate the specific standard population used when reporting adjusted rates.

Once the standard population has been selected, one is ready to calculate the adjusted rates. Example 6–1 (on page 98) illustrates the direct method of age adjustment and the interpretation of the results using a step-by-step procedure.

Exhibit 6–1 Examples of Derived Standard Populations for Use in the Direct Method of Rate Adjustment

1. This is the United States standard population. It is based on the relative age distributions of the 1940 enumerated census of the United States. Note that the population is arbitrarily set at one million, and the proportions of the 1940 population are applied to each age category.

Age	Number	Proportion
All ages	1,000,000	1.000000
Under 1 year	15,343	0.015343
1–4 years	64,718	0.064718
5–14 years	170,355	0.170355
15–24 years	181,677	0.181677
25–34 years	162,066	0.162066
35–44 years	139,237	0.139237
45–54 years	117,811	0.117811
55–64 years	80,294	0.080294
65–74 years	48,426	0.048246
75–84 years	17,303	0.017303
85 years and over	2,770	0.002770

2. This standard population is derived by combining the age-specific groups of two adult populations to form a new population distribution.

Population One

Age (years)	Population
20–29	3,000
30–39	2,500
40–49	2,500
50–59	1,500
60–69	900
70–79	650
80 and over	125

Population Two

Age (years)	Population
20–29	1,000
30–39	1,500
40–49	2,000
50–59	2,000
60–69	1,750
70–79	1,000
80 and over	250

Standard Population = Population One + Population Two

Age (years)	Population
20–29	3,000 + 1,000 = 4,000
30–39	2,500 + 1,500 = 4,000
40–49	2,500 + 2,000 = 4,500
50–59	1,500 + 2,000 = 3,500
60–69	900 + 1,750 = 2,650
70–79	650 + 1,000 = 1,650
80 and over	125 + 250 = 375
All ages	11,175 + 9,500 = 20,675

Reference: Hoyert, D. L., Kochanek, K. D., and Murphy, S. L. (1999). Deaths: Final Data for 1997. *National Vital Statistics Reports* 47(19). Hyattsville, MD: National Center for Health Statistics.

Example 6–1: Direct Method of Age Adjustment

For the two populations described below, calculate and compare the crude death rates, then adjust the crude rates for differences in age distribution using the direct method of age adjustment. Compare the results.

Population A

Age (years)	Population	Number of deaths
15–19	1,000	24
20–24	4,000	16
25–29	6,000	121
All ages	11,000	161

Population B

Age (years)	Population	Number of deaths
15–19	5,000	120
20–24	2,000	10
25–29	500	10
All ages	7,500	140

Solution:

Step 1: Calculate the crude death rates for the two populations using the formula in figure 5–2.

$$CDR = \frac{\text{Number of deaths during a specified time period}}{\text{Mid-interval population}} \times 10^n$$

Population A:

Number of deaths = 161; Total population = 11,000

Crude death rate = $(161 / 11,000) \times 10^n = 0.0146 \times 10^3 = 14.6$ deaths per 1,000 population

Population B:

Number of deaths = 140; Total population = 7,500

Crude death rate = $(140 / 7,500) \times 10^n = 0.0187 \times 10^3 = 18.7$ deaths per 1,000 population

Step 2: Compare the crude death rates by calculating the ratio of the crude death rates (R_C). R_C for population B to A is:

$$R_C = CDR_{pop.B} / CDR_{pop.A} = (18.7 \text{ per } 1,000) / (14.6 \text{ per } 1,000) = 1.3.$$

This means that the crude death rate for population B is about 1.3 times greater than that for population A.

Step 3: Determine the standard population for the rate adjustment. A common way of determining the standard population is to add the two populations being compared as shown below:

Age (years)	Population		
	A	B	Standard
15–19	1,000 +	5,000 =	6,000
20–24	4,000 +	2,000 =	6,000
25–29	6,000 +	500 =	6,500
All ages	11,000 +	7,500 =	18,500

Step 4: Calculate the age-specific rates for each population being compared.

Population A

Age (years)	Population	Number of deaths	*Age-specific rates*
15–19	1,000	24	24 / 1,000 = 0.024
20–24	4,000	16	16 / 4,000 = 0.004
25–29	6,000	121	121 / 6,000 = 0.020
All ages	11,000	161	

Population B

Age (years)	Population	Number of deaths	*Age-specific rates*
15–19	5,000	120	120 / 5,000 = 0.024
20–24	2,000	10	10 / 2,000 = 0.005
25–29	500	10	10 / 500 = 0.020
All ages	7,500	140	

Step 5: Multiply the populations of the respective age groups in the standard population by the age-specific rates for each population to determine the number of expected events in each case.

Standard Population

Age (years)	Population		Specific Rates for Population A		*Expected Deaths*
15–19	6,000	×	0.024	=	144
20–24	6,000	×	0.004	=	24
25–29	6,500	×	0.020	=	130
All ages	18,500				298

Standard Population

Age (years)	Population		Specific Rates for Population B		*Expected Deaths*
15–19	6,000	×	0.024	=	144
20–24	6,000	×	0.005	=	30
25–29	6,500	×	0.020	=	130
All ages	18,500				304

Step 6: Divide the total number of expected events in each population by the total standard population and determine the adjusted rates.

Population A: Age-adjusted rate = $(298 / 18,500) \times 10^n = 0.0161 \times 10^3 = 16.1$ per 1,000

Population B: Age-adjusted rate = $(304 / 18,500) \times 10^n = 0.0164 \times 10^3 = 16.4$ per 1,000

Step 7: Compare the adjusted rates visually or by calculating the ratio of the adjusted rates (R_A). R_A for population B to A is:

R_A = Adjusted rate$_{pop.B}$ / Adjusted rate$_{pop.A}$ = (16.4 per 1,000) / (16.1 per 1,000) = 1.0

This indicates that the age-adjusted rate in population B is virtually the same as that in population A. In other words, after adjustment for age the rates are essentially the same. The risk of death is similar in populations A and B after adjusting for age differences between the populations.

Step 8: Compare the ratio of adjusted rates (R_A) to the ratio of crude death rates (R_C) by calculating their ratio (R_A / R_C), known as the ratio of ratios.

The ratio of ratios indicates the degree of confounding by age. The more it departs from one, the greater the degree of confounding. Therefore, a ratio of, say, 0.95 or 1.1 indicates minimal confounding, while a ratio of 0.52 or 1.6 indicates substantial confounding.

$$R_A / R_C = 1.0 / 1.3 = 0.77$$

When comparing R_A and R_C the same populations must be represented in the numerators and denominators, respectively. For example,

$$\frac{R_A}{R_C} = \frac{\text{Adjusted rate}_{pop.B} / \text{Adjusted rate}_{pop.A}}{CDR_{pop.B} / CDR_{pop.A}}$$

Notice that the same population is represented in each numerator and in each denominator of the adjusted and the crude rates, respectively. One would not want to compare the ratio of the adjusted rates in populations B to A to the ratio of the crude rates in populations A to B. If the adjusted rate in population B is compared to the adjusted rate in population A for R_A, then the crude rate in population B should be compared to the crude rate in population A for R_C, and vice versa.

Answer: The crude death rates in the two populations were clearly different (Population B, 18.7 per 1,000, and Population A, 14.6 per 1,000). The ratio of the crude death rates was 1.3, indicating that the crude death rate in population B was 1.3 times greater than that in population A. After age adjustment, however, the difference almost disappeared (Population B, 16.4 per 1,000, and Population A, 16.1 per 1,000). The ratio of adjusted rates was 1.0, indicating that the age-adjusted rate in population B was the same as that in population A. In conclusion, the crude rates were significantly confounded by age, as indicated by the ratio R_A / R_C of 0.77. After adjusting for age, however, there was essentially no difference between the rates. Thus, the risk of death in populations A and B is the same after adjusting for age differences.

Comments:

1. In age adjustment, when $R_A \neq R_C$, we can say that differences in age distributions between the populations produced distortion (confounding) that affected the magnitude of the crude rates. Age adjustment corrects this distortion and, therefore, represents a more equitable way to make the comparison, assuming all other factors are equal. If there are other suspected confounding factors, these must also be controlled. If $R_A = R_C$, then age adjustment was unnecessary; there is no confounding. The irony here is that it is generally necessary to perform the adjustment in order to determine if it is really needed.

2. When the age-specific rates were calculated for the rate adjustment, the rates were computed as decimal fractions without a rate base. While this is not required, it makes the calculations easier since one never has to worry about what to do with the rate base. For example, in population B, the age-specific rate in the 25–29-year age group was determined to be $10 / 500 = 0.020$. This could have been reported as 20 per 1,000 using a rate base of 1,000. However, when this is multiplied by 6,000 in the standard population, one has to be careful to also divide the product by 1,000. In other words, it is not $20 \times 6,500 = 130,000$ deaths, but $(20 \text{ per } 1,000) \times 6,500 = 130$ deaths. Although this may seem obvious, the mistake, unfortunately, is not uncommon among beginners.

3. The rate base used in this example was 1,000. The reason 1,000 was used is because this is one of the conventional rate bases used with crude death rates (see figure 5–2), and the adjusted rates were being compared to the crude rates, so it is desirable to use the same rate base. The use of 100 also would have been acceptable, if not conventional, because the resulting rates would still have been greater than one per 100.

Use of the Indirect Method

The indirect method of age adjustment is used as an alternative to the direct method when not all of the specific rates can be calculated or when some of the specific rates are unstable. Like the direct method of age adjustment, the indirect method begins with the selection of a standard population. This is often the larger or more stable of the populations being compared. The next step is to calculate the age-specific rates in the standard population and then to multiply these rates by the respective age-specific groups in the **comparison population** (i.e., the smaller or less stable of the populations being compared) to arrive at the number of expected events in each age group. The total number of actual or observed events (OE) in the comparison population is then divided by the total number of expected events (EE) to obtain the **standardized mortality** (or **morbidity**) **ratio** (SMR). The SMR provides an indication of how much the rates differ after age adjustment. In essence, the SMR compares the crude rate to the expected rate in the comparison population based on the age-specific rates in the standard population; that is, SMR = [OE / N] / [EE / N], where N = the size of the comparison population. This formula can be simplified to:

(6.1)

$$SMR = OE / EE$$

An SMR of one implies that after age adjustment there is no difference in the adjusted rates, and an SMR less than or greater than one implies that the adjusted rates are different. The amount of difference depends on how far the SMR departs from one. The interpretation of the SMR is discussed further in example 6–2.

Example 6–2: Indirect Method of Age Adjustment

For the populations below, calculate and compare the crude death rates, then perform indirect age adjustment using one of the populations as the standard population. Report and interpret the SMR.

Population A

Age (years)	Population	Number of deaths
15–19	1,000	12
20–24	2,000	20
25–29	3,000	91
All ages	6,000	123

Population B

Age (years)	Population	Number of deaths
15–19	4,000	85
20–24	250	Not available
25–29	750	Not available
All ages	5,000	95

Solution:

Step 1: Calculate the crude death rates for the two populations using the formula in figure 5–2.

$$CDR = \frac{\text{Number of deaths during a specified time period}}{\text{Mid-interval population}} \times 10^n$$

Population A:

Number of deaths = 123; Total population = 6,000

Crude death rate = $(123 / 6,000) \times 10^n = 0.0205 \times 10^3 = 20.5$ deaths per 1,000 population

Population B:

Number of deaths = 95; Total population = 5,000

Crude death rate = $(95 / 5,000) \times 10^n = 0.0190 \times 10^3 = 19.0$ deaths per 1,000 population

Step 2: Compare the crude death rates. This can be done visually, or quantitatively by calculating the ratio of the crude rates (R_C). In the indirect method, *the crude rate for the comparison population must be in the numerator of R_C.* This means that we must determine which population is the standard population and which is the comparison population. Since the age-specific rates can only be calculated from population A, it must be the standard population. Therefore,

$$R_C = CDR_{comparison} / CDR_{standard} = CDR_{pop.B} / CDR_{pop.A} =$$

$$(19.0 \text{ per } 1,000) / (20.5 \text{ per } 1,000) = 0.93$$

This means that the crude death rate in population B (the comparison population) is about 93% of that in population A (the standard population). This is the same as saying that the CDR in population B is 7% smaller than that in population A.

Step 3: Calculate the age-specific rates in the standard population.

Standard Population (Population A)

Age (years)	Population	Number of deaths	*Age-specific rates*
15–19	1,000	12	12 / 1,000 = 0.012
20–24	2,000	20	20 / 2,000 = 0.010
25–29	3,000	91	91 / 3,000 = 0.030
All ages	6,000	123	

Step 4: Multiply the respective age-specific groups in the comparison population by the age-specific rates in the standard population to determine the number of expected events (i.e., deaths) in each age group. Sum the expected events in each age group to obtain the total number of expected events (EE) in the comparison population.

Comparison Population (Population B)

Age (years)	Population		Specific Rates from Standard Population		*Expected Deaths*
15–19	4,000	×	0.012	=	48.0
20–24	250	×	0.010	=	2.5
25–29	750	×	0.030	=	22.5
All ages	5,000				73.0

Step 5: Calculate the SMR using formula 6.1.

$$SMR = OE / EE = 95 / 73.0 = 1.3$$

Since the SMR $\neq$ 1, this indicates that the adjusted rates are different. Specifically, more deaths were observed (OE) than expected (EE) in the comparison population based on the age-specific rates in the standard population.

Step 6: Compare the SMR to the ratio of crude rates (R_C) by calculating their ratio.

$$SMR / R_C = 1.3 / 0.93 = 1.4$$

This ratio of ratios indicates whether the crude rates were confounded by differences in age distribution and, therefore, whether age adjustment was necessary. When the ratio of SMR to R_C equals one, there is no confounding by age, and thus age adjustment is not necessary; the crude rates can be fairly compared. However, when the ratio does not equal one, it indicates that age differences have confounded the comparison of crude rates and that age adjustment is necessary to correct for the confounding. In this case age adjustment was appropriate because there was confounding by age.

Answer: The SMR of 1.3 indicates that the adjusted rates were different after controlling for differences in age distribution. The ratio of SMR to R_C indicates that age differences between the populations being compared confounded the crude rates, and, therefore, age adjustment was appropriate.

Comments:

1. Calculating the ratio of the crude rates (R_C) is a simple but convenient way of determining quantitatively how much the crude rates differ. The greater the R_C departs from one, the greater the difference in the crude rates. In calculating R_C the crude rate of the comparison population should be in the numerator because it may later be compared to the SMR, whose numerator is the observed rate (i.e., the crude rate) of the comparison population. This assures an "apples to apples" comparison.

2. The standard population is usually the larger or more stable of the populations being compared. Population A is larger, and nothing suggests that it is unstable. If the number of events in one or more of the age categories was very small (i.e., less than 10) or if there were indications that the data were otherwise unstable, then we would not want to select it as a standard population. Also, when there are missing numbers of events in one or more age categories of a population, that population cannot be used as the standard population since not all the age-specific rates can be calculated, and the indirect method depends on the age-specific rates of the standard population. In this example, of the two populations only population A qualifies as a suitable standard population. Population B is not appropriate because of the missing number of deaths in two of the age categories. *It should be noted that the same criteria for using the indirect method are those for excluding a population as the standard.* If neither population qualifies as a standard, then another population could be chosen.

3. As in example 6–1, when the age-specific rates were calculated for the rate adjustment, the rates were computed as decimal fractions without a rate base. Once again, this makes the calculations easier since one never has to worry about what to do with the rate base later on.

4. The crude death rates in this example were relatively close (R_C = 19.0 per 1,000 / 20.5 per 1,000 = 0.93). The SMR provides an indication of how much the rates differ after age adjustment. In this example, the SMR = 1.3. Since this is different than 0.93, we conclude that there was confounding by age, and rate adjustment was appropriate prior

to making comparisons. Any time the SMR differs from R_C (i.e., SMR / $R_C \neq 1$), and especially where the difference is appreciable, we can say that age adjustment is necessary. In a sense, the SMR can be thought of as being somewhat analogous to the R_A (see example 6–1). However, as was stated previously, *when the SMR is compared to R_C, the numerator for R_C must always be the crude rate for the comparison population* (population B in this example). Once again, this is because the numerator for the SMR is based on the comparison population. Although we do not have two age-adjusted rates like we did with the direct method of adjustment, we do have the SMR. If the SMR = 1, there is no difference in the adjusted rates, but if the SMR $\neq$ 1, there is a difference in the adjusted rates. In this example, the adjusted rates were different, and the difference appeared to be in a direction opposite to what was suggested by the crude rates.

5. As with example 6–1, the rate base used was 1,000. The reason 1,000 was used is because this is one of the conventional rate bases used with crude death rates (see figure 5–2). The use of 100 would also have been acceptable, if not conventional, because the resulting rates would still have been greater than one per 100.

Concluding Remarks

In the *direct method* of age adjustment, the *same* age-specific groups in the standard population are multiplied by the *unconfounded* age-specific rates from each population being compared. Therefore, any differences in the resulting age-adjusted rates *must* be due to differences in age-specific rates between the populations (i.e., true differences) and *not* to differences in age distributions between the populations. Remember, both adjusted rates are based on the *same* population distribution (i.e., that of the standard population). Exhibit 6–2 summarizes the interpretation of adjusted rates when the direct method is used.

In the *indirect method* of age adjustment, the age-specific groups in the comparison population are multiplied by the *unconfounded* age-specific rates of the standard population to determine the number of expected events in the comparison population (i.e., those that would be expected to occur in the comparison population if there were no differences in the specific rates between the standard and the comparison populations). The number of observed events in the comparison population is then divided by the number of expected events. Since the number of observed and expected events are based on the *same* age distribution (i.e., that in the comparison population), any difference must be due to differences in the age-specific rates of the standard and comparison populations (i.e., true differences) and *not* to differences in age distributions between the populations. The interpretation of rate adjustment when the indirect method is used is also summarized in exhibit 6–2.

Exhibit 6–2 Interpretation of Findings from Rate Adjustment

Direct Method

If $R_A = R_C$, then there is *no* confounding by the factor(s) for which adjustment was performed. Hence, adjustment was unnecessary, and the crude rates can be fairly compared.

If $R_A \neq R_C$, then there *is* confounding by the factor(s) for which adjustment was performed. Hence, adjustment was necessary, and the crude rates should *not* be compared. The greater the ratio of ratios, R_A / R_C, departs from one, the greater the degree of confounding. Small differences may be due to random error and not statistically important. When $R_A \neq R_C$, only the adjusted rates should be compared.

R_A = the ratio of the adjusted rates, and R_C = the ratio of the crude rates. The respective numerators and denominators of these ratios must correspond to the same populations.

Indirect Method

If SMR = R_C, then there is no confounding by the factor(s) for which adjustment was performed. Hence, adjustment was unnecessary, and the crude rates can be fairly compared.

If SMR $\neq R_C$, then there is confounding by the factor(s) for which adjustment was performed. Hence, adjustment was necessary, and the crude rates should *not* be compared. The greater the ratio of ratios, SMR / R_C, departs from one, the greater the degree of confounding. Small differences may be due to random error and not statistically important. When the SMR $\neq R_C$, only the SMR should be used.

SMR = the standardized mortality ratio (or the standardized morbidity ratio if morbidity is the outcome of interest), and R_C = the ratio of the crude rates where the numerator is the crude rate in the comparison population, and the denominator is the crude rate in the standard population.

Note: If we assume a normal distribution, an approximate 95% confidence interval (CI) for the SMR can be calculated as follows:

$$\text{95\% CI} \cong \text{SMR} \pm 1.96 \sqrt{\text{SMR} / \text{EE}}$$

An adjusted rate for the comparison population can be calculated by multiplying the SMR by the crude rate in the standard population; however, multiple adjusted rates calculated by the indirect method cannot be directly compared to one another.

EE = the number of expected events in the comparison population based on the specific rates in the standard population.

References: Kahn, H. A., and Sempos, C. T. (1989). *Statistical Methods in Epidemiology.* New York: Oxford University Press; Stone, D. B., Armstrong, W. R., Macrina, D. M., and Pankau, J. W. (1996). *Introduction to Epidemiology.* Madison, WI: Brown and Benchmark.

Measures of Association

Measures of association in epidemiology determine the *strength* or *impact* of the relationship between specific exposures and outcomes. The most common way to make these comparisons is by the use of *ratios*; another method is to utilize *differences*.

Using Ratios to Measure Associations

A common measure of association in epidemiology is **relative risk** (RR), also known as the **risk ratio**. In the most basic sense, RR is the ratio of the **absolute risk** of a given outcome in the exposed group to the absolute risk of the same outcome in the unexposed group. *Absolute risk* is the probability that the outcome (e.g., disease) will occur in a given time period. It is commonly referred to simply as *risk* and is measured by the cumulative incidence rate (see chapter 5). Relative risk can be calculated as shown in the following formula, where IR_{C-e} is the cumulative incidence rate in the *exposed* group, and IR_{C-ue} is the cumulative incidence rate in the *unexposed* group.

(6.2)

$$RR = \frac{IR_{C-e}}{IR_{C-ue}}$$

Before attempting to calculate RR, it is essential to know the exposure under consideration. Usually this is readily apparent, but in some circumstances, where the exposure is represented by variables such as sex, age group, or a condition of not being exposed (e.g., not wearing a seat belt), this may not be so obvious. In the following hypothetical example of the calculation of RR, the exposure is environmental tobacco smoke (from smoking husbands). Assume that investigators conducted a prospective cohort study and found 100 deaths from heart disease among 22,500 nonsmoking spouses of nonsmoking husbands during a 13-year follow-up period. Meanwhile, 120 deaths from heart disease occurred among 20,000 nonsmoking spouses whose husbands smoked. The investigators were interested in seeing if environmental tobacco smoke increased the risk of mortality from heart disease in nonsmoking women.

Based on the findings, the $IR_{C-e} = (120 / 20,000) \times 10^n = 0.0060 \times 10^3 = 6.0$ deaths per 1,000, and the $IR_{C-ue} = (100 / 22,500) \times 10^n = 0.0044 \times 10^3 = 4.4$ deaths per 1,000. The RR = (6.0 per 1,000) / (4.4 per 1,000) = 1.4. This means that the nonsmoking spouses whose husbands smoked *were 1.4 times more likely to die* from heart disease than those whose husbands did not smoke. This is the same as saying that the risk of dying from heart disease among the spouses of smoking husbands is 40% higher than that among the spouses of nonsmoking husbands.[4] The percent change in a ratio measure of association, like the relative risk, from a baseline value of one is known as the **percent relative effect**, and it is calculated as follows:

(6.3 a and b)

> *For a ratio > 1*
>
> **(a)**   % Increased Change = (Ratio − 1) × 100
>
> *For a ratio < 1*
>
> **(b)**   % Decreased Change = (1 − Ratio) × 100

Therefore, using formula 6.3a, $(1.4 - 1) \times 100 = 0.4 \times 100 = 40\%$. *Percent relative effect* for a relative risk (risk ratio) is interpreted as the percent increased or decreased *risk* as noted above. When applied to other ratio measures of association the interpretation is somewhat different. Examples are discussed elsewhere in the text.

The relative risk provides an estimate of the increased or decreased risk of an outcome due to a particular exposure. There are several points that need to be kept in mind when interpreting a relative risk:

- Relative risk has no units and ranges in magnitude from 0 to infinity.

  RR = 1 implies *no increased risk* of the outcome due to the exposure.

  RR < 1 implies a *decreased risk* of the outcome due to the exposure (i.e., the exposure is protective).

  RR > 1 implies an *increased risk* of the outcome due to the exposure (i.e., the exposure is hazardous).

- The more the relative risk departs from 1, the stronger the association between the exposure and outcome.

  RR = 8.0, for example, implies a strong, positive association between the exposure and outcome.

  RR = 0.2 indicates a strong, inverse association between the exposure and outcome.

  RR = 1.2 implies a weak, positive association between the exposure and outcome (see figure 6–1 for rules of thumb in interpreting the magnitude of the RR).

- Relative risk does not measure absolute risk; therefore, a high RR is not necessarily associated with a high risk (i.e., cumulative incidence rate) of the outcome or vice versa.

  RR = 10 would result if IR_{C-e} = 90 per 100 and IR_{C-ue} = 9 per 100 or if IR_{C-e} = 10 per 1,000,000 and IR_{C-ue} = 1 per 1,000,000. In the former case, the risk is very high among the exposed, but in the latter case, the risk among the exposed is very small.

- Relative risk varies with time of observation.

  The longer susceptible people are observed, the more likely it is that they will succumb to the outcome of interest, thereby altering the RR. Thus, time period should be indicated when reporting a RR (e.g., in the above example the RR of 1.4 was based on 13 years of observation).

In interpreting RR from a public health perspective, one also needs to consider: (a) the severity of the outcome, and (b) the prevalence of the exposure. If, for example, the outcome is life threatening and the exposure is very prevalent, then even a slightly elevated RR could be a cause for concern. On the other hand, even a high RR for a serious disease may not garner much attention if the prevalence of exposed individuals is very small. Malignant mesothelioma, for example, is a rare type of terminal cancer that is very closely associated with occupational exposure to asbestos. Nonoccupational exposures to asbestos tend to be very low, however; hence, mesothelioma is not considered a significant health issue for the general public. It is a concern, however, for those working with asbestos-containing materials and for certain other groups who may be indirectly exposed to elevated levels (e.g., those living near asbestos mines or spouses of asbestos workers).

Type of Association		Relative Strength
Inverse	Positive	
0.71–0.99	1.01–1.50.	Weak Association
0.41–0.70	1.51–3.00.	Moderate Association
0.00–0.40	3.01 or more	Strong Association

Adapted and reprinted with permission from Monson, R. R. (1980). *Occupational Epidemiology*, copyright © CRC Press, Boca Raton, FL.

Figure 6–1 General rules of thumb for interpreting the magnitude of the relative risk and other ratio measures of association

Another closely related measure of association is the **rate ratio**. Rate ratios are commonly reported based on the results of cohort or other longitudinal studies. The rate ratio is the person-time incidence rate in the exposed group (IR_{P-T-e}) divided by the person-time incidence rate in the unexposed group (IR_{P-T-ue}). This can be expressed mathematically as:

(6.4)

$$\text{Rate Ratio} = \frac{IR_{P-T-e}}{IR_{P-T-ue}}$$

To illustrate the use of the rate ratio, consider the following observation based on an analysis of national injury data sets for 18–64 year olds: "overall injury mortality rates . . . for men were almost 3 times higher than those for women (overall rate: 68.7 vs 23.7 per 100,000 person-years). . . ."[5(p71)] This observation is based on the *rate ratio* (i.e., 68.7 per 100,000 person-years / 23.7 per 100,000 person-years = 2.9 ≅ 3). Since men are the exposed group in this example, women are the unexposed group. Also note that the injury mortality rates referred to are cause-specific mortality rates that represent the *incidence* of death due to injuries.

The interpretation of the rate ratio is similar to that of the relative risk except that reference is made to *rates* versus *risk* of outcome as inferred from the above quotation. Alternatively, we might have said, the rate at which men die of injuries is almost three times higher than the rate among women. This represents a moderate association between being male and dying from an injury as indicated in figure 6–1. Since time is incorporated into the denominators of the person-time incidence rates that are used to calculate the rate ratio, it is not necessary to indicate the period of observation for the rate ratio as it is with relative risk. It is still a good idea, however, to indicate the person, place, and time factors when reporting rate ratios if this information is not clear from the context of the study or report. When the risk of an outcome over the period of observation is low in both the exposed and unexposed groups (say, less than 5 per 100), the relative risk and rate ratio will approximate each other well.[6]

A third measure of association using ratios is the **odds ratio** (OR). This measure is most often associated with case-control studies, although it can be used with cohort and cross-sectional study designs as well. The derivation and interpretation of the OR varies somewhat depending on the specific study design.[7] In this chapter the OR will be discussed only with reference to case-control studies.

As its name indicates, the OR is a ratio of **odds**. Odds refer to the probability of an event occurring relative to it not occurring. For example, someone at a racetrack might remark that the odds of her horse winning the next race are three to one. What she means is that the probability that the horse will win is three times greater than the probability that it will lose. The probability the horse will win is 3 / 4. The probability that it will lose is 1 / 4. Therefore, the odds are (3 / 4) / (1 / 4) = 3 / 1. In case-control studies, the OR is the ratio of the odds of exposure among the cases to the odds of exposure among the controls. This is perhaps best illustrated using a 2 × 2 contingency table like the one presented below.

	Outcome Status	
Exposure Status	**Cases**	**Controls**
Exposed	a	b
Unexposed	c	d

As long as the data are set up in correspondence with this table, the odds of exposure among the cases are a / c, and the odds of exposure among the controls are b / d. Therefore, the odds ratio is:

(6.5)
$$OR = (a / c) / (b / d) = ad / bc$$

For example, in order to determine if cigarette smoking was related to stroke incidence, Ruth Bonita and her colleagues conducted a case-control study in the mid-1980s.[8] The exposure was cigarette smoking (smokers versus nonsmokers), and the outcome was stroke (present or absent). Their overall results were as follows:

	Outcome Status	
Exposure Status	**Cases**	**Controls**
Exposed	66	424
Unexposed	66	1,162

Based on these results, the OR = (66 × 1,162) / (424 × 66) = 76,692 / 27,984 = 2.7. That is, the odds of cigarette smoking among the cases were 2.7 times greater than the odds of cigarette smoking among the controls. As with the relative risk and other ratio measures of association, the more the OR departs from one, the greater the association between the exposure and outcome (see figure 6–1). When the outcome is relatively rare, the odds ratio approximates the relative risk, which approximates the rate ratio. In these cases, the OR is often interpreted in the same manner as the RR. Assuming this to be the case in the above example, we could say that the risk of stroke is 2.7 times more likely in cigarette smokers compared to nonsmokers. This is the same as saying that the risk of stroke is 170% higher in cigarette smokers versus nonsmokers based on formula 6.3a. This represents a moderately increased risk of stroke for cigarette smokers, all other factors being equal (see figure 6–1). The reasons for using the odds ratio and its interpretation in different circumstances are discussed in chapter 11.

Measures of association like the relative risk, rate ratio, and odds ratio can also be applied in situations where *levels* of exposure are not dichotomous (e.g., number of alcoholic drinks per day). In addition, it should be mentioned that these measures may need to be adjusted for potentially confounding factors as was true for crude rates. The odds ratio reported in the above example, for instance, represents a *crude* odds ratio that may need to be adjusted for differences in the distributions of age, hypertension status, alcohol use, and other potentially important variables between the case and control groups. This topic is discussed further in chapter 8. Another type of rate ratio, the *prevalence ratio*, sometimes used in cross-sectional studies, is discussed in chapter 10.

Using Differences to Measure Associations

An alternative to calculating ratios as measures of association is to determine differences. The **risk difference** is the arithmetic difference between the cumulative incidence rates in the exposed and unexposed groups, while the **rate difference** is the difference between the person-time incidence rates in the exposed and unexposed groups.

Ratios and differences are both measures of association, but they must be interpreted differently because they measure different things. A ratio reflects the *strength* of the association between an exposure and outcome. Therefore, it is useful in uncovering causative factors.[10] A difference, on the other hand, indicates *how much* of the outcome in the exposed group is associated with the exposure. Therefore, a large difference can indicate an *important* public health problem.[9] Differences cannot be used to predict corresponding ratios and vice versa. Together, however, they provide a comprehensive picture of the effect of an exposure on the occurrence of disease.[9]

Unlike ratio measures, which have no units, differences are usually expressed as cumulative or person-time incidence rates. In practice, ratios are often considered more useful because they have a common reference point of one, which represents no deviation between the rates. For example, a relative risk of three tells us instantly that the risk of the outcome in the exposed group is three times greater than that in the unexposed group, all other factors being equal. Similarly, a relative risk of one implies no difference in risk between the exposed and unexposed groups. With difference measures, the magnitude of the difference does not necessarily indicate the strength of the association between exposure and outcome because it is largely influenced by the size of the rate in the unexposed group. If this rate is large, then even a small, positive association between exposure and outcome can result in a large risk or rate difference. If the rate in the unexposed group is small, however, it will take a substantial association between the exposure and outcome to produce a large difference (see example 6–3).

Risk and rate differences make no assumptions about causality between exposure and outcome. If we assume that the exposure causes the outcome, difference measures take on added significance from a public health perspective. When causality is assumed, the *risk difference* becomes equivalent to what is known as **attributable risk** (AR), which is the amount of the absolute risk *in the exposed group* due (or attributable) to the exposure. Similarly, the *rate difference* becomes the **attributable rate**, which is the amount of the person-time incidence rate *in the exposed group* attributable to the exposure. Formulas for these measures are:

(6.6 a and b)

(a)	Attributable Risk (AR) or Risk Difference = $IR_{C\text{-}e} - IR_{C\text{-}ue}$
(b)	Attributable Rate or Rate Difference = $IR_{P\text{-}T\text{-}e} - IR_{P\text{-}T\text{-}ue}$

In theory, if a harmful exposure can be eliminated from a population, we would expect the incidence rate in the exposed group to decrease by the amount of the attributable risk or rate difference, whichever is applicable. This can be more conveniently stated as a percentage, known as the attributable risk or rate percent, respectively. The **attributable risk percent** (AR%) is calculated in the following manner:

(6.7)

$$AR\% = \frac{IR_{C-e} - IR_{C-ue}}{IR_{C-e}} \times 100$$

The **attributable rate percent** is calculated in the same manner, only using person-time incidence rates instead of cumulative incidence rates. An alternative method of calculating the *attributable risk percent* is:

(6.8)

$$AR\% = \frac{RR - 1}{RR} \times 100$$

This formula, which is easily derived from formula 6.7, uses the relative risk (RR) in the calculation. Since cumulative incidence rates cannot normally be calculated directly in case-control studies, this can be useful when the odds ratio is used to estimate the RR (e.g., when the outcome is rare). An analogous formula can be derived for the attributable rate percent by using the rate ratio in place of relative risk in formula 6.8. Example 6–3 illustrates the use and integration of both ratio and difference measures.

Example 6–3: Use and Interpretation of Ratio and Difference Measures

According to the U.S. Surgeon General, cigarette smoking is a cause of both lung cancer and coronary heart disease (CHD) in the United States. A study conducted in a northeastern county in the United States estimated the age-adjusted incidence rates in the county for 2001. The findings are indicated below.

	Incidence	
Population	Lung Cancer	CHD
Overall	60 per 100,000	240 per 100,000
Cigarette smokers	180 per 100,000	420 per 100,000
Non-cigarette smokers	20 per 100,000	180 per 100,000

Based on this information, calculate the appropriate ratio and difference measures of association and interpret the results.

Solution:

Step 1: Since the data in the problem are cumulative incidence rates, the appropriate ratio measure to calculate is the relative risk. This can be accomplished using formula 6.2. The exposure is cigarette smoking.

$$RR = IR_{C-e} / IR_{C-ue}$$
Lung cancer: RR = 180 per 100,000 / 20 per 100,000 = 9.0
CHD: RR = 420 per 100,000 / 180 per 100,000 = 2.3

Step 2: Since cigarette smoking is a cause of both lung cancer and CHD, the appropriate difference measure is the attributable risk (AR). This can be calculated using Formula 6.6a.

$$AR = IR_{C-e} - IR_{C-ue}$$
Lung cancer: Attributable Risk = 180 per 100,000 – 20 per 100,000 = 160 per 100,000
CHD: Attributable Risk = 420 per 100,000 – 180 per 100,000 = 240 per 100,000

Step 3: We can also calculate the attributable risk percent (AR%) using formula 6.7, but this is not required based on the problem.

$$AR\% = \frac{IR_{C\text{-}e} - IR_{C\text{-}ue}}{IR_{C\text{-}e}} \times 100$$

Lung cancer: AR% = (160 per 100,000 / 180 per 100,000) × 100 = 88.9%

CHD: AR% = (240 per 100,000 / 420 per 100,000) × 100 = 57.1%

Answer: Based on the county studied, the RR indicates that cigarette smoking is more strongly associated with lung cancer than with CHD. The risk of lung cancer is nine times greater among cigarette smokers than non-cigarette smokers, while the risk of CHD is only 2.3 times greater among cigarette smokers than nonsmokers. The attributable risk, however, shows that more CHD is caused by cigarette smoking in the county than lung cancer, all other factors being equal (240 cases per 100,000 compared to 160 cases per 100,000, respectively).

Comments:

1. Of the three epidemiologic measures illustrated in this example, the relative risk (RR) is perhaps the easiest to comprehend. The RR of lung cancer in the county due to cigarette smoking was very strong, while the relative risk of CHD was moderate (see figure 6–1). The more the RR departs from one, the greater the association between the exposure and the outcome. Based on the data in the example, county residents who smoked cigarettes were nine times more likely to develop lung cancer compared to non-cigarette smokers, and 2.3 times more likely to develop CHD. Thus, cigarette smoking increased the risk of lung cancer by 800% and CHD by 130%, respectively (formula 6.3a).

2. The attributable risk can be more difficult to comprehend than the relative risk. However, there is a simple logic to attributable risk, which is illustrated here using the data on lung cancer. First, it is important to recognize that even though cigarette smoking is considered a cause of lung cancer, some individuals will develop lung cancer even if they do not smoke. Therefore, the cumulative incidence rate of 180 per 100,000 among cigarette smokers includes cases of lung cancer due to cigarette smoking *as well as* to other causes (e.g., cigar or pipe smoking or occupational exposure to asbestos or radon). The risk among the non-cigarette smokers (20 per 100,000), however, *must* be due to causes other than cigarette smoking, since these individuals do not smoke cigarettes. When we subtract the risk due to "other causes" (i.e., the background risk) from the risk among cigarette smokers we are left with the attributable risk, that is, the risk of lung cancer *among cigarette smokers* due only to cigarette smoking. In the example this was 160 per 100,000. Theoretically, if cigarette smokers in the county gave up smoking cigarettes, their risk would drop to that of non-cigarette smokers or to 20 per 100,000. This does not take into account the nature of the disease process, however. We know, for example, that lung cancer risk does not revert to that of nonsmokers once someone quits smoking cigarettes. The decline in risk is more gradual and never reaches the level of nonsmokers.

3. The magnitude of the attributable risk does not indicate the strength of an association between the exposure and outcome since it is largely influenced by the cumulative incidence rate (i.e., risk) in the unexposed group. Notice that cigarette smoking increases the risk of development of lung cancer (RR = 9.0) substantially more than CHD (RR = 2.3). Because of the high risk of CHD in the unexposed group (180 per 100,000), however, even a small association (RR = 2.3) can account for a large attributable risk (240 per 100,000). It takes a very strong association, however, to produce a large difference if the risk in the unexposed group is low as in the case of lung cancer (RR = 9.0, AR = 160 per 100,000, and $IR_{C\text{-}ue}$ = 20 per 100,000).

4. The AR% for lung cancer (88.9%) indicates that almost 89% of the incidence of lung cancer among cigarette smokers in the county is due to cigarette smoking. This tells us that cigarette smoking is a major cause of lung cancer. All other factors account for only 11% of the incidence of lung cancer among cigarette smokers in the county. The AR% for CHD is 57.1%. Therefore, about 57% of the incidence of CHD among cigarette smokers in the county is due to cigarette smoking, and about 43% is due to other factors. This tells us that cigarette smoking is an important cause of CHD but that other factors are also important. This may explain the higher incidence of CHD compared to lung cancer among the non-cigarette smokers in the county.

Population Attributable Risk

Two other related and useful difference measures are *population attributable risk* and *population attributable risk percent*. Unfortunately, these terms, and those used for attributable risk and attributable risk percent and their counterparts using person-time incidence rates, have not been standardized in the epidemiologic literature. Therefore, you may encounter many other terms meaning the same thing. Usually, the context in which they are used will help you discern which measures are being applied. Population attributable risk percent, for example, has been referred to as attributable fraction, attributable fraction (population), attributable proportion, etiologic fraction, etiologic fraction (population), and attributable risk percent (population). Sadly, there is no universal consensus as to which are the more acceptable terms. Also, although it should be, a distinction is often not made between measures employing cumulative incidence rates and those using person-time incidence rates.

Population attributable risk (Pop AR) measures the amount of absolute risk in a defined population due to a given exposure. This is the same as saying it represents the *excess risk* (that beyond background risk) attributable to the exposure. Whereas attributable risk measures the excess risk in the *exposed group* in a population, population attributable risk measures the excess risk in the *entire defined population* regardless of exposure status. Like attributable risk, Pop AR assumes causality between the exposure and outcome. It is calculated as follows:

(6.9)

$$\text{Pop AR} = IR_{C\text{-}p} - IR_{C\text{-}ue}$$

where $IR_{C\text{-}p}$ is the cumulative incidence rate in the *population*. $IR_{C\text{-}p}$ should not be confused with $IR_{C\text{-}e}$, which represents the cumulative incidence rate in the exposed group only. Using data on lung cancer from example 6–3, the Pop AR = 60 per 100,000 – 20 per 100,000 = 40 per 100,000. This is the absolute risk of lung cancer *in the population* that is attributable to cigarette smoking.* The Pop AR says theoretically that if cigarette smoking could be

---

* Technically, the population attributable risk represents a population-based risk (e.g., the risk of lung cancer in the entire population due to cigarette smoking in the population), whereas the attributable risk represents an individual-based risk (i.e., the risk of lung cancer in cigarette smokers due to their cigarette smoking).

eliminated from this population, we would expect the overall cumulative incidence rate of lung cancer to drop by 40 per 100,000 (from 60 per 100,000 to 20 per 100,000). This is less than the attributable risk calculated earlier (160 per 100,000). In fact, the population attributable risk will always be less than the attributable risk in a given population as long as the exposure increases the risk of the outcome, since unlike the exposed group, the total population also contains unexposed persons who are at lower risk of the outcome.[10]

The **population attributable risk percent** (Pop AR%) is perhaps more indicative of the impact of the exposure than the population attributable risk. There are two basic ways to calculate this measure:

(6.10 a and b)

$$\text{(a)} \quad \text{Pop AR\%} = \frac{IR_{C\text{-}p} - IR_{C\text{-}ue}}{IR_{C\text{-}p}} \times 100$$

$$\text{(b)} \quad \text{Pop AR\%} = \frac{P_e\,(RR - 1)}{P_e\,(RR - 1) + 1} \times 100$$

Using formula 6.10a and applicable data in example 6–3, the Pop AR% = [(60 per 100,000 – 20 per 100,000) / 60 per 100,000] × 100 = (40 per 100,000 / 60 per 100,000) × 100 = 66.7%. Hence, hypothetically speaking, if cigarette smoking could be eliminated from this population, we would expect a 66.7% decrease in the cumulative incidence rate of lung cancer. In the second formula, P_e is the proportion of the exposed individuals in the population (i.e., the proportion of cigarette smokers). If the proportion is 0.25, then the Pop AR% = {0.25 (9 – 1) / [0.25 (9 – 1) + 1]} × 100 = (2 / 3) × 100 = 66.7%.

The population attributable risk percent has tangible public health significance. It can be used to determine the potential benefit of controlling different harmful exposures in a population as long as they can be considered to have causative roles in the outcome. For example, hypertension and cigarette smoking are both causative factors for stroke. Bonita and her colleagues found that the population attributable risk percents for hypertension and cigarette smoking were nearly identical in a case-control study conducted in Auckland, New Zealand.[8] Overall, 36% of the strokes in the population could be attributed to hypertension, and 37% could be attributed to cigarette smoking. From a public health perspective, limited resources should be directed to controlling those exposures that contribute the most to a given outcome. In this example, one would expect to achieve similar reductions in strokes by controlling either hypertension or cigarette smoking. However, if one exposure was associated with a much higher population attributable risk percent than another, then public health professionals could decide whether more resources might be used in controlling that exposure because of the greater potential benefits to the population. The relative difficulty in controlling a factor would be another consideration, of course. The population attributable risk and the population attributable risk percent, and their counterparts, the *population attributable rate* and the *population* *attributable rate percent*,* can therefore serve as useful public health policy tools for health administrators by indicating the potential health benefits to be achieved by reducing the causes of a given outcome in a population.

Tests of Statistical Significance

When two rates are compared, say, by ratios or differences, one often wonders whether an observed difference is large enough to be statistically significant. This assumes that the rates have been calculated from samples of populations and, therefore, are subject to possible **sampling error**, the random variation that can result when using sample statistics to estimate population parameters.[11] When two sample rates are found to be statistically different, it suggests that the difference is unlikely due to sampling error and, therefore, probably represents a real difference between the population rates. Of course, we can never be totally certain that differences are real when comparing sample statistics, but we can estimate the probability of sampling error. If this probability is small, it gives us confidence that the difference is probably a real one. This topic is covered in more detail in chapter 8.

An alternative to testing for statistical significance is to calculate a confidence interval (discussed in chapter 5) for the measure of association. The confidence interval method is often preferred since it not only gives us a probable range for a measure of association, but it also tells us whether any difference is statistically significant. Thus, if a measure of association is calculated and indicates a difference, we can either test to see if the difference is statistically significant (unlikely due to sampling error) or calculate a confidence interval to get an idea of the probable range of the population measure, and if desired, also determine whether or not the difference is statistically significant. The use of confidence intervals over statistical testing has gained many proponents in epidemiology, and confidence intervals are frequently the preferred way of reporting results in many epidemiologic, public health, and biomedical journals. Nevertheless, statistical testing is still used and has its adherents. Therefore, it is prudent to be familiar with both methods.

Measures of association can be developed for comparisons of crude, specific, or adjusted rates. One must be very cautious, however, when comparing crude rates for reasons cited earlier in this chapter. When rates are compared for different cities, counties, countries, and so forth, the exposure of interest is place of residence. For example, when comparing the HIV infection rates in Los Angeles and New York, we can assume that those living in Los Angeles represent the exposed group, and those not residing in Los Angeles (i.e., those living in New York) represent the unexposed group. Similarly, in comparing rates in the same location at different times, we can assume that the exposure is represented by one of the time periods, and the other time period corresponds to the unexposed group. For instance, the age-adjusted death

---

* The population attributable rate and population attributable rate percent are calculated like the population attributable risk and the population attributable risk percent but using applicable person-time incidence rates instead of cumulative incidence rates. They are interpreted as excess rates versus risks, however.

rate for Alzheimer's disease was reported to be 2.7 per 100,000 in 1996 and 1.3 per 100,000 in 1984.[12] The relative risk of dying of Alzheimer's disease in 1996 versus 1984 is 2.7 per 100,000 / 1.3 per 100,000 = 2.1, assuming all other factors are equal. We could perform a test of statistical significance to see if this relative risk is statistically different from 1.0 (1.0 represents no increased risk), or we could develop a confidence interval for the relative risk to determine the probable range of the population relative risks. We could do something similar based on rate ratios.

The methods for determining measures of association in this chapter have involved comparisons of **independent rates**. Independent rates are those that do not include any of the same events in the numerators. A case or death included in the numerator of one rate is not included in the numerator of another.[13] Methods of calculating confidence intervals for various measures of association, as well as methods of testing for significant differences for *independent rates*, are discussed in chapters 10–13, which deal with specific study designs.

Methods of testing for significant differences between independent rates differ, however, from those for **dependent rates**, which are those in which some of the events in the numerators are the same. This occurs when one rate is based on a subgroup of the population used to calculate the other rate or when the rates are based on the same population but during overlapping time periods. An example is comparing the incidence rate of diabetes in Boston with that for Massachusetts. Since Boston is a part of Massachusetts, cases that occur in Boston are already represented in the state rate. If the rate is high in Boston, it will have the effect of increasing the overall rate in Massachusetts. In other words, the rate in Massachusetts *depends* to some extent on the rate in Boston. Similarly, if the rate in Boston for 2001 is compared to the Boston rate for 2000–2002, some overlap occurs. The events that took place in 2001 will be included in the numerator of the 2000–2002 rate. Therefore, the 2001 rate depends on the 2000–2002 rate and vice versa.

A method for testing for significant differences for *dependent rates* has been discussed by Dever.[13] This method can be applied to both prevalence and incidence rates, including mortality rates, as long as they are dependent. Because this procedure assumes normality, the number of events in each sample should be relatively large (ideally 100 or more). A formula for calculating the level of statistical significance, along with an annotated example (6–4), is presented below.

(6.11)

$$z = (r_S - r_L) \sqrt{n / (r_L - r_L^2)}$$

In this formula, r_S is the rate calculated from the smaller population, r_L is the rate calculated from the larger population, and n is the actual denominator used in calculating r_S. The symbol z refers to a **z-score**, a type of transformed score based on the standardized normal distribution.

You may recall from basic statistics that for a two-tailed test of significance if $z \geq \pm 1.96$, then the difference between the rates is considered statistically significant at $p \leq 0.05$. If $z < \pm 1.96$, then the difference is not considered statistically significant ($p > 0.05$). The **p-value**, which measures the probability that the difference is due to sampling error, is discussed further in chapter 8. In general, the greater the absolute value of z ($|z|$), the smaller is the value of p. The smaller the value of p, the more likely the difference is real, all other factors being equal. For further information on z-scores and statistical testing, consult any introductory statistics textbook.

Example 6–4: Testing for Significant Difference for Dependent Rates

The National Center for Health Statistics reported recently that the annual infant mortality rate in the U.S. among all mothers of Hispanic origin was 6.0 per 1,000 live births.[1] The rate among Hispanic mothers who were of Mexican descent was 5.8 per 1,000. Given that there were 709,767 live births among all mothers of Hispanic origin in the U.S. that year, and 499,024 of these were among mothers of Mexican descent, determine if the difference between the two rates is statistically significant. Assume the rates were calculated from samples of the populations.*

Solution: The statistical difference between the rates can be calculated using formula 6.11.

$$z = (r_S - r_L) \sqrt{n / (r_L - r_L^2)}$$

$r_S = 5.8$ per 1,000; $r_L = 6.0$ per 1,000; and $n = 499{,}024$, therefore,

$$z = (0.0058 - 0.0060) \sqrt{499{,}024 / (0.0060 - 0.0060^2)}$$

$$= -0.0002 \sqrt{499{,}024 / 0.0060}$$

$$= -0.0002 \, (9{,}119.80) = -1.82$$

Since $|1.82| < |1.96|$, the rates are not statistically different ($p > 0.05$)

Comments:

1. The rates are *dependent* since the number of infant deaths among mothers of Mexican descent is included in the number of infant deaths among all Hispanic mothers. In other words, the numerator of the rate for one group is included in the numerator for the other.

2. The rate in the smaller sample is 5.8 infant deaths per 1,000 live births, and the rate in the larger sample is 6.0 infant deaths per 1,000 live births. Sample size is determined by the number of live births, since this represents the relevant denominator for the infant mortality rate. The denominator used in calculating the smaller rate is 499,024 live births. In calculating z, it is *necessary* to place the rates on a per person or per person-time unit basis, whichever is being used. If this is *not* done, then $r_L - r_L^2$ will always be a negative number, and the square root cannot be computed for negative numbers. The negative z-score only reflects that r_L is larger than r_S and otherwise has no special importance.

3. The value of r_L^2 in this case is very small. Therefore, the difference between r_L and r_L^2 is negligible and actually disappears after rounding.

---

* It is not actually necessary to assume that rates are calculated from samples of a population to perform statistical significance testing. Since populations are dynamic; that is, since they are always changing, rates based on entire populations are also subject to sampling error. Therefore, it is appropriate to test population rates for statistical significance.[1]

4. Because the obtained z-score is less than ±1.96, we can say that the difference between the rates is *not* statistically significant. The corresponding p-value is greater than 0.05. This means that we would expect the magnitude of the observed difference to be due to sampling error more than 5% of the time. The 0.05 level is the conventional level of significance, and p-values above 0.05 imply that the probability of sampling error is too high to conclude that the population rates are likely to be different. Though widely accepted and used, a p-value of 0.05 is completely arbitrary. Based on the results in this example, we conclude that the rates are too close to say that there is a statistically significant difference. Had the difference between the rates been larger so that $z \geq \pm 1.96$, we would have concluded that the difference between the rates was statistically significant since the value of p would have been ≤ 0.05, indicating that sampling error could be expected to account for the observed difference only 5% or less of the time.

Summary

- Crude rates are overall or summary rates for a defined population, but they are often distorted (confounded) by differences in the underlying population distributions, especially age, that can bias the comparisons. Adjusted rates are statistically derived summary rates that remove the distortion so as to permit fair, unbiased comparisons among summary rates.

- There are two basic methods of rate adjustment—the direct and indirect methods. The direct method uses the specific rates in the populations to be compared to develop adjusted rates based on a standard population. The indirect method uses the specific rates in the standard population to develop a standardized mortality (or morbidity) ratio. The direct method is usually used unless specific rates in the populations are unstable or unavailable.

- Measures of association in epidemiology tell the strength or the impact of an association between a given exposure and an outcome. Common ratio measures of association are the relative risk (risk ratio), rate ratio, and odds ratio. These measures assess the strength of an association, and the more they depart from one, the stronger the association. Common difference measures include attributable risk and attributable risk percent. These measures assess the impact of eliminating a given exposure among exposed persons assuming that the exposure is causative. Population attributable risk and population attributable risk percent determine the impact of eliminating a given exposure among the entire defined population regardless of exposure status.

- Tests of statistical significance require that we know whether the rates being compared are independent or dependent. A method for testing the statistical difference between dependent rates provides a z-score that can be readily interpreted for significance assuming a standardized normal distribution. The p-value corresponding to the z-score tells us the likelihood that the observed difference is due to sampling error. If the p-value is equal to or less than 0.05, we can conclude that the difference is statistically significant and is probably real, all other factors being equal.

New Terms

absolute risk	independent rates	rate difference
adjusted rates	indirect method	rate ratio
age adjustment	measures of association	rate standardization
age standardization	odds	relative risk
attributable rate	odds ratio	risk difference
attributable rate percent	p-value	risk ratio
attributable risk	percent relative effect	sampling error
attributable risk percent	population	specific rates
comparison population	attributable risk	standard population
confounding	population attributable	standardized morbidity ratio
crude rates	risk percent	standardized mortality ratio
dependent rates	rate adjustment	z-score
direct method		

Study Questions and Exercises

1. Meadville and Barton are two small communities in the Northeast. The overall unintentional injury rates among 15–29 year olds are similar in both communities, but the age distributions among the 15–29 year olds are quite different. Use the direct method to age adjust the unintentional injury rates in the two populations based on the data in the table below. The standard population should be derived from a combination of the two populations. Compare and interpret your results. Also, explain why direct adjustment is the most appropriate method of age adjustment in this example.

	Meadville			Barton		
Age	Population	No. Injuries	Age-specific rate	Population	No. Injuries	Age-specific rate
15–19	200	14	0.070	1,000	20	0.020
20–24	1,200	36	0.030	100	14	0.140
25–29	800	12	0.015	400	12	0.030
All ages	2,200	62		1,500	46	

2. Streamland and Castleton represent two relatively young populations in the same state. Both cities are similar economically and culturally. Using the data in the table below, calculate and compare the crude death rates in the two cities. Next, adjust the rates by age. Are the age-adjusted rates different, and why or why not? Was age a confounding factor in the comparison of the crude rates, and why or why not?

	Streamland			Castleton		
Age	Population	No. Deaths	Age-specific mortality rate	Population	No. Deaths	Age-specific mortality rate
0–9	2,000	18	0.009	3,000	15	0.005
10–19	3,500	11	0.003	5,500	12	0.002
20–29	4,500	20	0.004	1,000	N.A.*	N.A.
30–39	6,000	12	0.002	3,000	N.A.	N.A.
40–49	1,500	12	0.008	2,500	18	0.007
50–59	1,000	25	0.025	1,500	14	0.009
60 +	1,500	42	0.028	2,500	15	0.006
All ages	20,000	140		19,000	105	

*N.A. = Not available

3. A prospective cohort study of 18,540 men was designed to determine the relationship of hypertension and cigarette smoking to cardiovascular disease (CVD) deaths. After five years of follow-up, the study produced the following results:

Subgroup	Number	CVD Deaths
Cigarette smokers	4,205	339
Non-cigarette smokers	14,335	422
Total	18,540	761
Hypertensives	3,297	305
Nonhypertensives	15,243	456
Total	18,540	761

Based on the data provided, determine: (a) the relative risk of CVD death due to cigarette smoking and hypertension, respectively, (b) the percent relative effect for cigarette smoking and hypertension, respectively, (c) the attributable risk percent for cigarette smoking and hypertension, respectively, and (d) the population attributable risk percent for cigarette smoking and hypertension, respectively. In each case, indicate what your answer means in words. Which factor appears to be more important as a cause of CVD deaths in this population, and why?

4. Eighteen new cases of HIV infection were reported among men, 20–29 years of age, in Howard County last year. It is estimated that 6,398 men in this age group were free of HIV at the beginning of last year. Altogether, 33 new cases of HIV infection were reported in the 20–29-year age group last year. Given that there were 6,113 women free of HIV at the beginning of last year, determine whether or not the cumulative incidence rate of HIV infection among men is significantly different from that for both sexes combined in the 20–29-year age group in Howard County last year.

References

1. MacDorman, M. F., and Atkinson, J. O. (1999). Infant Mortality Statistics from the 1997 Period Linked Birth/Infant Death Data Set. *National Vital Statistics Reports* 47(23). Hyattsville, MD: National Center for Health Statistics.
2. Hoyert, D. L., Kochanek, K. D., and Murphy, S. L. (1999). Deaths: Final Data for 1997. *National Vital Statistics Reports* 47(19). Hyattsville, MD: National Center for Health Statistics.
3. U.S. Census Bureau (2000). Population Estimates for the U.S. Regions, Divisions, and States by 5-year Age Groups and Sex: Time Series Estimates, July 1, 1990 to July 1, 1999 and April 1, 1990 Census Population Counts. Population Estimates Program, Population Division, U.S. Census Bureau, Washington, DC (Internet Release Date: March 9, 2000). Available: http://census.gov/population/estimates/state/st-99-08.txt (Access date: March 22, 2000.)
4. Rothman, K. J. (1986). *Modern Epidemiology.* Boston: Little, Brown and Company.
5. Cubbin, C., LeClere, F. B., and Smith, G. S. (2000). Socioeconomic Status and the Occurrence of Fatal and Nonfatal Injury in the United States. *American Journal of Public Health* 90(1): 71–77.
6. Kelsey, J. L., Thompson, W. D., and Evans, A. S. (1986). *Methods in Observational Epidemiology.* New York: Oxford University Press.
7. Last, J. M., ed. (1995). *A Dictionary of Epidemiology.* New York: Oxford University Press.
8. Bonita, R., Scragg, R., Stewart, A., Jackson, R., and Beaglehole, R. (1986). Cigarette Smoking and Risk of Premature Stroke in Men and Women. *British Medical Journal* 293: 6–8.
9. Brownson, R. C., Remington, P. L., and Davis, J. R. (1998). *Chronic Disease Epidemiology and Control,* 2nd ed. Washington, DC: American Public Health Association.
10. Hennekens, C. H., and Buring, J. E. (1987). *Epidemiology in Medicine.* Boston: Little, Brown and Company.
11. Vogt, W. P. (1993). *Dictionary of Statistics and Methodology.* Newbury Park, CA: Sage.
12. Hoyert, D. L., and Rosenberg, H. M. (1999). Mortality from Alzheimer's Disease: An Update. *National Vital Statistics Reports* 47(20). Hyattsville, MD: National Center for Health Statistics.
13. Dever, G. E. A. (1984). *Epidemiology in Health Services Management.* Rockville, MD: Aspen.

CHAPTER SEVEN

Association and Causation

Learning Objectives

▸ Describe and give examples of spurious, noncausal, and causal associations in epidemiology, including the reasons spurious and noncausal associations occur.

▸ Discuss six criteria for judging potential causal associations, including the advantages and limitations of each criterion.

▸ Distinguish among the types of causal associations, including those based on classifications of necessary and/or sufficient causes and direct or indirect causes, respectively.

▸ Explain the importance of determining causal associations in epidemiology.

▸ Define cause, Hill's postulates, predisposing or enabling factors, and threshold.

Overview

A statistically significant association between an exposure and outcome is a starting point for evaluating cause-effect relationships. Apparent associations can be spurious, noncausal, or causal in nature. Identifying causal associations is important in designing effective disease prevention and control programs. Criteria developed by Sir Austin Bradford Hill and others can be adapted to evaluate associations for possible causality. These criteria take into account the temporal sequence, strength of the association, consistency of the findings, dose-response relationships, biological plausibility, and experimental evidence. There are various ways to classify causes depending on the role they play in disease causation. Types of causes include necessary and sufficient causes as well as direct and indirect causes.

Introduction

One of the primary goals of epidemiology is to discover the causes of morbidity and mortality in human populations. This goal has immense practical significance for health professionals because a better understanding of the causes of morbidity and mortality often leads to more effective prevention and control measures and thus to a reduction in the incidence, prevalence, or severity of disease.

The search for causes of morbidity and mortality usually begins when a statistically significant association is found between an exposure and outcome. A statistical association implies that the exposure is associated with a change in the *probability* of the outcome. It does not necessarily mean, however, that the exposure *causes* the outcome.[1] In order to be considered a **cause**,* a change in the exposure *must produce* a corresponding change in the outcome.[2] Removal of the exposure does not have to result in the elimination of the outcome, however. For example, though cigarette smoking is considered a cause of lung cancer, some nonsmokers still contract lung cancer. Therefore, even if cigarette smoking could be completely eliminated from a population, it would not result in the elimination of lung cancer. It would, however, have a dramatic effect on reducing the incidence of lung cancer over time. To summarize briefly, an association means it is *more or less likely* that the outcome will occur in the presence of the exposure, while causation means that changes in the exposure *will result* in corresponding changes in the outcome. The remainder of this chapter focuses on developing a deeper understanding of the differences between association and causation.

Types of Association

Statistically significant associations between exposures and outcomes may be categorized into three types:

- Spurious associations
- Noncausal associations
- Causal associations

Spurious Associations

Spurious associations are *false* associations. These usually result from sampling error or bias. For example, as mentioned in chapter 6, an association is generally considered statistically significant if $p \leq 0.05$. This means that we should have at least 95% confidence that the association is real, assuming no significant flaws in study design, conduct, or analysis. Nonetheless, we would still predict that as many as five times out of 100 the association would be due to sampling error. Thus, even statistically significant associations that result from well-executed epidemiologic studies can sometimes be spurious.

---

* There are many terms relating to or derived from the term *cause*. These include causation, causality, etiology, cause-effect, causal, causative, and so forth. These are not defined separately in this chapter, but each has as its root the basic definition of cause as defined herein.

Inderjit S. Thind, for example, conducted an ecological study of the association between dietary intake and cancer using a sample of 60 countries. He found a number of significant statistical associations, including some that were biologically implausible and which he thought to be spurious. In his discussion of the findings, he reiterated a common concern in broad-based studies where large numbers of statistical tests of significance are performed. Thind cautioned the readers by stating, "The . . . large numbers of correlations . . . with significant associations occurring purely by chance, suggest extreme care in assessing the role of specific dietary items as risk factors and using the results as the basis for public policy."[3(p162)]

Spurious associations may also arise from sources of bias. **Bias**, which is discussed in chapter 8, is a type of systematic (nonrandom) error in the design, conduct, or analysis of epidemiologic studies, such as the use of flawed measurement techniques, differential recall among study and comparison groups, or selection of comparison groups that are really not comparable. Bias can be quite insidious. Consider a hypothetical case-control study of the relationship between exposure to low-frequency electromagnetic fields, such as those generated by electric power lines, electric blankets, and electric alarm clocks, and the incidence of childhood leukemia. The cases consist of patients from area hospitals newly diagnosed with childhood leukemia, and the controls are those of similar age, sex, and racial/ethnic background who had been randomly selected from the communities served by the hospitals. The parents of cases and controls are then queried about their children's exposure to low-frequency electromagnetic fields. The parents of the cases may be more likely to recall their children's exposures than those of the controls since they are probably more motivated to remember past exposures that might help explain their children's leukemia than are the parents of the controls. If this is true, the study could result in a positive, but *spurious*, association between exposure to low-frequency electromagnetic fields and the incidence of childhood leukemia.

Noncausal Associations

Noncausal associations are real associations, but they are *not* causal associations. That is, a change in the exposure does not necessarily result in a change in the outcome. Noncausal associations usually represent *secondary* associations due to confounding factors. The association exists because the exposure is associated with another factor that in turn is associated with the outcome. A whimsical example is provided by Max Michael III, W. Thomas Boyce, and Allen J. Wilcox.[4] Dr. Al Betzerov conducted a prospective cohort study to test his hypothesis that gambling causes cancer. He chose two neighboring states, one where gambling was legal and the other where it was not. He then followed randomly selected samples of subjects from each state matched by age, sex, urban/rural differences, and family income for 10 years. At the conclusion of the study, he noted a statistically significant positive association between gambling and cancer. Specifically, the residents of Nevada had a higher rate of cancer than those from Utah. The association, although real, was *not* one of cause-effect. Unfortunately for Dr. Betzerov, one of the states he chose was Utah. Utah is a state composed of a large number of Mormons, who have very different lifestyles from typical Nevada residents, who are not Mormons. The fact that the Mormon Church requires its adherents to abstain from tobacco and alcohol explains this association. The association between gambling and cancer was a *secondary* association due to confounding by alcohol and tobacco use, which are higher in Nevada than in Utah. In other words, gambling is associated with alcohol and tobacco use, which are directly linked to cancer. Therefore, although gambling itself does not cause cancer, its association with causes of cancer produces a secondary, but noncausal, association with cancer. This type of association can also be considered spurious in that it can lead to an erroneous conclusion.

Noncausal associations may also exist when the defined exposure results from the outcome. Hypertension, for example, may result from kidney disease. Thus, there may be an association between the two, but in this example, hypertension would not be considered a cause of kidney disease because the exposure does not *precede* the outcome and therefore cannot alter its frequency. This type of hypertension is generally referred to as secondary hypertension to differentiate it from primary hypertension, which can cause kidney damage.

Causal Associations

Causal associations are those in which changes in the exposure produce changes in the outcome. In epidemiology, we cannot prove causal associations because it is impossible to account for all the other factors that might play some role in an association, especially in observational studies where there may be many unrecognized, and therefore uncontrolled, variables. Well-designed experimental epidemiologic studies can come much closer to establishing causation than observational studies, but even in these studies there may be other factors of which the investigator is unaware. Since no two humans beings are exactly alike in their makeup or reactions to external stimuli, one cannot always be assured that even randomized groups of people are perfectly comparable. Even laboratory experiments with mice rely on well-defined strains to minimize intraspecies differences that can invalidate the results of an experiment.

A given association may not be clearly spurious, noncausal, or causal. This is because sampling error can never be completely eliminated as a possible reason for an association in an epidemiologic study based on samples, although it can be greatly minimized. Similarly, it would be extremely difficult to discount any possibility of bias in a study. The same can be said for possible confounding. Thus, the job of the epidemiologist is to determine which type of association is more likely, and this is not always an easy task.

Since our main concern is identifying causal relationships when they exist, we need some guidance in determining whether an association is likely to be a causal one. In practice, the determination of a cause–effect relationship is based on a careful review and judgment of all relevant information available, and never on the basis of one or two studies alone. It is somewhat like trying a criminal case where there are no eyewitnesses to the crime. The prosecutor has to rely on circumstantial evidence to convince a jury beyond a reasonable doubt that the defendant is guilty. It was based on a thorough review of major epidemiologic and non-epidemiologic studies that in 1964 the Surgeon General of the U.S. Public Health Service determined that cigarette smoking is a cause of lung cancer.[5]

Criteria for Assessing Causation

In 1965, Sir Austin Bradford Hill, Professor Emeritus of Medical Statistics with the University of London, delivered a landmark address where he outlined nine criteria that could be used to determine if statistical associations were likely to represent causal associations.[6] His reasoning built on the earlier work of others, such as John Stuart Mill, who in 1856 had defined several canons from which causal relationships could be deduced.[1] Over the years many authors have articulated or added to Hill's basic criteria, which have become known as **Hill's postulates**. Using these as a general guide, the following six criteria should be helpful in deciding whether statistical associations are likely to represent causal associations. In the end, the process of determining causation, however, is largely subjective except for the first criterion.

- **Correct temporal sequence.** In order for an exposure to be a cause of an outcome, it must *precede* the outcome. Of all the criteria used to judge whether an association is causal or not, this is the only one that is considered *absolutely essential*. Exposures that occur concurrently with an outcome or subsequent to an outcome cannot be considered causes because they do not alter the frequency of the outcome. Determining if exposure precedes outcome can be a problem in cross-sectional studies where exposure and outcome are assessed concurrently. For example, in a cross-sectional study designed to determine if there is a relationship between the prevalence of excess body weight and osteoarthritis, it may not be clear which factor came first. Thus, the correct temporal sequence cannot be established reliably.

- **Strength of the association.** In general, the stronger an association, the more likely it is a causal association. When the relative risk or rate ratio is high, for example, it is less likely that the association can be explained away by unrecognized or subtle sources of bias or confounding. Compared to nonsmokers, those who smoke and are exposed to high levels of asbestos in their jobs have a fifty- to ninetyfold increased risk of lung cancer. It seems improbable that these factors are not causative. Even if some bias or confounding exists, it is unlikely that it would account for the entire relationship. This is not to say that small associations cannot also be causal in nature. This is one reason why several criteria are needed to judge causality.

- **Consistency of the association.** When other investigators studying different populations at different times in different places using different methodologies obtain similar findings with regard to an association, it increases the probability that the association is causal. In concluding that cigarette smoking is a cause of lung cancer, the Advisory Committee to the Surgeon General of the United States cited diverse epidemiologic and other studies showing a strong relationship between smoking and lung cancer.[5]

- **Dose-response relationship.** In general, if increased exposure leads to a greater frequency of the outcome, then this is suggestive of a causal relationship. Heavy smokers, for example, have been shown to be at a higher risk of lung cancer than light smokers. In fact, a linear dose-response relationship between smoking and lung cancer can be demonstrated based on the number of cigarettes smoked per day. The absence of a dose-response relationship does not necessarily mean that an association is noncausal, however. A threshold may exist. A **threshold** is a level of exposure that must be reached before effects become apparent. Below the threshold, there are no observed effects. Copper, which may be found in small quantities in drinking water, demonstrates a threshold; that is, copper has no adverse effects until it reaches a certain level. In fact, in very small quantities it is an essential mineral needed for proper growth and development. On the other hand, a dose-response relationship could be due to a strong confounding factor that closely follows an exposure.[7] Once again, several criteria should be considered in making a judgment of causation.

- **Biological plausibility.** The basic question here is, does the association make biological sense? Is the association credible based on our understanding of the natural history of the disease or possible pathogenic mechanisms? When Thind found significant associations for protein, fat, and caloric intake and certain forms of leukemia, he could offer no biological evidence to support the associations, thereby casting doubt on their authenticity.[3] Failure to make biological sense, however, does not necessarily negate the possibility of a causal association. In some cases, our understanding of the biological mechanisms may be incomplete, and what does not make sense today may make sense sometime in the future. From a contemporary vantage point, it seems difficult to understand why the theory of contagion was considered controversial as an explanation for the spread of epidemics during the Middle Ages.

- **Experimental evidence.** Having experimental evidence to support an association between an exposure and an outcome strengthens the case for a causal association. Well-designed randomized controlled trials and randomized community trials can provide strong corroboration of a suspected causal association. This is because these study designs virtually eliminate selection bias and confounding. Of course, the degree of control possible in epidemiologic experiments is not to the same level as that in animal studies. Nevertheless, they can be powerful tools when establishing causation. Evidence from nonepidemiologic experiments can also be used in judging cause–effect relationships. Because of the limited circumstances in which experimental studies can be conducted with humans, some associations will not be testable in this manner. We would not perform a randomized controlled trial on the effects of microwave radiation on cataract development, for example, because such a study would be unethical even if some were willing to volunteer for the study.

The following list ranks the major types of epidemiologic studies in descending order of the degree to which identical findings of a statistically significant association are likely to demonstrate a causal association.

1. Randomized Controlled Trial
2. Randomized Community Trial
3. Prospective Cohort Study
4. Retrospective Cohort Study
5. Case-Control Study
6. Cross-Sectional Study
7. Ecological Study
8. Descriptive Study

The relative rankings actually reflect the probability of encountering unrecognized bias, confounding, or other errors within the specific study designs. It also assumes that the studies have been planned appropriately and conducted to minimize errors; a poorly designed experimental study can provide less convincing evidence of causality than a well-designed observational study. It should be kept in mind, however, that causality is never determined on the basis of one study alone.

Figure 7–1 summarizes the overall decision-making process for deciding whether or not an association is causal. The process begins by asking if the observed statistical association appears to be spurious. If this is unlikely (e.g., minimal sampling error or bias), the next question is whether or not it appears to be noncausal. If this is not likely (e.g., no obvious confounding and exposure does not follow outcome), then the criteria for judging causality can be examined, and a conclusion can be reached based on the overall weight of the evidence.

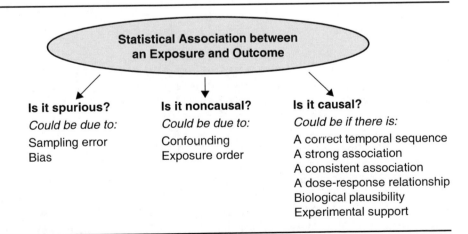

Figure 7–1 Deciding whether an association is causal

Types of Causes

With communicable diseases the concept of causation appears to be relatively straightforward. However, as discussed in chapter 3, this apparent simplicity can be deceiving. Not everyone exposed to *Mycobacterium tuberculosis* (the bacterium implicated in tuberculosis), for example, develops tuberculosis. A number of host and environmental factors must also be considered. Similarly, not everyone exposed to cold germs gets a cold. In fact, the more we learn about causation, the more complex it seems. With many noncommunicable diseases, especially chronic conditions like arthritis, mental illness, Alzheimer's disease, multiple sclerosis, cerebral palsy, cardiovascular disease, diabetes, and so forth, the causal pathways can be extremely complex. Multifactorial etiology (see chapter 2) is the rule rather than the exception for most health-related problems.

Necessary and Sufficient Causes

To get a better understanding of causality as it is used in epidemiology it is helpful to look at different types of causes. A **necessary cause** is an exposure that is *required* for a particular outcome to occur, and, therefore, it is always associated with that outcome. If the exposure is absent, the outcome cannot occur. A **sufficient cause** is an exposure that by itself will produce a particular outcome, but it may not be the only cause of the outcome. The outcome, therefore, may occur without the exposure if it is also caused by other exposures. These two classifications of causes give rise to four possible scenarios described by John Last.[1]

		Necessary	
Sufficient		**Yes**	**No**
Yes		A	C
No		B	D

Combination A represents a **necessary and sufficient cause**. This is a cause that is required to produce the outcome *and* which is able to cause the outcome by itself. This can be represented by:

Exposure X → Outcome Y

where Exposure X is the specified cause, and Outcome Y is the specified outcome.

Necessary and sufficient causes are not very common in the real world. One example of a condition that results from a necessary and sufficient cause is lead poisoning. Lead is *necessary* to produce lead poisoning, and it is also *sufficient*. The rabies virus might also be considered a necessary and sufficient cause of human rabies. It is *not* essential that a necessary and sufficient cause always produces the outcome. Observations have shown, for example, that not everyone infected with the rabies virus contracts the disease even if they have not been immunized.[8] Nevertheless, anyone who contracts rabies must have the virus (i.e., it is necessary), and no other known cause must be present for the disease to occur (i.e., it is sufficient). It is important to emphasize, however, that as knowledge of disease causation expands, classifications may need to be revised. We may learn in the future, for example, that some causes thought to be necessary and sufficient would be better classified in another way. At one time many believed that cancer was caused by a single factor, still undiscovered. Today we recognize its multifactorial etiology.

Combination B in the above table represents a **necessary but not sufficient cause**. This is a cause that is required to produce a specified outcome *but* is *not* able to cause the outcome by itself. Other causes are necessary for the outcome to occur. This can be represented by:

Exposure X + Other Causes → Outcome Y

Alcoholism is a disease in which alcohol consumption is a necessary but not sufficient cause of the disease. Alcohol is definitely necessary for alcoholism to develop, but other factors, including genetic, social, behavioral, and environmental factors, also appear to be necessary for the disease to manifest itself.

Combination C represents a **not necessary but sufficient cause**. This is a cause that is *not* required to produce a specified outcome *but* when present is able to cause the outcome by itself. This means that there are other causes of the specified outcome. A not necessary but sufficient cause may be represented by:

Exposure X → Outcome Y; Exposure Z → Outcome Y

where Exposure Z is some other cause of Outcome Y.

Ionizing radiation at high doses will cause sterility in men. Heavy exposure to certain pesticides will do the same. In this example, Exposure X is ionizing radiation, Exposure Z is a specific pesticide, and Outcome Y is sterility in men. Thus, sterility in men has more than one cause. Both ionizing radiation and certain pesticides are capable of causing sterility in men (at high doses).

Combination D denotes a **not necessary and not sufficient cause**. This is a cause that is *not* required to produce the specified outcome *and* when present is *not* able to cause the outcome by itself. Hence, there are other causes of the specified outcome. A not necessary and not sufficient cause is known as a **contributory cause**. It can be represented by:

Exposure X + Other Causes → Outcome Y; Exposure Z → Outcome Y

Where Exposure Z is another cause of Outcome Y.

Not necessary and not sufficient causes are very common causes of chronic diseases. For example, a sedentary lifestyle is not necessary and not sufficient to cause coronary heart disease (CHD). It is not required for CHD development, nor is it sufficient to cause CHD by itself. It is, however, a contributory cause of CHD, and when present with other contributory causes, such as high blood cholesterol, family history of heart disease, hypertension, cigarette smoking, and so forth, may lead to the development of CHD. That is, the frequency of CHD will be higher in groups with these factors than in groups without them.

In epidemiology causation is determined by what occurs in groups of people or populations as opposed to what occurs in any particular individual. We know, for example, based on the Framingham Heart Study that people who live certain lifestyles die more frequently from coronary heart disease. From the group data, we can make predictions about individuals based on their lifestyle habits, but we cannot expect that the predictions will always be correct. For example, everyone seems to know someone who smoked four packs of cigarettes a day, had high blood pressure, and drank like a fish, but lived until 103. Undoubtedly, this person met an "untimely" death when his bungee cord broke. The exception, however, does not make the rule.

Direct and Indirect Causes

Causal associations can also be classified as direct or indirect. A **direct causal association** (or **direct cause**) can be thought of as representing a causal pathway in which there are *no* intermediate steps, while an **indirect causal association** (or **indirect cause**) involves one or more intervening factors.[9] For example, in a direct causal association, X causes Y, where X is the causative exposure, and Y is the outcome. In an indirect causal association, I causes X, which in turn causes Y. While I is a direct cause of X, it is an *indirect* cause of Y. Since I causes X, and X causes Y, it follows that I causes Y based on the definition of cause. A change in I will result in a change in X, which in turn will result in a change in Y. Thus, I is an indirect cause of Y.

Indirect causes can include a variety of **predisposing or enabling factors** that precede the direct cause. For example, excessive heat applied to the skin is the direct cause of burns, but the exposure to the heat may be influenced by a dangerous working environment or failure to follow certain safety precautions, which might be considered indirect causes of burns. Also, the human immunodeficiency virus (HIV) is said to be the direct cause of AIDS, but factors that facilitate contracting HIV include sharing syringes and promiscuous sexual behaviors. In practice, controlling the predisposing or enabling factors should result in a decrease in the outcome. *Predisposing* or *enabling factors* are often referred to as *risk factors*, which, as noted previously, may or may not be causal in nature. When used in connection with indirect causes, it is assumed that they represent causal factors.

Whatever classification scheme is used, most health-related problems can be determined to have multiple causes. This multifactorial etiology, which has been referred to often in this text, presents a challenge to epidemiologists who are concerned with unraveling the determinants of disease and to the health professionals whose efforts are directed toward disease prevention and control. As our knowledge of the natural history of health problems expands, the models of causation and the methods of intervention will continue to undergo change.

Causes of Death

Before concluding this chapter, it should be interesting to look at the *true* causes of the major health problems in the United States as represented by their cause-specific mortality rates. In a recent publication, the National Center for Health Statistics listed in descending order of importance the leading overall causes of death in the United States.[10] The top 10 on this list were:

1. Heart disease (271.6 deaths per 100,000 population)
2. Cancer (201.6 deaths per 100,000 population)
3. Cerebrovascular diseases (59.7 deaths per 100,000 population)
4. Chronic obstructive pulmonary diseases (40.7 deaths per 100,000)
5. Accidents and adverse effects (35.7 deaths per 100,000 population)
6. Pneumonia and influenza (32.3 deaths per 100,000 population)
7. Diabetes mellitus (23.4 deaths per 100,000 population)
8. Suicide (11.4 deaths per 100,000 population)
9. Renal diseases (9.5 deaths per 100,000 population)
10. Chronic liver disease and cirrhosis (9.4 deaths per 100,000 population)

Although the causes of these deaths are manifold, J. Michael McGinnis and William H. Foege[11] identified nine factors that presumably account for about half of the total deaths, including deaths due to HIV infection, which was the tenth leading cause of death when McGinnis and Foege published their findings some years earlier. The nine causes McGinnis and Foege identified were: tobacco, diet and activity patterns, alcohol, microbial agents, toxic agents, firearms, sexual behavior, motor vehicles, and illicit use of drugs. What is most revealing about this list is that all of these factors can be modified through the implementation of primary prevention programs. Of course, there must be a willingness to commit the necessary resources and establish priorities to deal with these problems if they are to be managed effectively.

Summary

- Statistical associations between exposures and outcomes can be of three types—spurious, noncausal, or causal. Spurious associations are false associations that are usually due to sampling error or bias. Noncausal associations usually result from confounding, although they can also occur when the exposure is the result of the outcome instead of vice versa. Causal associations are ones in which a change in the exposure results in a corresponding change in the outcome.

- Because it is not possible to prove causation, it is helpful to have reliable criteria upon which to judge a statistical association in terms of its likelihood of being causal. A final decision regarding causation should be based on all relevant information and not just on the basis of one or two studies. Six criteria, derived from Hill's postulates, should help in determining whether an association is likely to be causal. These criteria are correct temporal sequence, strength of the association, consistency of the association, dose-response relationship, biological plausibility, and experimental evidence. Of the six criteria, only correct temporal sequence is required for an association to be considered causal. The others are highly suggestive of causation, however, especially when all or most of them are met.

- Causes can be classified as to whether they are necessary and/or sufficient or whether they are direct or indirect. A necessary cause is one that is required to produce an outcome, while a sufficient cause is one that can produce an outcome by itself (i.e., in the absence of other known causes). The most common types of causes are those that are not necessary and not sufficient. These are known as contributory causes and are the causes that account for most chronic diseases. Indirect causes include a variety of predisposing or enabling factors that precede the direct cause of an outcome. Controlling indirect causes can reduce the incidence of the outcome and is sometimes easier than controlling the direct cause.

New Terms

bias	dose-response	noncausal association
biological plausibility	relationship	not necessary and not
causal association	experimental evidence	sufficient cause
cause	Hill's postulates	not necessary but
consistency of	indirect causal association	sufficient cause
the association	indirect cause	predisposing or
contributory cause	necessary and	enabling factor
correct temporal	sufficient cause	spurious association
sequence	necessary but not	strength of the association
direct causal association	sufficient cause	sufficient cause
direct cause	necessary cause	threshold

Study Questions and Exercises

1. For each of the following statements indicate whether the results are more likely to be due to a spurious association, a noncausal association, or a causal association. Also, explain the reasons for your answers.

   a. A case-control study revealed that there was a moderate to strong association between coffee consumption and deaths from coronary heart disease. Other studies have shown that those who drink coffee are more likely to smoke than those who do not drink coffee.

   b. A prospective cohort study showed that women who exercise regularly were less likely to contract cancer than women who exercised only occasionally or not at all. The exercise group was selected from women attending a fitness center, and the comparison group was selected from women attending a weight-loss clinic.

c. A large randomized controlled trial showed that folic acid supplementation by prospective mothers significantly reduced the incidence of neural tube defects in their offspring. This finding was confirmed in subsequent studies.

d. A large exploratory epidemiologic study examined the possible relationship of 25 different lifestyle behaviors to teenage suicide. One of the findings was a positive association between bicycle helmet use and suicide ($p = 0.05$) that had not been previously reported in the literature.

2. On bottles of wine and other alcoholic beverages, it states, "According to the Surgeon General, women should not drink alcoholic beverages during pregnancy because of the risk of birth defects." Discuss the evidence that alcohol consumption causes birth defects using the six criteria for causation discussed in this chapter. For each criterion, describe the degree to which the evidence supports a conclusion of causation and the reasons for your response. In answering this question it may be necessary to consult a review of epidemiologic literature on alcohol consumption and birth defects.

3. Provide an example other than one used in this chapter of a necessary and sufficient cause, a necessary but not sufficient cause, a not necessary but sufficient cause, and a not necessary and not sufficient cause of disease, respectively. Also indicate why your examples are appropriate.

4. Give two examples, respectively, of direct and indirect causes of disease and justify your choices.

References

1. Last, J. M., ed. (1995). *A Dictionary of Epidemiology*. New York: Oxford University Press.
2. Valanis, B. (1992). *Epidemiology in Nursing and Health Care*. Norwalk, CT: Appleton and Lange.
3. Thind, I. S. (1986). Diet and Cancer—An International Study. *International Journal of Epidemiology* 15(2): 160–162.
4. Michael, M. III, Boyce, W. T., and Wilcox, A. J. (1984). *Biomedical Bestiary: An Epidemiologic Guide to Flaws and Fallacies in the Medical Literature*. Boston: Little, Brown, and Company.
5. U.S. Department of Health, Education, and Welfare (1964). *Smoking and Health: Report of the Advisory Committee to the Surgeon General of the Public Health Service*. USPHS Publication No. 1103. Washington, DC: U.S. Government Printing Office.
6. Hill, A. B. (1965). The Environment and Disease: Association or Causation? *Proceedings of the Royal Society of Medicine* 58: 295–300.
7. Brownson, R. C., Remington, P. L., and Davis, J. R. (1998). *Chronic Disease Epidemiology and Control*, 2nd ed. Washington, DC: American Public Health Association.
8. Chin, J., ed. (2000). *Control of Communicable Diseases Manual*, 17th ed. Washington, DC: American Public Health Association.
9. Jekel, J. F., Elmore, J. G., and Katz, D. L. (1996). *Epidemiology, Biostatistics, and Preventive Medicine*. Philadelphia, PA: W. B. Saunders Company.
10. Hoyert, D. L., Kochanek, K. D., and Murphy, S. L. (1999). Deaths: Final Data for 1997. *National Vital Statistics Reports* 47(19). Hyattsville, MD: National Center for Health Statistics.
11. McGinnis, J. M., and Foege, W. H. (1993). Actual Causes of Death in the United States. *Journal of the American Medical Association* 10(270): 2207–2212.

CHAPTER EIGHT

Assessing the Accuracy of Epidemiologic Studies

Learning Objectives

▸ Compare and contrast internal and external validity.

▸ Distinguish between selection and measurement bias.

▸ Describe at least four specific types of selection and measurement bias, respectively.

▸ Differentiate between differential and nondifferential misclassification.

▸ Explain confounding and each of the requirements for confounding to occur.

▸ Identify specific methods to minimize bias and confounding.

▸ Describe the types of random error that affect the precision of study findings.

▸ Define accuracy, type I and type II errors, positive and negative bias and confounding, power, convenience and probability samples, and statistical significance.

Overview

The accuracy of an epidemiologic study depends on the validity and precision of the findings. Internal validity is the degree to which the findings are free of systematic errors due to bias or confounding. Bias can pose a serious threat to internal validity and usually occurs in the study design or data collection phases of a study. It includes selection and measurement bias. Selection bias results from the manner in which subjects are selected or retained in a study, while measurement bias results from misclassification of subjects with regard to exposure or outcome status. Confounding is another source of systematic error caused by a mixing of effects between an exposure and an incidental variable that is not equally distributed between the study and comparison groups. Precision is affected by random measurement and sampling errors. The external validity of a study represents the degree to which the findings can be generalized to populations other than the target population. Accurate findings are a prerequisite for external validity.

Introduction

The search for truth is always concerned with exposing error,
since error clouds the truth and can lead to false conclusions.

In an ideal world, all epidemiologic studies would be designed, conducted, analyzed, and interpreted in a manner that eliminated all errors. Although the ideal can never be fully realized, it must be a goal of epidemiologists to see that errors in epidemiologic studies are minimized to the extent possible. Likewise, those who read and use the epidemiologic literature need to be careful when and how they apply the findings. This latter point is especially important when epidemiologic findings are used to support the development or adoption of health-related programs and policies. Though rare, there have been incidents where flawed epidemiologic research has been used to develop expensive programs or establish policies or procedures that have been counterproductive or detrimental.

The Meaning of Accuracy

The **accuracy** of an epidemiologic study indicates the extent to which the study findings are free of errors. Accuracy has two major components—**validity** and **precision**. Briefly, validity is concerned with the degree of *systematic error* in a study, while precision is concerned with the degree of *nonsystematic error*. Sources of systematic (nonrandom) error include selection bias, measurement bias, and confounding, while sources of nonsystematic (random) error include random measurement error and sampling error. These terms are defined and discussed in the sections that follow. Figure 8–1 on page 139 shows the components of accuracy and the sources of error that can threaten it.

Validity

There are two types of validity—internal and external. **Internal validity** represents the degree to which the results of a study are true for the target population (defined in chapter 5). Internal validity is threatened by sources of systematic error. **Systematic error** denotes nonrandom flaws in study design, conduct, or analysis that can have the effect of uniformly increasing or decreasing the magnitude of the measure of association between an exposure and outcome. Therefore, systematic error can lead to either artificially elevated or artificially reduced risk, rate, or odds ratios. The two primary reasons for systematic error—*bias* and *confounding*—will be discussed in the following sections.

External validity, also known as **generalizability**, represents the degree to which the results of a study are relevant for populations other than the target population. For example, can the findings of an epidemiologic study conducted on white, male physicians in the United States be generalized to all adult males in the U.S.? Similarly, can the findings be applied to all

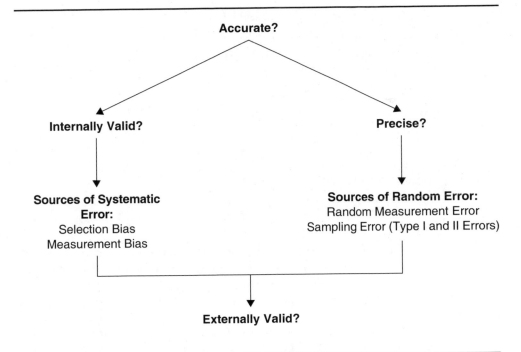

Figure 8–1 Assessing the findings of epidemiologic studies (or "the house upon which accuracy is built")

adults in the U.S. regardless of their race/ethnicity or sex? These questions have to do with the external validity of a study. Unfortunately, there is no simple formula for determining external validity. A judgment has to be made as to whether the findings would make sense in other populations. This judgment can always be challenged and may have to be defended. When the authors of a large randomized controlled trial in Scandinavia found that long-term treatment with simvastatin (a cholesterol-lowering drug) significantly increased the survival of patients with coronary heart disease, it did not seem like much of a stretch to assume that the findings might also apply to coronary heart disease patients in other parts of the world.[1] It would be questionable, however, on the basis of this study alone, to assume that simvastatin would have the same effect on healthy populations. Additional research on groups free from coronary heart disease would need to be conducted.

Of the two types of validity, internal validity is *more important* than external validity, since it does not make sense to generalize findings that are *not* internally valid.[2] As a result, internal validity needs to be evaluated carefully before one even considers the external validity of a study. The findings of the Scandinavian Simvastatin Survival Study discussed above were considered reasonably valid internally, thus permitting generalization of the findings to populations other than the one studied.[1]

Bias

Bias, which was defined in chapter 7 as a type of systematic (nonrandom) error in the design, conduct, or analysis of epidemiologic studies, falls into two major categories:

- *Selection bias*
- *Measurement bias*

Either form of bias can lead to spurious associations and, therefore, can present serious problems in the interpretation of epidemiologic findings. Bias can also be classified as *positive* or *negative*. While **positive bias** overestimates the magnitude of a measure of association (e.g., relative risk), **negative bias** underestimates it.

Selection Bias

Selection bias refers to systematic error in a study resulting from the manner in which the subjects are selected or retained in the study. This error can occur when the characteristics of the subjects selected for a study differ systematically from those in the target population[3] or when the study and comparison groups are selected from different populations. For example, selection bias can occur in a cross-sectional study when a **convenience sample** (as opposed to a **probability sample**)* is employed, in a case-control study when cases and controls differ with regard to factors related to the study exposure, or in a cohort study when the exposed and unexposed groups vary in their susceptibility to the study outcome due to factors other than the study exposure. Selection bias can also occur in cohort and experimental studies after the subjects have been selected due to systematic withdrawal or losses to follow-up. Withdrawals or losses to follow-up occur when subjects fail to complete the study for various reasons. In short, selection bias can occur in any type of epidemiologic study, although it is more common in case-control studies because cases and controls are often selected on the basis of *different* criteria, which in turn may be related to the frequency of exposure.[2]

Selection bias is problematic because it can result in an over- or underestimation of the true magnitude of the relationship between an exposure and an outcome. In fact, in some situations selection bias produces an apparent association when none exists, or it conceals a real association. The potential for selection bias is not always easily recognized. To avoid selection bias investigators need to be very careful that the subjects are representative of the target population, that the study and comparison groups are similar except for the variables being investigated, and that subject losses are kept to a minimum. Exhibit 8–1 provides a hypothetical example of selection bias in a case-control study.

---

* Convenience samples are nonrandom samples selected for expedience. They are usually chosen because they are readily available, but they may not be representative of the target population from which they were selected. Probability samples are those in which everyone in the target population has a *known* probability of being selected. In a randomly selected sample, which is a type of probability sample, everyone in the population has an *equal* probability of being selected.[4]

Exhibit 8–1 Example of Selection Bias

An investigator hypothesized that coffee drinking is associated with angina pectoris. To test his hypothesis, he designed a case-control study where the cases were drawn from patients attending a heart clinic staffed by cardiologists. The controls, who had no medical history of angina, were drawn from another clinic in the same community that specialized in the treatment and management of ulcers. The patients were matched by age and sex. The results of the investigation were as follows:

Subjects

Coffee Drinkers	Cases	Controls
Yes (1 or more cups/day)	160	100
No (less than 1 cup/day)	90	150

OR = 2.7, p < 0.001

The odds ratio (OR) appears to indicate that coffee drinking is significantly associated with angina pectoris, all other factors being equal. However, all other factors are probably not equal. Since the controls came from a different clinic than the cases, it is possible that they may have been systematically different from the cases in ways that could affect the study results. Patients attending the ulcer clinic are likely to have reduced or stopped their coffee drinking on physician recommendations due to the irritation it can cause when one has an ulcer. Therefore these controls are less likely to be coffee drinkers than other possible controls. The OR, then, is probably overstated due to selection bias. In fact, when the study was repeated using patients in the local community hospital, where the controls represented a variety of diagnoses unrelated to angina, no significant association was found between coffee drinking and angina pectoris.

Subjects

Coffee Drinker	Cases	Controls
Yes (1 or more cups/day)	140	130
No (less than 1 cup/day)	110	120

OR = 1.2, p > 0.05

The selection bias in the original case-control study occurred because the cases and controls were systematically different from each other with regard to a factor related to the study exposure (i.e., the presence of ulcers).

Common Types of Selection Bias

Many types of selection bias have been identified in the literature. Some of the more common ones are described below.

Berkson's bias, named after Dr. Joseph Berkson who first described it in the 1940s, is a type of selection bias that can occur in hospital-based case-control studies. The bias results when the *combination* of the study exposure and outcome increases or decreases the chance that cases will be admitted to the hospital.[5] In most circumstances, this chance is increased. Thus, the exposure among hospitalized patients will normally be systematically higher in the case versus the control group, thereby inflating the true magnitude of the measure of association (e.g., making the odds ratio appear stronger than it actually is). This is an example of positive bias since the magnitude of the measure of association is overestimated.

Berkson's bias can be illustrated in the following example: Suppose that an investigator wanted to test the hypothesis that unmanageable hypertension is related to transient ischemic attacks (TIAs) at a time before the relationship between hypertension and stroke had been scientifically confirmed. The investigator planned a case-control study in a major community hospital using TIA patients as the cases and a randomly selected group of patients with other diagnoses as the controls. If the presence of unmanageable hypertension *and* a TIA made hospitalization more likely than a TIA alone, perhaps due to physician suspicion of an increased potential for stroke or because of the presence of two serious conditions, we would expect the case group to have a higher proportion of patients with unmanageable hypertension than the control group *due solely to hospital admission practices*. This would lead to an inflated measure of association between unmanageable hypertension and TIAs due to selection bias.

Another form of selection bias is **prevalence–incidence bias**. This type of bias can occur in cross-sectional and case-control studies when asymptomatic, mild, clinically resolved, or fatal cases are inadvertently excluded from the case group because the selected cases are examined some time after the disease process has already begun (i.e., looking at prevalent versus incident cases).[3] This bias exists if the association would have been different had the early cases been included in the sample. A cross-sectional study of the relationship between drug use and depression, for example, could result in an inflated association between the two study variables if the causes of undetected mild depression or severe depression resulting in suicide were actually due to factors *other* than drug use. Had the subjects with mild or severe depression been included in the analysis, perhaps no association, or at least a weaker association, would have been found. This type of selection bias can also occur in other types of analytic studies.[6]

The **healthy worker effect** is a type of selection bias that can arise in cohort studies when the outcomes among workers are compared to general population samples. For instance, imagine a prospective cohort study testing the hypothesis that working in nuclear power plants is associated with increased mortality from all causes. The study group is selected from all those working in nuclear power plants in northern Illinois, and the comparison group is a randomly selected sample of residents of northern Illinois with similar age, sex, and racial/ethnic characteristics. It is likely that the magnitude of the measure of association would underestimate the true association between working in nuclear power plants and mortality. The reason is that workers as a whole tend to be healthier than the general population. This is because one must have a certain level of health to work and hold a job, and the general population is composed of both healthy and unhealthy individuals, including those whose health problems prevent them from working. Thus, the members of the study group in this example are less likely to die prematurely than those in the comparison group *independent* of exposure to the nuclear power industry. The consequence is likely to be a *negative bias* in the study results. To avoid the bias it would have been better to use a similar occupational group for the comparison (e.g., those working in fossil fuel plants).

The healthy worker effect is a common example of the broader category of **membership bias** that says that those who belong to an organized group (e.g., the military, athletic associations, civic groups, religious organizations) tend to differ systematically with regard to their health status from the general population.[3] That is, they tend to be healthier and, thus, less prone to morbidity and premature mortality.

Volunteer bias is another type of selection bias. It is due to the fact that those individuals who take part in epidemiologic studies tend to be systematically different from those who do not. For example, one study found that volunteers are likely to be better educated, more active in community affairs, less likely to smoke, and more concerned about health matters than nonvolunteers.[7] If these or other characteristics of volunteers are related to the frequency of the study exposure or susceptibility to the study outcome, they can produce associations that are systematically different from those in the target population, leading to selection bias. If they are not related to the study exposure or outcome, they will not bias the study, although they may affect the external validity of the study.

Volunteer bias was revealed in a randomized controlled trial comparing the efficacy of lipid-lowering drugs to a placebo. The five-year mortality rate for those receiving the drug clofibrate was 15.0 per 100 among those judged to be compliant with the study regimen and 24.6 per 100 among those who were considered noncompliant. The death rates among those taking the placebo, however, showed a similar divergence. Among the compliant group, the five-year mortality rate was 15.1 per 100 compared to 28.2 per 100 in the noncompliant group. Apparently, *compliance* itself, as revealed by the results in the placebo group, had a positive effect on the outcome. This was most likely due to the fact that those who voluntarily comply tend to be systematically different from those who do not.[7, 8]

Volunteer bias is also a type of **response bias** because it can occur when those who respond to questionnaires (volunteers) are systematically different from those who do not respond (nonvolunteers).[5] Descriptive studies of sexual behaviors using preprinted surveys in magazines are notoriously biased, since: (a) only readers of the magazine are likely to respond, and (b) the respondents are more likely to be those with liberal attitudes toward sex. In general, response rates of less than 80% may signal potential selection bias. In these cases it is prudent to try to establish the reasons for nonresponses. If the nonrespondents are systematically different from the respondents, this could mean the study findings are biased.[6]

Loss to follow-up bias is a form of selection bias that may occur when there are significant losses to follow-up in ongoing cohort and experimental studies. If the final sample is systematically different from the original or target population with regard to exposure frequency or outcome susceptibility, then spurious associations can result. As a general rule of thumb, losses should be no more than 20% to minimize the potential for selection bias. Also, as is the case for assessing potential response bias, it is a good idea to compare the study results with the results among those who dropped out or were otherwise lost to follow-up whenever possible.[6] If there are significant differences between these groups, it suggests that the findings may have been biased.

Measurement Bias

Measurement bias, also referred to as **information** or **observation bias**, is systematic (nonrandom) error in classifying subjects with regard to exposure or outcome status.[5] This is sometimes due to inaccurate measurements. For example, suppose in a study of the effects of hypertension on heart disease, a nurse performs blood pressure measurements on the subjects using a faulty sphygmomanometer that always records blood pressures on the high side. This will result in some misclassification on exposure status, with some normotensives being classified as hypertensives. The result is measurement bias. Notice, however, that inaccurate measurements lead to measurement bias only because they are *systematic* (*nonrandom*). If the nurse had used a normal sphygmomanometer, but occasionally made mistakes in recording the results so that some blood pressures were recorded higher and some lower than the actual values, this is *not* considered measurement bias because the mistakes would be *random* and, on average, could be expected to cancel each other out. In fact, this is considered *random measurement error*, which is discussed later in this chapter. Measurement bias is systematic error, that is, *one-sided* error. Therefore, it causes the applicable measure of association to be either overstated or understated from its true value.

Measurement bias results from two major types of misclassification—*differential* and *nondifferential*. **Differential misclassification** occurs when the extent of misclassification is different between the study and comparison groups. For example, in a case-control study if more cases are *mistakenly* classified as being exposed than controls, then the misclassification is differential. Similarly, in a cohort study if the exposed group is more likely to be *mistakenly* classified as having developed the outcome than the unexposed group, then again the misclassification is differential.

Nondifferential misclassification occurs when the degree of misclassification between study and comparison groups is uniform, that is, when there is an equal frequency of incorrect classifications on exposure status among those with and without the outcome or on outcome status among those with or without the exposure. Nondifferential misclassification may occur when the criteria for exposure or outcome are estimated for practical reasons. For example, the exposure, "passive smoking," can be difficult to measure directly in an epidemiologic study, so a proxy measure, "the time subjects spend with smokers," may be used instead.[9] This measure, however, can lead to errors in classification of actual exposure experiences since some smokers may choose not to smoke in the presence of nonsmokers. The degree of misclassification in this example, however, is unlikely to be different on the basis of outcome status. Therefore, nondifferential misclassification is the likely result. To summarize briefly, nondifferential misclassification arises when measurement errors with regard to exposure are independent of outcome status or when measurement errors with regard to outcome are independent of exposure status, respectively.[9]

It is important to distinguish between differential and nondifferential misclassification since they produce different effects on the measures of association. Like selection bias, *differential* misclassification leads to over- or underestimation of the true magnitude of the measure of association. If the cases in a case-control study are more likely to be misclassified as being exposed compared to the controls, then the study will likely *overestimate* the magnitude of the odds ratio (i.e., produce positive bias). If, on the other hand, the controls are more likely to be misclassified as being exposed than the cases, the study will likely *underestimate* the magnitude of the odds ratio (i.e., produce negative bias).

Unlike differential misclassification, *nondifferential* misclassification results in a *dilution* of the measure of association.* That is, the measure of association is biased toward the **null value**, the value that represents no association between the exposure and outcome (e.g., a relative risk of one or a risk difference of zero). Therefore, nondifferential misclassification can result in the apparent absence of an association when in fact an association exists. While differential misclassification can lead to either underestimation or overestimation of an association, nondifferential misclassification invariably biases the association toward the null value. Figure 8–2 on page 146 provides examples of the effects of differential and nondifferential misclassification on epidemiologic study results.

Common Types of Measurement Bias

While selection bias occurs primarily in the *design stage* of a study, measurement bias occurs chiefly in the *data collection* phase.[3] Some common types of measurement bias are described below.

Recall bias is a type of measurement bias that is very common in case-control studies. It results from the fact that cases often remember past exposures better than controls. This usually happens because cases tend to spend time reflecting on the possible causes of their disease or because they are more motivated than controls to learn if particular factors increased their risk of getting a particular disease. As an example, consider the following hypothetical study: An investigator is trying to determine if there is a relationship between eating fried potatoes and stomach cancer. He hypothesizes that eating fried potatoes increases the risk of stomach cancer because of some specific chemical changes taking place in the potatoes during the frying process. To test his hypothesis, he designs a case-control study. As part of the study, he asks each subject to estimate their average monthly intake of fried potatoes over the previous 15 years, including the use of fried potatoes in casseroles. It is likely that the cases would recall and report their potato eating habits more accurately than the controls, who have less vested interest in

---

* There are some exceptions to this rule. For example, when there are more than two exposure categories (e.g., low, moderate, and high), it may be possible that the estimate of the measure of association can be under- or overestimated. For more information on this topic, see Norell.[9]

Differential Misclassification

100 exposed subjects ────────▶ 20 cases, 80 noncases

100 unexposed subjects ────────▶ 10 cases, 90 noncases

RR = 2.0

100 exposed subjects ────────▶ 30 cases, 70 noncases

100 unexposed subjects ────────▶ 10 cases, 90 noncases

RR = 3.0

Note: The first set of figures represents the results of a hypothetical prospective cohort study assuming correct classification of the study (the exposed) and comparison (the unexposed) groups with regard to outcome status. The second set of figures shows the effects of differential misclassification. In this example, the exposed subjects were more likely to be mistakenly classified as cases than the unexposed subjects, resulting in an inflated RR.

Nondifferential Misclassification

100 exposed subjects ────────▶ 20 cases, 80 noncases

100 unexposed subjects ────────▶ 10 cases, 90 noncases

RR = 2.0

100 exposed subjects ────────▶ 30 cases, 70 noncases

100 unexposed subjects ────────▶ 20 cases, 80 noncases

RR = 1.5

Note: The first set of figures represents the results of a hypothetical prospective cohort study assuming correct classification of the study (the exposed) and comparison (the unexposed) groups with regard to outcome status. The second set of figures shows the effects of nondifferential misclassification. In this example, the exposed subjects were equally likely to be mistakenly classified as cases as the unexposed subjects, resulting in a dilution of the RR toward 1.0.

Figure 8–2 Examples of differential and nondifferential misclassification using results of a hypothetical cohort study

the study outcome. If eating fried potatoes is related to stomach cancer, and the controls systematically underestimate their consumption, this could lead to an overestimation of the association between eating fried potatoes and developing stomach cancer. Recall bias can also occur in cross-sectional studies when subjects are asked to recall past events.

Interviewer bias is a type of measurement bias that can arise in all types of epidemiologic studies. It can occur in case-control studies when the investigators are aware of the subjects' outcome status, and this awareness influences how they solicit, record, or interpret information on exposure.[3] The bias may be conscious or unconscious and can occur when investigators probe more intensely for exposure information from cases than controls. Examples include seeking clarification from cases or asking follow-up questions that are not part of the study protocol, providing more time for cases than controls to respond to questions, and emphasizing certain words or phrases differently for cases than for controls.[10] Interviewer bias can occur in other types of studies whenever there are systematic differences in obtaining data between study and comparison groups.

Diagnostic suspicion bias usually occurs in cohort studies when knowledge of the subjects' exposure status leads to systematic differences in the procedures for diagnosing the outcome.[6] As an example of this type of measurement bias, consider a prospective study designed to determine if family-related stress in childhood is associated with adult chronic fatigue syndrome. Chronic fatigue syndrome is a controversial diagnosis for a persistent, noncurable condition that is characterized by extreme fatigue, low-grade fever, muscles aches and pains, and other vague symptoms. Say those with a high-degree of family-related stress during childhood constituted the exposed group and those with minimal family-related stress were the unexposed group. If a clinician believed the study hypothesis and was aware of the subjects' exposure status, he or she might be more likely to diagnose chronic fatigue syndrome among those in the exposed versus the unexposed group even if the reported symptoms were similar, thus leading to positive measurement bias.

Exposure suspicion bias is another type of measurement bias. It can occur in case-control studies when knowledge of the subjects' outcome status influences how exposure is assessed. For example, if investigators know or think they know the cause of a particular disease, then this knowledge may affect the degree to which they search for the suspected exposure in the case and control groups. They may, for instance, make a more intense search among cases than controls in a case-control study, leading to an overestimation of the effect (i.e., a positive bias). Exposure suspicion bias has been demonstrated in studies of thyroid cancer among children where intensive inquiries have led to substantially higher reported rates of exposure to irradiation than more routine inquiries.[6]

Controlling Bias

Selection and measurement biases are best controlled by *prevention* during the design, data collection, and execution phases of a study. This means that potential sources of bias must first be recognized as potential threats to the internal validity of a study. Once they are recognized, measures must be taken to see that their potential is minimized to the extent possible. This generally will be easier to accomplish in experimental than observational studies, but the goal must always be to eliminate bias in a study. Various procedures have been developed to minimize different types of bias. These include using randomly selected samples where possible, standardizing measurement instruments and protocols, using objective means of verifying exposures and outcomes (e.g., laboratory tests), blinding investigators as to the status of study subjects on either exposure and/or outcome as appropriate, and aggressively following up subjects who withdraw from a study so as to determine their exposure and outcome status. Some of these measures will be reviewed in chapters 10–13 where specific study designs are discussed.

Confounding

Confounding, which was first defined in chapter 6, is a distortion in the degree of association between an exposure and an outcome due to a mixing of effects between the exposure and an incidental factor, which is known as the **confounding factor** or **confounder** for short.[11] Like bias, confounding represents systematic error and threatens the internal validity of an epidemiologic study since it can lead to false conclusions regarding the true relationship between an exposure and outcome. Confounding can either overestimate or underestimate the true magnitude of the measure of association between an exposure and outcome. When the effect of a confounder overestimates the magnitude of a measure of association, it is said to be a **positive confounder**. Conversely, if the confounding factor leads to underestimation of the magnitude of the measure of association, it is said to be a **negative confounder**. Depending on the nature of its relationship with the exposure and outcome, a confounder can even distort associations to such an extent that a positive association appears negative or no association appears as an association.[11]

For an incidental factor to be a confounder, it must satisfy the following conditions (see figure 8–3):

1. It must be associated with the exposure,
2. It must be an independent risk factor for the outcome,
3. It must *not* be an intermediate step in the causal chain between the exposure and outcome, and
4. It must be present to a greater or lesser degree in the study group versus the comparison group.

With regard to the last requirement, it is important to understand that confounding occurs because the confounder is *unequally distributed* between the study and comparison groups. If the factor is equally distributed between the groups, no confounding will take place, even if the first three requirements are met. It is also possible that an incidental factor may cause confounding in one study but not in another. This is because the distribution of the variable may differ from one study to another.

Because we normally do not know what factors actually will confound any given association, many epidemiologists suggest that all suspected or known risk factors for the outcome, especially if they are known to be associated with the exposure, should be considered **potential confounders**. In any event, as was the case with rate adjustment (chapter 6), it is only after the fact that we learn whether or not confounding was present and to what degree. If adjusting the measure of association for a potential confounder alters its magnitude, then the factor must have been a confounder. The degree of confounding is indicated by the extent to which the magnitude of the measure of association is affected. If there is no effect, then there is no confounding.

Because the topic of confounding can itself be confounding in the more common use of the term, it should help to provide an example before we go any further. Several studies have shown a positive association between ciga-

Is the exposure-outcome association confounded by an incidental factor?

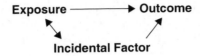

For confounding to occur:

1. The exposure and the incidental factor must be associated.
2. The incidental factor must be a risk factor for the outcome.
3. The incidental factor cannot be an intermediate step in the causal chain between the exposure and outcome.
4. The incidental factor must be present to a greater or lesser degree in the study group versus the comparison group.

If there is confounding, any association between the exposure and outcome will be partially or entirely explained by the confounding factor. Controlling for the confounding factor (incidental factor) will therefore eliminate the effect of confounding by that factor.

Figure 8–3 The presence of confounding

rette smoking and motor vehicle injuries.[12] A potential confounder of this association, however, is alcohol consumption. Cigarette smoking and alcohol consumption are associated with each other as any trip to a bar will substantiate (unless there is legislation prohibiting smoking), and alcohol consumption is a well-documented independent risk factor for motor vehicle injuries. Furthermore, it is unlikely that alcohol consumption is part of a causal chain between cigarette smoking and motor vehicle injuries based on current knowledge. Therefore, alcohol consumption is considered a *potential confounder*. Now, assume a case-control study finds a positive association between cigarette smoking and motor vehicle injuries. If the case group contains significantly more drinkers than the control group, we cannot be sure whether the association is really due to cigarette smoking. Part or all of the association between cigarette smoking and motor vehicle injuries could be due to alcohol consumption. Even if cigarette smoking is *not* associated with motor vehicle injuries, it could appear to be so because of its association with alcohol consumption. On the other hand, even if cigarette smoking is associated with motor vehicle injuries, the association could be overstated because of an excess number of drinkers among the case group. In fact, when alcohol consumption is controlled in studies of the association between cigarette smoking and motor vehicle injuries, the measure of association decreases but still remains significant.[12] Thus, alcohol appears to be a positive confounder (i.e., one that overstates the magnitude of the measure of association).

Another example concerns a study of coffee consumption and myocardial infarction in women.[13] In this case-control study, the investigators found an elevated risk of myocardial infarction in the heaviest coffee drinkers even after adjusting for cigarette smoking and other potential confounders. It seems likely though that women who drink large amounts of coffee on a daily basis probably have highly stressed lives that could increase their risk of myocardial infarction. Stress levels, however, were not evaluated as potential confounders, yet they could meet the criteria for confounding.

Controlling Confounding

To assure the validity of epidemiologic studies confounding needs to be controlled. Whereas selection bias occurs primarily in the design stage of a study and measurement bias in the data collection stage, confounding takes place mainly in the analysis phase.[3] Confounding can be controlled, however, in *either* the design or analysis stages of a study. In the design stage, *restriction*, *matching*, or *random allocation* may be used to reduce the potential for confounding. In the analysis stage, various statistical procedures can be applied to adjust or control for potential confounding after the fact, as mentioned previously. These methods include *stratification* and *multivariable analysis* and are discussed in subsequent chapters dealing with the specific epidemiologic study designs.

Restriction involves limiting the study subjects to those with certain characteristics. For example, if the sample is limited to women only, then differences in sex cannot confound an association. Similarly, if a study of the effect of cigarette smoking on motor vehicle injuries is limited to nondrinkers, then alcohol consumption cannot possibly confound an association between these variables. Other factors, such as risk taking, however, may still be confounders. Obviously, restriction as a method of controlling confounding has its limits. If many potential confounders exist, the study would have to be so restricted that it might be difficult to find a sufficient number of participants. Also, restriction can limit the external validity of a study. A study restricted to women, for example, may not be generalizable to populations including men.

Matching attempts to produce study and comparison groups that are similar with regard to potential confounders. **Pair matching**, for example, uses study and comparison subjects who have the same characteristics on selected variables. This is illustrated in a case-control study that pair matches for age, sex, and smoking status. For each case, a corresponding control is selected with the same characteristics. Thus, if the first case selected is between 20 and 24 years old, a male, and a nonsmoker, then a control is selected who is also between 20 and 24 years old, a male, and a nonsmoker, and so on. The individually matched cases and controls are treated as pairs in the analysis phase (see chapter 11).

Like restriction, matching has its limits. Matching on more than four or five characteristics can become very tedious because many potential subjects may have to be considered in finding ones who meet the criteria. It would be very difficult, for instance, to locate many 55–59-year-old males who have type AB negative blood and live at home taking care of triplets. Another disadvantage of matching is a loss of information. For example, if one subject in a matched pair does not respond to a study questionnaire, the other paired subject has to be excluded from the analysis. Also, the variables for which matching was performed cannot be examined for their relationship to the study outcome.[8] Thus, if one matches for age, its role cannot be examined in the study.

Another form of matching, known as **frequency matching**, relies on obtaining similar frequencies of the matched variables in the study and comparison groups. For example, if 25% of the subjects in the exposed group in a prospective cohort study are females, and if sex is considered a potential confounder, then the investigator seeks to obtain 25% females in the unexposed group. The goal of frequency matching is to assure that the study and comparison groups are similar with respect to the distribution of potential confounders. Frequency matching, however, does not assure as precise a comparison as pair matching, and some subgroups created during the analysis phase may differ substantially in the frequencies of potential confounders; therefore, it is still important to adjust for potential confounding in studies using frequency matching.

In randomized controlled trials, and some community trials, confounding is controlled in the design stage by *random allocation*. Random allocation refers to the assignment of study subjects to either experimental or control groups using random methods. This technique tends to eliminate confounding by increasing the probability that the groups being compared are similar with regard to the distribution of incidental factors that might confound an association. Random allocation is discussed further in chapter 13.

Precision

As was stated at the outset of this chapter, there are two major components of accuracy. One of these is validity, which is jeopardized by sources of bias and confounding. The other is precision, which is affected by sources of **random error** (see figure 8–1). As a matter of fact, *precision* can be defined as the degree to which random error is absent,[9] and random error can be thought of as variability due to chance.[5] Thus, a precise finding from an epidemiologic study will be one that is *unlikely* due to chance. Random errors can occur while obtaining and recording individual measurements (known as **random measurement error**) and from *sampling error*.

Random Measurement Error

With regard to measurements, we all tend to make some mistakes when obtaining or recording information, especially large quantities of data. For example, in recording the age and sex of 10,000 participants in a cross-sectional study, even a careful recorder of the data will invariably enter some incorrect values. As long as there is no *pattern* to the mistakes, the errors are considered random and tend to cancel each other out in the long run.

Random measurement errors can affect the precision of a measure of association, but because they are *just as likely* to increase or decrease a value, no bias is introduced. Remember, bias is one-sided, thus it always moves the measure of association in a specific direction depending on the direction of the bias. Using a relative risk as an example, assume we derive a RR = 1.5 from an analytic study. It would be impossible to know whether this estimate over- or understates the correct value due to random measurement error unless we can identify all the specific measurement errors made, which is highly improbable. With selection and measurement bias, however, if we can identify the likely source of the bias, we may be able to determine the probable effect on the measure of association. For example, if we can identify a negative bias, we can assume the RR has been understated. Random measurement errors can be minimized by making multiple measurements on the same subjects and then by computing averages, cross-checking data with others, and designing instruments and data-entry programs that only allow certain values or types of information to be collected or entered.

Sampling Error

Sampling error is the random variation that can result when using sample statistics to estimate population parameters (chapter 6). This is another type of random error that can compromise precision, and hence the accuracy of epidemiologic studies. This type of error arises from the fact that a sample will never be a perfect representation of the target population. Therefore, there is always the probability that findings based on a sample will not match those in the target population. Sampling error is represented by types: *type I error and type II error*.

Type I error is the probability of finding an association in a sample when none exists in the target population. It is measured by the p-value. If the p-value is high, it suggests that an observed association is *likely* due to sampling error. A p-value of 0.85, for example, says that the probability of a type I error is 85%. In other words, 85 times out of 100 one would expect the observed association to be due to sampling error. The lower the p-value, the less likely that sampling error accounts for an observed association. A p-value of 0.001 says that only 1 out of 1,000 times would a given association be expected to be due to sampling error. By convention, p-values less than or equal to 0.05 are considered **statistically significant** (unlikely due to sampling error), and p-values greater than 0.05 are considered **not statistically significant** (likely due to sampling error). The choice of the cutoff, known as the **alpha level** (α), is arbitrary, however, and some may choose to use a lower value (e.g., 0.01) to judge statistical significance.

P-values are affected by sample size and the magnitude of the association. Since larger samples tend to be more like the target population, increasing sample size can reduce sampling error. Thus, increasing sample size has the effect of decreasing the p-value, thereby increasing the precision of the measurement. Another factor that affects the p-value is the magnitude of the association. When the magnitude of an association is very large, the association is likely to be real (i.e., unlikely to be due to sampling error). It is important to realize that p-values tell us nothing about the strength of the association, just whether an observed association is likely or unlikely to be due to sampling error. The strength of an association is determined by the measure of association (e.g., RR or OR).

Type II error is the probability of *not* finding an association in a sample when one exists in the target population. It is measured by the **beta level** (β). The smaller the beta level, the less chance of a type II error and greater the **power** of the study, that is, the probability of detecting an association *if* one really exists.[5] Power $= 1 - \beta$, or, expressed as a percentage, $(1 - \beta) \times 100$. Thus, beta and power are inversely associated. Because power is largely affected by sample size, studies with inadequate sample size have insufficient power to detect real associations (i.e., they are more subject to type II error). Therefore, if *no* association is found in a study *with small sample size*, it is possible that the result is due solely to a lack of power. This type of result is often regarded as *inconclusive*. In other words, if no statistical association is found *and* the sample size is small, one should consider the finding inconclusive due to insufficient power. To minimize the chance of type II error, it is recommended that a study have at least 80% power, or a corresponding beta level of no more than 0.20. Although most epidemiologists are more concerned about making a type I error (finding an association when none exists) than a type II error (not finding an association when one exists), both types of errors are important and need to be minimized if the study results are to be precise.

Confidence Intervals

The effect of sampling error on the precision of a measure of association can be evaluated by a confidence interval. If the confidence interval is relatively narrow, it suggests the measure of association is relatively precise. Conversely, if the interval is relatively wide, it intimates a relatively imprecise measure of association. For example, if RR $= 2.5$ and the 95% CI $= 2.1 - 2.9$, we would be very confident that we have a fairly precise estimate of the association, barring major measurement errors. On the other hand, if the RR $= 2.5$ and the 95% CI $= 0.6 - 19.5$, we would say that the measure of association appears very imprecise. It is important to realize, however, that the confidence interval tells us nothing about whether or not the measure of association is valid. If the effects of bias and confounding can be considered minimal in a particular study, and the 95% confidence interval for the measure of association is relatively narrow, then we can be reasonably sure that we probably have an accurate measure of association. This also assumes random measurement errors are minimal or cancel each other out.

Partly because significance testing is based on an arbitrary cutoff point, many epidemiologists favor the use of confidence intervals. A confidence interval for a risk, rate, or odds ratio containing a value of one represents a nonsignificant finding, while a confidence interval not containing a value of one represents a significant finding. Thus, confidence intervals can be used to test statistical significance, but this is not their appeal since many who favor confidence intervals do not care to do significance testing anyway. The usefulness of the confidence interval lies in the fact that it contains information not available from significance testing. For one thing, the confidence interval gives us a range of possible values for the measure of association. A RR = 3.4 (95% CI = 0.7 – 15.1) tells us that while the point estimate of the population RR is 3.4, we are 95% confident that the true population RR ranges from 0.7 to 15.1. Furthermore, as stated earlier, we can see from this broad range that the point estimate is relatively imprecise, and, therefore, we would not want to stake too much on the population RR being 3.4. A RR = 2.6 (95% CI = 2.1 – 3.0), on the other hand, suggests a relatively precise point estimate, and we would be relatively confident using 2.6 as our population estimate of the RR knowing that we probably have not under- or overestimated it by too much. Of course, there is still a 5% chance that the true value is really outside this range (i.e., we are, after all, using a 95% confidence interval). Oh, the verities of probability! Certainty is just not part of the game plan when samples are used to estimate population measures. A decision-making outline based on the results of significance testing is shown in exhibit 8–2. Figure 8–1 also lists the major components of accuracy that need to be addressed in assessing a statistical association.

Exhibit 8–2 A Framework for Evaluating the Effect of Sampling Error on an Association

Is p ≤ 0.05?	Is p > 0.05?
1. If YES, the association is *statistically significant*. The probability of a type I error is equal to or less than 5%, which is the traditional cutoff point.	1. If YES, the association is *not statistically significant*. The probability of a type I error is more than 5%, which is the traditional cutoff point.
2. Sampling error is an *unlikely* explanation for the observed level of association.	2. Sampling error is a *reasonable* explanation for the observed level of association.
3. The *smaller* the p-value, the *less* likely sampling error explains the association.	3. The *larger* the p-value, the *more* likely sampling error explains the association.
4. *If* the sample size is *very large*, most associations will be significant, so the association should be judged for its *practical significance*.	4. *If* the sample size is *small*, the association should be considered *inconclusive* due to low study power. Confidence intervals can provide clues to a probable association.
• Practical significance is a subjective determination that depends on the clinical importance of the association.	• A relatively *narrow* confidence interval implies a *precise* finding, and thus there probably is no missed association.
• In determining practical significance one should consider the incidence of the outcome and the prevalence of the exposure. If either or both are rare, and the measure of association is weak, there may be no practical significance.	• A relatively *wide* confidence interval implies an *imprecise* finding, and thus an association may have been missed due to low power.

Summary

- The accuracy of a study depends on having valid and precise findings. Validity can be internal or external. Internal validity is the degree to which study results are true for the target population, that is, free from bias or confounding. External validity, also known as generalizability, is the degree to which study results are relevant for populations other than the target population. Of the two forms of validity, internal validity is more important since it does not make sense to generalize findings that are not internally valid.

- There are two major categories of bias—selection bias and measurement bias. Selection bias can result when the characteristics of the subjects selected for a study differ systematically from those in the target population or when the study and comparison groups are selected from different populations. Examples of selection bias include Berkson's bias, prevalence-incidence bias, the healthy worker effect, volunteer bias, and loss to follow-up bias. Measurement bias can result from systematic (nonrandom) misclassification of subjects on exposure or outcome status. Major types of measurement bias include recall bias, interviewer bias, diagnostic suspicion bias, and exposure suspicion bias.

- Confounding is systematic error that results from a mixing of effects between an exposure and an incidental factor. The incidental factor must be associated with the exposure, a risk factor for the outcome, not a part of the causal chain between the exposure and outcome, and unequally distributed between the study and comparison groups.

- Precision is the degree to which random error is absent. Major sources of random error include random measurement error and sampling error. Careful planning can minimize random measurement errors. Sampling error can result in type I and type II errors, which can be minimized by increasing sample size. The precision of a specific measure of association can be judged by viewing its confidence interval. Narrow intervals imply greater precision.

New Terms

accuracy
alpha level (α)
Berkson's bias
beta level (β)
confounder
confounding factor
convenience sample
diagnostic suspicion bias
differential
   misclassification

exposure suspicion
   bias
external validity
frequency matching
generalizability
healthy worker effect
information bias
internal validity
interviewer bias
loss to follow-up bias

matching
measurement bias
membership bias
negative bias
negative confounder
nondifferential
   misclassification
not statistically
   significant
null value

observation bias	prevalence-incidence	restriction
pair matching	bias	selection bias
positive bias	probability sample	statistically significant
positive confounder	random error	systematic error
potential confounder	random measurement	type I error
power	error	type II error
precision	recall bias	validity
	response bias	volunteer bias

Study Questions and Exercises

Each of the following problems contains a potential error that could affect the accuracy of the results. Using the key below, indicate the most likely source of error in each problem based solely on the information provided. Also, give a detailed rationale for your answers, including the specific type of selection or measurement bias, confounding, or sampling error where possible.

A. Selection bias   C. Confounding

B. Measurement bias   D. Sampling error

____ 1. The authors of a cross-sectional study hypothesized that lack of regular exercise is associated with obesity in children. Their study of 12 children in Michigan, however, failed to show a significant association between exercise habits and obesity (p = 0.11).

____ 2. In a case-control study of the relationship between intravenous drug use and HIV infection, the investigators discovered after the study that the case group had tended to underreport their drug use due to fears arising from previous convictions for drug-related violations. Underreporting was not a problem in the control group, however, which was not under medical supervision at the time.

____ 3. A prospective cohort study followed 8,542 women for 10 years to determine if alcohol consumption increased the risk of breast cancer. No significant association was found. Twelve thousand women had been enrolled in the study at its initiation, but 3,458 had withdrawn during the 10-year period. A follow-up of spouses, friends, and relatives of the women who withdrew revealed that more than 60% of them had developed breast cancer and that nearly 84% were regular drinkers.

____ 4. A case-control study was designed to test whether persons exposed to certain types of pesticides during early childhood were more likely to develop neurological problems in later adulthood. The results were statistically significant. The cases consisted of those with severe but treatable neurological disorders, and the controls consisted of those without any diagnosed neurological disorders. Both the cases and controls were asked detailed questions about their pesticide exposures during early childhood.

___ 5. A large epidemiologic study found that elderly adults with dementia were more likely to develop liver cancer than those without dementia. The investigators, however, could offer no plausible biological mechanism for the association between dementia and liver cancer.

___ 6. An epidemiologist reported the following conclusion from a large randomized controlled trial during a national meeting: "Daily use of 500 milligrams of vitamin C for a period of one year was associated with a reduced frequency of upper respiratory infections in children under 10 years of age (RR = 0.9, 95% CI = 0.6 - 1.7)."

___ 7. In a large hospital-based case-control study of smoking and lung cancer, controls consisted of patients with noncancerous chronic pulmonary diseases, such as chronic bronchitis and emphysema. The investigators were surprised to find that the association between smoking and lung cancer was relatively weak (RR = 1.4, p < 0.05).

___ 8. Three hundred cases and 600 controls were selected among mothers for a case-control study to see if maternal coffee consumption was related to low birth weight in the mothers' babies. Data were collected on past coffee consumption patterns for the mothers and on cigarette smoking, a known risk factor for low birth weight. The overall association between maternal coffee consumption and low birth weight was reported to be strong (OR = 3.4). When the data were later reanalyzed and adjusted for cigarette smoking, however, the association was found to be nonexistent (OR = 1.0).

___ 9. The investigators of a prospective cohort study collected blood samples from the participants at the beginning of the study and froze them for later analysis. A subsequent nested case-control study was conducted to determine if blood levels of certain hormones were associated with Alzheimer's disease. The previously stored blood samples were analyzed for the cases and controls. It was later determined that the samples had degenerated during the storage period because of a failure to maintain consistent temperatures.

___10. An epidemiologist examines the association between the use of diet pills and migraine headaches using a case-control study design. His subjects are outpatients at a large community hospital. He finds that those using diet pills are more likely to complain of migraines, but he also discovers that those who have migraine headaches and use diet pills are more likely to be referred to the community hospital for outpatient diagnostic testing than those who have migraines but are not using diet pills.

References

1. The Scandinavian Simvastatin Survival Study Group (1994). Randomised Trial of Cholesterol Lowering in 4444 Patients with Coronary Heart Disease: The Scandinavian Simvastatin Survival Study (4S). *The Lancet* 344(8934): 1383–1389.
2. Hennekens, C. H., and Buring, J. E. (1987). *Epidemiology in Medicine*. Boston: Little, Brown and Company.

3. Choi, B. C. K., and Noseworthy, A. L. (1992). Classification, Direction, and Prevention of Bias in Epidemiologic Research. *Journal of Occupational Medicine* 34(3): 265–271.
4. Vogt, W. P. (1993). *Dictionary of Statistics and Methodology.* Newbury Park, CA: Sage.
5. Last, J. M., ed. (1995). *A Dictionary of Epidemiology.* New York: Oxford University Press.
6. Sackett, D. L. (1979). Bias in Analytic Research. *Journal of Chronic Diseases* 32: 51–63.
7. Streiner, D. L., Norman, G. R., and Blum, H. M. (1989). *PDQ Epidemiology.* Toronto: B. C. Decker.
8. Elwood, J. M. (1988). *Causal Relationships in Medicine: A Practical System for Critical Appraisal.* New York: Oxford University Press.
9. Norell, S. E. (1995). *Workbook of Epidemiology.* New York: Oxford University Press.
10. Szklo, M., and Nieto, F. J. (2000). *Epidemiology: Beyond the Basics.* Gaithersburg, MD: Aspen.
11. Rothman, K. J. (1986). *Modern Epidemiology.* Boston: Little, Brown and Company.
12. Oleckno, W. A. (1988). Is Smoking a Risk Factor for Accidental Injuries? *Health and Hygiene* 9: 56–60.
13. La Vecchia, C., Gentile, A., Negri, E., Parazzini, F., and Franceschi, S. (1989). Coffee Consumption and Myocardial Infarction in Women. *American Journal of Epidemiology* 130(3): 481–485.

CHAPTER NINE

Screening for Disease Detection

Learning Objectives

▸ Explain the purpose, value, and common types of screening.

▸ Calculate, compare, and interpret sensitivity, specificity, positive and negative predictive values, accuracy of the screening test, false positive and false negative rates, and Cohen's kappa.

▸ Compare and contrast the consequences of false positive and false negative results.

▸ Distinguish among method variability, subject variability, and observer variability.

▸ Describe the benefits and risks of screening programs.

▸ Discuss the potential sources of bias in evaluating the efficacy of screening.

▸ Define validity and precision of a screening test, true positives and negatives, gold standard, reliability, screening level, and yield.

Overview

The purpose of screening is to detect disease before it becomes manifest so that it can be treated early leading to a better prognosis. Types of screening include mass screening, selective screening, multiphasic screening, and case finding. The validity of screening tests is measured by their sensitivity and specificity, which represent their ability to classify correctly the presence or absence of disease. Other useful measures are positive and negative predictive value, which are affected by sensitivity and specificity and the prevalence of the disease. The precision of a screening test is compromised by method, subject, and observer variability. Since screening programs have benefits and risks, many factors should be considered before they are undertaken. Some of these factors include the importance of the problem, the accuracy and practicality of the test, and the accessibility, acceptability, and effectiveness of follow-up tests and treatment. Screening programs should be rigorously evaluated to avoid lead time bias, length bias, and volunteer bias.

Introduction

Screening for disease detection has become very common in our culture. Infants are routinely screened for phenylketonuria (PKU), a congenital, hereditary disorder in amino acid metabolism that can lead to mental retardation. School children are typically screened for diminished visual acuity, and free blood pressure screening is available at many pharmacies and public health departments. In addition, health fairs usually offer a variety of free or low-cost screening tests for health and disease, and some large corporations and public organizations offer their employees periodic screening for various diseases. Physicians and other health care providers also perform a number of routine screening tests and usually recommend additional tests at various life stages or for certain high-risk groups.

Screening for disease detection can be defined as a relatively quick means of detecting *potential* disease before it has become manifest. Screening does *not* establish a diagnosis but helps to identify individuals who appear to have a given disease and who should, therefore, undergo further testing to determine if the disease is actually present. A positive urine test for diabetes, for example, does not necessarily mean someone has diabetes. Further testing would be required to establish a diagnosis. Screening for disease detection is valuable where early identification of a disease leads to more effective treatment and a better prognosis for the individual. Examples include screening for breast, colorectal, and cervical cancer and screening for hypertension, diabetes, and rubella.

Depending on its intent, screening can take place at different stages in the natural history of disease and can represent different levels of prevention (chapter 3). Screening for disease detection seeks to identify individuals in the *stage of presymptomatic disease*. Thus, it can be considered a mode of *secondary prevention* (see figure 3–4). Screening can also be used to identify risk factors for disease. In a technical sense, this type of screening usually is aimed at those in the *stage of susceptibility*. Hence, it represents a method of *primary prevention*. Cholesterol screening, for example, is used routinely to identify individuals at increased risk of heart disease. While the focus of this chapter is on *screening for disease detection*, many of the same principles also apply to screening for risk factors. The major difference is one of intent, and in fact, few authors make a distinction between the two.

Types of Screening

Screening for disease detection is often categorized into one of the following four types:

- **Mass screening.** This form of screening is aimed at large population groups that vary widely in their risk of the disease.[1] Screening for PKU is an example of mass screening directed at newborns. Screening for visual impairment in elementary schools is another example of mass screening. In both cases everyone in the group is screened regardless of the probability of having the disease or condition.

- **Selective screening.** This form of screening is applied only to groups at *high risk* for the disease. Screening for elevated blood lead levels among inner-city children is an example of selective screening. So is screening for tuberculosis among prison inmates. Selective screening would be expected to detect more potential cases of a given disease than mass screening because of the difference in risk profiles between the populations being screened. Selective screening is sometimes referred to as **targeted screening.**[2]

- **Multiphasic screening.** This type of screening employs multiple screening tests at the same time. Thus, it may be used to detect the possibility of more than one disease or condition.[3] Premilitary exams, for example, may use multiphasic screening to test for possible diabetes, hypertension, and hearing impairment.

- **Case finding.** This type of screening occurs in a clinical setting when patients visit their physician (or other health care provider) for general consultation or unrelated problems, and the physician *takes the opportunity* to request one or more routine screening tests. Unlike mass or selective screening where individuals with abnormal test results are generally referred for follow-up, case finding places the responsibility for follow-up on the physician performing or supervising the screening tests. Therefore, case finding is more likely to result in follow-up than other types of screening.[1] Many individuals identified as having elevated blood pressure during a mass screening, for example, may not seek the recommended follow-up, but a physician finding elevated blood pressure during a routine examination will ordinarily schedule additional tests. Examples of case finding include screening for cervical cancer using Pap tests, heart abnormalities using an electrocardiogram, weight changes using a calibrated scale, and diabetes using blood tests or urine samples. In addition, optometrists and ophthalmologists routinely screen patients for glaucoma. Case finding has also been referred to as **opportunistic screening.**[4]

Accuracy of Screening Tests

As discussed in chapter 8, accuracy has two major components—validity and precision. Thus, screening tests are *accurate* to the extent that they are *both* valid and precise. In this context, the **validity of a screening test** refers to the degree to which the screening test does what it is designed to do (i.e., detect those who have the disease and those who do not). The **precision of a screening test** refers to its reliability, that is, its consistency from one application to the next. Because of the importance of these concepts, the *validity* and *precision* of screening tests are discussed separately in the following two sections.

Validity of Screening Tests

Many screening tests are designed to produce positive or negative results. A positive test implies that the disease *is likely* to be present, and follow-up diagnostic tests are therefore advisable. A negative test implies that the disease is *unlikely* to be present, and follow-up diagnostic tests are therefore not indicated. Unfortunately, screening tests vary in how well they detect the presence or absence of disease. To measure the validity of a screening test, a pre-selected group is normally tested with a **gold standard**, that is, a definitive diagnostic test, to determine who has and does not have the disease. The screening test is also administered, and the results are compared for congruence. This can lead to four possible outcomes—*true positives, false positives, true negatives,* and *false negatives*. **True positives** are individuals in the group who test positive on the screening test and who have the disease. **False positives** are individuals in the group who test positive on the screening test but do not have the disease. Correspondingly, **true negatives** are those who test negative on the screening test and who do not have the disease, and **false negatives** are those who test negative on the screening test but have the disease. For simplicity, a 2 × 2 contingency table can be used to summarize the four possible outcomes of a screening test based on the results of the gold standard.

True Disease Status

Screening Test	Positive	Negative	Total
Positive	True Positives (TP)	False Positives (FP)	TP + FP
Negative	False Negatives (FN)	True Negatives (TN)	FN + TN
Total	TP + FN	FP + TN	TP + FP + FN + TN

Although all four possible outcomes (TP, FP, FN, and TN) are used to measure the validity of a screening test, two of these outcomes (i.e., FP and FN) are the keys to validity. If there were no false positives or false negatives, the screening test would have 100% validity. Therefore, increasing the validity of screening tests has to do with minimizing the number of false positives and false negatives. There are several approaches to determine the validity of screening tests. These are discussed below.

Sensitivity and Specificity. The validity of a screening test is usually measured in terms of *sensitivity* and *specificity*. **Sensitivity** is a measure of the ability of a screening test to identify correctly those *with* the disease, while **specificity** is a measure of the ability of a screening test to identify correctly those *without* the disease.[5] Sensitivity and specificity usually are calculated in percents and are determined by comparing the screening results with those of a definitive diagnostic test or *gold standard*. For example, the sensitivity and specificity of a new screening test for coronary heart disease could be measured by comparing the screening results on a sample of volunteers to the results obtained by angiograms, which represent the gold standard for the diagnosis of coronary heart disease. Drawing on the above contingency table, these measures are calculated as follows:

(9.1)

$$Sensitivity\ (\%) = [TP\ /\ (TP + FN)] \times 100$$

(9.2)

$$Specificity\ (\%) = [TN\ /\ (FP + TN)] \times 100$$

Ideally, we would like to have screening tests with 100% sensitivity and specificity.[5] This way, the screening test would be able to identify correctly all those with the disease and all those without the disease. Unfortunately, this usually is not possible because most screening tests are based on continuous measures that rely on relatively arbitrary cutoff points, known as **screening levels**, for classifying participants as positive or negative.[6] Screening questionnaires designed to detect clinical depression, for example, often depend on an overall score to indicate the likelihood of depression. The score used as the cutoff can affect the sensitivity and specificity of the test. If a relatively *low* score is used to classify someone as clinically depressed, then the test will have high sensitivity but only by sacrificing specificity. In other words, most clinically depressed individuals will be classified correctly because of the low standard, but many who are not clinically depressed will be misclassified as depressed (i.e., will be false positives). Similarly, if the screening level is set too *high*, the test will have low sensitivity because many clinically depressed individuals will be missed (i.e., will be false negatives). The specificity, however, will be high because most people without clinical depression will be classified correctly. This concept is illustrated in figure 9–1. Screening level C in the diagram represents a compromise that minimizes losses in sensitivity and specificity. If sensitivity were considered more important than specificity in a particular application, then screening level A would be a better choice. If, on the other hand, specificity were considered more important than sensitivity, screening level B would be the best choice. In general, increasing the sensitivity of a screening test tends to decrease its specificity and vice versa.

As should be clear from the preceding discussion and formulas 9.1 and 9.2, the number of *false negatives* affects the *sensitivity* of a screening test, and the number of *false positives* affects the *specificity*. Sensitivity would be 100% if there were no false negatives, and specificity would be 100% if there were no false positives. Therefore, in deciding whether sensitivity may be more or less important than specificity in a particular screening application, one should weigh the potential consequences of identifying more false negatives than false positives and vice versa. Table 9–1 lists some of these potential consequences.

Misclassification on screening tests can also occur for reasons other than where the screening level is set. Notable examples are the presence of other health conditions or use of medications that interfere with the test and individual characteristics that tend to vary from one measurement to the next (e.g., blood pressure). With regard to individual characteristics, a screening test for blood pressure could result in classifying a normotensive individual as hypertensive if there was a transitory increase in blood pressure at the time of the test.

As indicated earlier, determining actual disease status requires a *definitive* diagnosis. Screening tests are *presumptive* only; they are not definitive. Nevertheless, screening can result in early detection of disease, which often results in more effective treatment and better prognosis, and, therefore, it is a valuable public health tool.

Positive and Negative Predictive Value.   Two other measures related to the validity of a screening test are the predictive values of positive and negative tests. **Positive predictive value** is the percent of those who test posi-

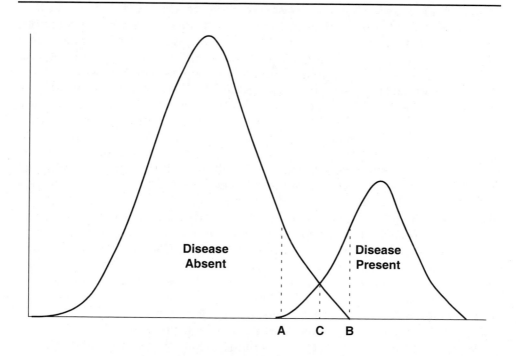

Which screening level is best?

A: Maximizes sensitivity but reduces specificity

B: Maximizes specificity but reduces sensitivity

C: Minimizes losses in both sensitivity and specificity

Figure 9–1 Selecting the screening level for a screening test

---

Table 9–1 Potential Consequences of False Positive and False Negative Test Results in a Screening Program

Screening Results	Potential Consequences
False Positives	• Overuse of health care resources due to increased referrals • Anxiety associated with the fear of having a serious disease (e.g., cervical cancer) • Inconvenience due to the additional time and expense for follow-up diagnostic tests (e.g., breast cancer) • Increased health risks from some diagnostic tests (e.g., angiograms for coronary heart disease)
False Negatives	• Delayed medical attention that for some diseases could result in permanent disability or death (e.g., PKU, breast cancer) • Increased disease transmission when the disease is communicable (e.g., tuberculosis)

---

tive for the disease on a screening test and who actually have the disease. **Negative predictive value** is the percent of those who test negative on a screening test and who actually do *not* have the disease. Unlike sensitivity and specificity, positive and negative predictive values are dependent on the *prevalence* (chapter 5) of the disease in the population being screened. For fixed levels of sensitivity and specificity, the higher the prevalence of the disease, the greater the positive predictive value and the lower the negative predictive value. Based on the four possible screening outcomes (see contingency table on page 162), these measures are calculated as follows:

(9.3)

$$\text{Positive Predictive Value (PPV; \%)} = [\text{TP} / (\text{TP} + \text{FP})] \times 100$$

(9.4)

$$\text{Negative Predictive Value (NPV; \%)} = [\text{TN} / (\text{FN} + \text{TN})] \times 100$$

(9.5)

$$\text{Prevalence Rate (\%)} = [(\text{TP} + \text{FN}) / (\text{TP} + \text{FP} + \text{FN} + \text{TN})] \times 100$$

Because of their relationship to prevalence, the predictive values of a screening test can be useful in deciding whether or not to use a particular screening test in a specific population.[7] Even a test with relatively high sensitivity and specificity may have poor positive predictive value if the prevalence of the disease is low. Thus, the same screening test is more likely to have a higher positive predictive value in applications involving *selective screening* compared to those involving *mass screening*, simply because populations at higher risk are more likely to have a higher prevalence of the disease. Negative predictive value, on the other hand, will tend to be higher in applications involving mass versus selective screening due to an expected lower prevalence of the disease in general populations.

Positive and negative predictive values are important characteristics of a screening test, especially positive predictive value. Sometimes new screening tests with high levels of sensitivity and specificity show good positive predictive value in clinical settings but then very poor positive predictive value when they are used in general populations. This is due to the difference in the disease prevalence rates between the two populations. Unless a screening test has a relatively high positive predictive value, it may be questionable for a physician to order potentially risky and expensive follow-up tests based on a positive screening result. This is because many of those testing positive will turn out not to have the disease (i.e., will be false positives). Some of the relationships among sensitivity, specificity, and predictive value are illustrated in table 9–2 and in examples that appear later in this chapter. As revealed by the formulas for positive and negative predictive value (formulas 9.3 and 9.4), when the number of false positives is high, the positive predictive value will be low, and when the number of false negatives is high, the negative predictive value will be low. Some of the potential consequences of false positives and negatives are shown in table 9–1.

Other Related Measures. The **accuracy of the screening test** is a measure of the validity of a screening test that indicates the percent agreement between the screening test and a corresponding definitive diagnostic test or gold standard.[2] Although this measure is named *accuracy of the screening test*, it only measures validity. Thus, it should not be confused with the more general terminology, accuracy of a screening test, which is comprised of both validity and precision. The accuracy of the screening test represents a *weighted average* of the sensitivity and specificity. Thus, mathematically, the accuracy of the screening test is: (sensitivity × proportion with the disease) + (specificity × proportion without the disease). The accuracy of the screening test thus summarizes the overall validity of the screening test in one value. It does not, however, provide as much detail as separate calculations of sensitivity and specificity and, therefore, is reported less frequently. Like the other validity measures, the *accuracy of the screening test* can be derived from a combination of the four possible screening outcomes referred to earlier:

(9.6)

$$\text{Accuracy of the Screening Test (\%)} = [(TP + TN) / (TP + FP + FN + TN)] \times 100$$

Other less used measures related to validity are the **false negative rate** and the **false positive rate**, which are described in table 9–2. These are the counterparts of sensitivity and specificity, respectively. In fact, sensitivity is also known as the **true positive rate**, while specificity is also known as the **true negative rate**.[6] The sum of sensitivity (i.e., the true positive rate) and the false negative rate is 100%. The same is true for specificity (i.e., the true negative rate) and the false positive rate.[8] Table 9–2 also summarizes some of the effects of increasing sensitivity and specificity on the false negative and false positive rates.

Table 9–2 Effects of Changes in Sensitivity, Specificity, and Prevalence on Predictive Value and Other Measures

Increasing . . .	Effect
Sensitivity	• Increases the negative predictive value • Decreases the false negative rate*
Specificity	• Increases the positive predictive value • Decreases the false positive rate**
Prevalence	• Increases positive predictive value • Decreases negative predictive value

*The *false negative rate* (FNR) is the percent of those with the disease that are false negatives (i.e., those who test negative but have the disease). This is calculated as follows:

$$\text{FNR (\%)} = \frac{\text{Number of false negatives}}{\text{Number of true positives} + \text{Number of false negatives}} \times 100$$

**The *false positive rate* (FPR) is the percent of those without the disease that are false positives (i.e., those who test positive but do not have the disease). This is calculated as follows:

$$\text{FPR (\%)} = \frac{\text{Number of false positives}}{\text{Number of false positives} + \text{Number of true negatives}} \times 100$$

Example 9–1: Validity of Screening Tests

A new screening test for thyroid cancer was administered to 1,000 adult volunteers at a large medical center complex in Europe. The results showed that 152 out of 160 diagnosed cases of thyroid cancer were correctly identified by the screening test. Also, of the 840 individuals without thyroid cancer, the screening test correctly identified 714. Based on this information, calculate the test's sensitivity, specificity, and positive and negative predictive values. Also, calculate the prevalence rate of thyroid cancer in this population and the accuracy of the screening test.

Solution:

Step 1: To assist in calculating the requested measures, it is helpful first to put the data in the form of a 2 × 2 contingency table as follows:

True Disease Status

Screening Test	Positive	Negative	Total
Positive	152 (TP)	126 (FP)	278
Negative	8 (FN)	714 (TN)	722
Total	160	840	1,000

Note that the data provided in the problem are sufficient to complete the above contingency table. Since 152 of the *diagnosed cases* of thyroid cancer were correctly identified by the screening test, they represent the true positives. True positives are those who test positive and have the disease. This group is depicted in the upper left portion of the contingency table. The number of false negatives (those who test negative but have the disease) is not given in the problem but can be determined by subtracting the number of true positives from the total number with the disease, which is provided in the problem (i.e., $160 - 152 = 8$). This group appears in the lower left portion of the table. There were 714 people who were correctly identified as not having the disease. These represent the true negatives, which are those who test negative and do not have the disease. They are found in the lower right portion of the contingency table. The number of false positives, those who test positive but do not have the disease, is not given in the problem but can be calculated by subtracting the number of true negatives from all those without the disease (i.e., $840 - 714 = 126$). This group can be found in the upper right portion of the table. The remaining marginal totals and the grand total can be calculated once the boxes of the contingency table have been completed. The column totals and the row totals should both equal the total number of persons screened (the grand total), which in this case is 1,000 (i.e., $160 + 840 = 1,000$ and $278 + 722 = 1,000$).

Step 2: Based on the applicable formulas and the data in the above contingency table calculate the requested measures.

Sensitivity $= [TP / (TP + FN)] \times 100 = [152 / (152 + 8)] \times 100 = (152 / 160) \times 100 = 95.0\%$

Specificity $= [TN / (FP + TN)] \times 100 = [714 / (126 + 714)] \times 100 = (714 / 840) \times 100 = 85.0\%$

Positive Predictive Value $= [TP / (TP + FP)] \times 100 = [152 / (152 + 126)] \times 100 = (152 / 278) \times 100 = 54.7\%$

Negative Predictive Value $= [TN / (FN + TN)] \times 100 = [714 / (8 + 714)] \times 100 = (714 / 722) \times 100 = 98.9\%$

Prevalence Rate $= [(TP + FN) / (TP + FP + FN + TN)] \times 100 = [(152 + 8) / (152 + 126 + 8 + 714)] \times 100 = (160 / 1,000) \times 100 = 16.0\%$

Accuracy of the Screening Test $= [(TP + TN) / (TP + FP + FN + TN)] \times 100 = [(152 + 714) / (152 + 126 + 8 + 714)] \times 100 = (866 / 1,000) \times 100 = 86.6\%$

Answer: The sensitivity of the screening test is 95.0%, and its specificity is 85.0%. Its positive predictive value is 54.7%, and its negative predictive value is 98.9%. The prevalence of thyroid cancer in the screened population is 16.0% (16.0 cases per 100 people), and the accuracy of the screening test in this population is 86.6%.

Comments:

1. Based on the screening test results, this is a very sensitive test. It is able to identify correctly 95% of those with the disease. The specificity of the test is not quite as good, however, since the test is only able to identify correctly 85% of those without the disease. The ideal sensitivity and specificity are each 100%. The overall validity of the screening test, as measured by the accuracy of the screening test, is 86.6%. This is a weighted average of the sensitivity and specificity.

2. The positive predictive value of this screening test is low. Of those who test positive for the disease, only 54.7% actually have the disease. This means that many false positives are identified. The reason is the relatively low prevalence of the disease. The negative predictive value, however, is very high. Of those who test negative for the disease, 98.9% actually do not have the disease. Thus, less than 2% of those who test negative for the disease are false negatives.

3. Sensitivity can be thought of as the *true positive rate*.[6] As mentioned above, it is the counterpart of the *false negative rate*, and together they equal 100%. Therefore, since the sensitivity is 95.0% in this problem, the false negative rate is 100% − 95.0% = 5.0%.

4. The specificity can be thought of as the *true negative rate*.[6] Its counterpart, the *false positive rate*, can be calculated as follows: 100% − 85.0% = 15.0%, since the specificity is 85.0%.

Example 9–2: Validity of Screening Tests

The same screening test for thyroid cancer described in example 9–1 was repeated in another population of 1,000 adult volunteers. This time, of 40 diagnosed cases, 38 were detected by the screening test. Of 960 persons without the disease, the screening test correctly identified 816. Based on these data, calculate the sensitivity, specificity, and positive and negative predictive values of the test. Also calculate the prevalence of thyroid cancer and accuracy of the screening test. Compare the results to those in example 9–1 and explain any differences.

Solution:

Step 1: As in example 9–1, a 2 × 2 contingency table showing the frequency of each of the four possible outcomes of a screening test can be developed from the data provided in the problem. Some minor calculations must be performed to fill in missing data.

True Disease Status

Screening Test	Positive	Negative	Total
Positive	38 (TP)	144 (FP)	182
Negative	2 (FN)	816 (TN)	818
Total	40	960	1,000

Step 2: Based on the applicable formulas and the data in the contingency table calculate the requested measures.

$$\text{Sensitivity} = [TP / (TP + FN)] \times 100 = [38 / (38 + 2)] \times 100 = (38 / 40) \times 100 = 95.0\%$$
$$\text{Specificity} = [TN / (FP + TN)] \times 100 = [816 / (144 + 816)] \times 100 = (816 / 960) \times 100 = 85.0\%$$
$$\text{Positive Predictive Value} = [TP / (TP + FP)] \times 100 = [38 / (38 + 144)] \times 100 =$$
$$(38 / 182) \times 100 = 20.9\%$$
$$\text{Negative Predictive Value} = [TN / (FN + TN)] \times 100 = [816 / (2 + 816)] \times 100 =$$
$$(816 / 818) \times 100 = 99.8\%$$
$$\text{Prevalence Rate} = [(TP + FN) / (TP + FP + FN + TN)] \times 100 =$$
$$[(38 + 2) / (38 + 144 + 2 + 816)] \times 100 = (40 / 1,000) \times 100 = 4.0\%$$
$$\text{Accuracy of the Screening Test (\%)} = [(TP + TN) / (TP + FP + FN + TN)] \times 100 =$$
$$[(38 + 816) / (38 + 144 + 2 + 816)] \times 100 = (854 / 1,000) \times 100 = 85.4\%$$

Answer: The sensitivity of the screening test is 95.0%, and its specificity is 85.0%. Its positive predictive value is 20.9%, and its negative predictive value is 99.8%. The prevalence of thyroid cancer in the screened population is 4.0% (4.0 cases per 100 people), and the accuracy of the screening test in this population is 85.4%. Comparing this problem to that in example 9–1, the sensitivity and specificity are identical; however, there are differences for the positive predictive value, negative predictive value, prevalence rate, and the accuracy of the screening test. The explanation for these differences is as follows:

1. As mentioned previously in this chapter, the predictive value of a screening test is affected by the prevalence of the disease for which screening is undertaken. In this example, the prevalence rate of thyroid cancer is only one-fourth of that in example 9–1 (4.0% vs.16.0%). At the same levels of sensitivity and specificity, a lower prevalence rate means a reduced positive predictive value and an increased negative predictive value.

2. Compared to example 9–1, the positive predictive value in this example decreased by more than half of its previous value (i.e., from 54.7% to 20.9%). The change in the negative predictive value was not as dramatic. It increased only slightly from 98.9% to 99.8%. In other words, the ability of the screening test to determine who actually has the disease among those testing positive was significantly compromised by a lower prevalence rate of the disease, which had the effect of only marginally increasing the test's ability to determine who did not have the disease among those testing negative. The reason for the smaller effect on negative predictive value is the relatively large number of people without the disease. Since in both populations the vast majority of the participants do not have thyroid cancer, most people testing negative will be true negatives. Thus, the ratio of true negatives to all individuals testing negative (i.e., the negative predictive value) will be high in both cases.

3. The accuracy of the screening test was similar in both examples, showing only a slight decrease from example 9–1 to 9–2. Since the accuracy of the screening test represents a *weighted average* of the sensitivity and specificity, it is influenced in these examples more by specificity than sensitivity. This is the case because the proportion of those with the disease is much smaller than the proportion of those without the disease. Remember that the accuracy of a screening test is the same as: (sensitivity × proportion with disease) + (specificity × proportion without disease). For the present example this is: (95% × 0.04) + (85% × 0.96) = 85.4%. For example 9–1, the equivalent measure is (95% × 0.16) + (85% × 0.84) = 86.6%. The proportion of those with the disease is the same as the prevalence rate of the disease expressed as a proportion, and the proportion of those without the disease is the 1 – the prevalence rate expressed as a proportion.

Precision of Screening Tests

Precision is also known as **reliability**, which is the degree of consistency or stability in the results of a measure from one use to the next.[9] In the context of screening tests, a precise test is one that produces consistent or stable results. A screening test for breast cancer that is sometimes positive and sometimes negative for the same individual when there has been no change in disease status or other factors would *not* be considered a very precise test.

The most common types of precision errors made in screening tests are those due to *method variability, subject variability,* and *observer variability.* **Method variability** has to do with the test itself. If the test itself produces inconsistent results under similar circumstances, it suffers from method variability. This can be due to several factors, such as chemical changes in the reagents used to produce the test results. Some screening tests, for example, rely on chemical reagents that have a limited shelf life. Once beyond the expiration date, the test results may be unreliable.

Subject variability can occur due to physiological changes taking place in the subject being tested. A screening test for anxiety disorder, for example, may produce different results in the same individual from one test to the next depending on the subject's current level of stress, which may be due to unrelated factors. Also, blood pressure readings can vary over the course of a day, leading to inconsistent results.

Observer variability can be of two general types—*intraobserver variability* and *interobserver variability*. **Intraobserver variability** occurs when the person who interprets the results of a screening test comes to different conclusions when successive tests are performed on the *same individual* at different times but under similar circumstances. Say a college student is inadvertently exposed to tuberculosis while vacationing in Mexico and has a tuberculin skin test performed when he returns home. When a nurse later observes the site of the student's skin test, she indicates that the result is negative. The student learns later that day that a friend who vacationed in the same area has just been diagnosed with tuberculosis. Feeling anxious, he returns to the nurse who now indicates that the test is positive (so much for relieving his anxiety!). This is an example of intraobserver variability. This type of variability can be evaluated by giving one observer two or more test results for each individual being tested and correlating the results for each individual. Low intraobserver variability is said to exist if the individual's results are relatively consistent with each other (i.e., there is a high degree of correlation between the test results).

Interobserver variability occurs when different observers of the same test result come to different conclusions about disease status. If the vacationing college student had gone to a nurse who indicated a negative test result and then to another nurse who concluded that the test was positive, interobserver variability would have occurred. The amount of interobserver variability can be evaluated by measuring the proportion of nonrandom agreement between two or more observers using a statistic known as **Cohen's kappa**.[10] Exhibit 9–1 illustrates the use of kappa (κ) to assess interobserver variability based on a hypothetical example using screening test results for cervical cancer. The closer kappa is to one, the better the agreement between the observers, and hence the lower the interobserver variability. In the example the kappa is 0.58 indicating a moderate level of agreement between the observers after accounting for expected agreement due to chance. As a rule of thumb, a kappa greater than 0.75 is considered excellent, and a kappa less than 0.40 is considered poor. Anything between is moderate to good.[11]

The precision of screening tests usually can be improved by standardizing test procedures, training screeners and observers, and monitoring the administration and evaluation of screening tests.[5] In general, the less a screening test depends on subjective interpretation, the more precise it will be.

Exhibit 9–1 Illustration of the Measurement of Interobserver Variability Using Cohen's Kappa

Problem:

Assume that as part of a quality control program a primary care physician sends the results of all routine Papanicolaou screening tests (Pap tests) to a clinical laboratory. At the laboratory two pathologists independently read the Pap tests to determine if the screening results are positive or negative for cervical cancer. The results of the independent assessment after one year have been placed in a 2 × 2 contingency table as follows:

Results from Pathologist B

Results from Pathologist A	Positive	Negative	Total
Positive	25 (a)	12 (b)	37 (a + b)
Negative	15 (c)	230 (d)	245 (c + d)
Total	40 (a + c)	242 (b + d)	282 (a + b + c + d)

Solution:

Cohen's kappa is calculated as follows: $\boxed{\kappa = (P_o - P_e) / (1 - P_e)}$ where,

$P_o = [(a + d) / (a + b + c + d)]$, and $P_e = [(a + b)(a + c) + (b + d)(c + d)] / (a + b + c + d)^2$.

P_o is the proportion of times agreement occurs between the observers, and P_e is the proportion of times agreement is expected between the observers due to chance. For the above problem, κ is calculated as follows:

$$P_o = [(25 + 230) / 282] = (255 / 282) = 0.90$$

$$P_e = [(37)(40) + (242)(245)] / 282^2 = (1,480 + 59,290) / 79,524 = 60,770 / 79,524 = 0.76$$

Therefore, $\kappa = (0.90 - 0.76) / (1 - 0.76) = 0.14 / 0.24 = 0.58$

Interpretation:

Cohen's kappa, which ranges from 0 to 1, measures the proportion of *nonrandom* agreement between two or more observers. Unlike some other measures of agreement, kappa corrects for chance (random) agreement. In the above example the proportion of agreement between the pathologists is 0.90. However, a significant proportion of this agreement is probably due to chance. The proportion of agreement after chance is taken into account is just 0.58. This indicates that there is a substantial amount of interobserver variability at the laboratory. For a quick overview of Cohen's kappa, see Norman, G. R., and Streiner, D. L. (1994). *Biostatistics: The Bare Essentials*. St. Louis: Mosby.

To Screen or Not to Screen

The benefits of a screening program can be reduced morbidity and mortality and improved quality of life. Nevertheless, screening programs, especially mass screening, can be expensive and time consuming. They may require valuable resources for marketing, training, test administration, referral for follow-up examinations, and program evaluation. In addition, screening programs may include risks, such as having little or no impact on disease outcome, missing cases due to too many false negative results, and unnecessary referrals subsequent to false positive results (see table 9–1).

Because there are both benefits and drawbacks to screening, several factors need to be considered before a screening program is initiated. Some of the more important factors are:

- *Nature of the disease.* The disease should generally be a significant public health problem that can be detected *before* symptoms develop. The disease should also be one that the public views as important enough to submit to screening and one that is likely to yield enough cases for the screening program to be cost effective. The **yield** of a screening program is the number of new cases diagnosed and treated as a result of screening.[5] Based on the foregoing, the disease should have a relatively high prevalence in its presymptomatic stage.

- *Nature of the screening test.* The screening test itself should be accurate (valid and precise), relatively quick and simple to apply, easily interpreted, safe, acceptable to those being screened, and relatively inexpensive.

- *Nature of the follow-up tests.* Follow-up tests must be available to confirm the suspected diagnosis. These tests should be readily accessible, accurate, generally safe, and acceptable to those with presumed disease from the standpoint of comfort and cost.

- *Nature of the treatment.* The treatment must be available, accessible, and acceptable to patients, and it must be more effective than if it or another treatment were initiated at a later stage of the disease. In other words, the treatment should result in a significantly better prognosis when the disease is treated in its early stages before symptoms arise.

Some of the diseases and conditions for which one or more types of screening have proven valuable include neonatal hypothyroidism, hypertension, breast cancer, cervical cancer, syphilis, gonorrhea, cystic fibrosis, Tay-Sachs disease, colorectal cancer, diabetes, tuberculosis, diminished visual acuity, hearing impairment, elevated cholesterol, lead poisoning, HIV infection, Down's syndrome, iron deficiency anemia, PKU, neural tube defects, and obesity.[3, 7]

The importance attached to screening for disease detection in the United States was emphasized many years ago by passage of the landmark Breast and Cervical Cancer Mortality Prevention Act of 1990. This comprehensive legislation has helped to spawn a nationwide effort to increase accessibility to breast and cervical cancer screening services for medically underserved women by means of state grants for screening, referrals and follow-up care, public education, training for health professionals, quality assurance, and program evaluation.[12] Although significant progress has been made, it is widely recognized within the public health community that much work still needs to be done if these and other serious chronic diseases are to be prevented or controlled to the extent possible.[13, 14]

Evaluating the Efficacy of Screening

In chapter 1, *efficacy* was defined as the benefits of a treatment, procedure, or service among those who use it compared to those who don't.[1, 6] The efficacy of screening then can be measured by the degree to which it benefits those who are screened compared to those who are not. Perhaps the most convincing way to evaluate the efficacy of screening is through a randomized controlled trial comparing the cause-specific mortality rates between those undergoing screening for a particular disease and those not undergoing screening. If the cause-specific mortality rates are significantly lower in the screened group compared to the unscreened group, then the efficacy of the screening would appear to have been established, all other factors being equal. Most evaluations of the efficacy of screening are not based on randomized controlled trials, however, often because of costs, feasibility, or ethical limitations.[15] More often than not, evaluations of screening utilize observational methods or other nonrandomized designs that are more subject to potential sources of bias, such as *volunteer bias*, *lead time bias*, and *length bias*.

As inferred in chapter 8, volunteer bias can occur because those who participate in screening programs tend to differ systematically from those who do not in terms of factors that may increase survival time. For example, volunteers appear to be better educated, less likely to smoke, and more concerned about their health than nonvolunteers.[16] Thus, comparisons of screened and unscreened groups may suffer from a positive bias. An exception may be those who seek out screening because of a family history or other predisposition for the disease. In this case, the survival rates may be decreased even if the screening is efficacious because of the increased risk among the participants in the screening group.[15] This could introduce a negative bias in the comparison.

Another type of bias that may affect the evaluation findings of screening programs is **lead time bias**. To understand this type of bias one has to first comprehend the concept of **lead time**, which is the extra time obtained to treat a disease because of earlier than usual detection.[6] Applied to screening, *lead time* is the extra time gained by detecting a disease in the presymptomatic stage versus detecting it in the clinical stage due to overt signs or symptoms. To the extent that lead time produces a better outcome with regard to the disease, screening is beneficial because it increases lead time. *Lead time bias* occurs when survival time is overestimated due an earlier diagnosis that does *not* improve prognosis.

To illustrate lead time bias say that a new screening test is being promoted for lung cancer. The test allows an individual to detect potential lung cancer one year earlier than when lung cancer is normally detected due to signs and symptoms of the disease. If patients with lung cancer normally die within an average of 18 months after the usual time of diagnosis, the screening test would increase this time to 30 months (12 months + 18 months = 30 months). However, unless treatment at this earlier stage is *more* effective in increasing survival, there will be no benefit from earlier detection. While patients will tend to die 30 months after diagnosis instead of 18 months, the survival time has not really changed.

As another example, consider two individuals of the same age who presumably contracted lung cancer at the same time. One person is diagnosed at age 49 with the help of the new screening test but still dies at age 51½. The other person is subsequently diagnosed with lung cancer at age 50 after reporting symptoms to a physician. He later dies from the cancer at age 51½. Though the first person was diagnosed earlier, there was no difference in survival time. Both died at exactly the same age. In other words, screening did not improve the prognosis. Thus, lead time bias can result when the supposed increase in survival time is only due to earlier detection and not to a better prognosis.

A study that compares survival times between screened and unscreened groups in order to evaluate the efficacy of screening and does not consider the concept of lead time may be subject to lead time bias. Charles H. Hennekens and Julie E. Buring[15] suggest two methods to minimize this type of bias. The first is to compare *age-specific death rates* between the screened and unscreened populations rather than survival times. The other is to take lead time into account when comparing survival experience. In the earlier example for lung cancer, the 30-month *survival rate* (see chapter 5) in the screened population could be compared to the 18-month survival rate in the unscreened population. This way average lead time has been considered in the comparison. Another way to do this would be to take the typically reported five-year survival rate and add the estimated lead time for the screened group before comparing the results to the five-year survival rate in the unscreened group. Unless steps are taken to deal with potential lead time bias, this type of error is likely to make a screening program appear more efficacious than it really is.

Length bias is another type of bias that may occur in the evaluation of screening programs. It is possible because: (a) a given disease may progress at different rates, and (b) individuals with slowly progressing disease tend to have a better prognosis. When the proportion of individuals with disease that progresses slowly (i.e., disease that remains in the presymptomatic stage longer) is disproportionately higher in the screened than in the unscreened group, length bias can occur. This is a natural tendency since rapidly progressing diseases are less likely to be caught in the preclinical stages of a disease.

Length bias can lead to an overly optimistic view of the value of screening. Breast cancer, for example, progresses at different rates and can be detected early by mammography. If cases of slow-growing, nonaggressive breast tumors, however, tend to be more frequent among those who are screened for the disease than among those who are not, as was suggested recently by a team of researchers from the Yale University School of Medicine,[17] length bias could distort the results of an evaluation of screening efficacy by producing a positive bias. In other words, it would make the association between screening and outcome appear more favorable than it really is. Even if mammography screening is an effective means of preventing mortality due to breast cancer, length bias could make it appear more so, thereby compromising the validity of the comparison. Unfortunately, failure to recognize this and other forms of bias has led to overconfidence in the efficacy of some screening programs.

Summary

- Screening for disease detection is a relatively quick way of detecting potential disease in a population before it has become manifest. There are four basic types of screening—mass screening aimed at general populations, selective screening aimed at high-risk populations, multiphasic screening using two or more screening tests at the same time, and case finding or opportunistic screening initiated by health care practitioners during routine examinations.

- The validity of screening tests is usually measured by their sensitivity and specificity, that is, their ability to identify correctly those with and without the disease, respectively. The positive and negative predictive values of screening tests are related measures that indicate how many of those testing positive or negative, respectively, actually have or do not have the disease. These and related measures can be calculated only if the number of true and false positives and true and false negatives can be determined. This depends on having a definitive diagnostic test, or gold standard, for comparison purposes.

- The precision of a screening test has to do with the consistency or stability of the results. The three most common precision errors are due to method variability, subject variability, and observer variability. Precision can usually be improved by standardizing test procedures, training screeners and observers, and monitoring test administration and evaluation.

- Screening programs have benefits and risks. Therefore, before a screening program is initiated consideration should be given to several factors, including the public health significance of the disease, the accuracy and practicality of the screening test, and the accessibility, acceptability, and effectiveness of follow-up tests and treatment.

- The efficacy of screening is best determined by randomized controlled trials where potential biases can be rigorously controlled. Common biases that can occur in nonrandomized studies of screening efficacy include volunteer bias, lead time bias, and length bias.

New Terms

accuracy of the screening test
case finding
Cohen's kappa
false negative
false negative rate
false positive
false positive rate
gold standard
interobserver variability
intraobserver variability
lead time
lead time bias

length bias
mass screening
method variability
multiphasic screening
negative predictive value
observer variability
opportunistic screening
positive predictive value
precision of a screening test
reliability
screening for disease detection

screening level
selective screening
sensitivity
specificity
subject variability
targeted screening
true negative
true negative rate
true positive
true positive rate
validity of a screening test
yield

Study Questions and Exercises

1. A new screening test for glaucoma produced the following results:

True Disease Status

Screening Test	Positive	Negative
Positive	87	14
Negative	16	362

Based on these data, calculate the test's sensitivity, specificity, positive predictive value, negative predictive value, and the accuracy of the screening test, respectively. Interpret your findings. Would you recommend that this test be used to screen for glaucoma in general populations, and why or why not?

2. Each of the following statements refers to a particular screening measure. Identify the measure referred to for each item using the following key.

A. Sensitivity
B. Specificity
C. Positive predictive value
D. Negative predictive value

E. False positive rate
F. False negative rate
G. Accuracy of the screening test

___ a. Eighteen percent of those with diagnosed coronary heart disease tested negative on a screening test for the disease.

___ b. Of the 125 individuals testing positive for illegal drug use, 91.2% were using illegal drugs.

___ c. Seventy-five percent of those with diabetes had positive screening tests.

___ d. Three thousand women were screened for cervical cancer. Of the 3,000, follow-up diagnostic tests revealed that 75 of those testing positive had cervical cancer, and 2,600 of those testing negative did not have cervical cancer.

___ e. Seven percent of those without breast cancer had positive mammography screening tests for breast cancer.

___ f. Only 36% of those with positive blood tests for *Helicobacter pylori*, a presumptive cause of gastric ulcers, had diagnostic evidence of gastric ulcers.

___ g. Sixty-three percent of the men testing negative on the prostate specific antigen test for prostate cancer were free of prostate cancer.

___ h. Four hundred children without hearing impairments were tested using a standard screening test for hearing. Eighty-seven percent tested negative for hearing impairments.

3. Indicate whether each of the following statements is true or false (T or F). For each false statement, indicate why it is false.

___ a. The degree of sensitivity of a screening test is a result of the number of false positives.

___ b. For given levels of sensitivity and specificity, the higher the prevalence of the disease, the greater the negative predictive value.

___ c. The true positive rate is synonymous with sensitivity.

___ d. Cohen's kappa measures the amount of intraobserver variability of a screening test.

___ e. The yield of a screening program is equal to the number of individuals screened.

___ f. Lead time bias occurs when survival time is overestimated due to an earlier diagnosis that improves prognosis.

___ g. Length bias is possible when a disease progresses at different rates and when individuals with less aggressive forms of the disease have a better prognosis.

References

1. Fletcher, R. H., Fletcher, S. W., and Wagner, E. H. (1988). *Clinical Epidemiology: The Essentials*, 2nd ed. Baltimore: Williams and Wilkins.
2. Friis, R. H., and Sellers, T. A. (1999). *Epidemiology for Public Health Practice*, 2nd ed. Gaithersburg, MD: Aspen.
3. Jekel, J. F., Elmore, J. G., and Katz, D. L. (1996). *Epidemiology, Biostatistics, and Preventive Medicine*. Philadelphia: W. B. Saunders Company.
4. Beaglehole, R., Bonita, R., and Kjellström, T. (1993). *Basic Epidemiology*. Geneva: World Health Organization.
5. Mausner, J. S., and Kramer, S. (1985). *Mausner & Bahn Epidemiology—An Introductory Text*. Philadelphia: W. B. Saunders Company.
6. Last, J. M., ed. (1995). *A Dictionary of Epidemiology*. New York: Oxford University Press.
7. Valanis, B. (1992). *Epidemiology in Nursing and Health Care*. Norwalk, CT: Appleton and Lange.
8. Wassertheil-Smoller, S. (1990). *Biostatistics and Epidemiology: A Primer for Health Professionals*. New York: Springer-Verlag.

9. Vogt, W. P. (1993). *Dictionary of Statistics and Methodology*. Newbury Park, CA: Sage.
10. Cohen, J. (1960). A Coefficient of Agreement for Nominal Scales. *Educational and Psychological Measurement* 20: 37–46.
11. Landis, J. R., and Koch, G. G. (1977). The Measurement of Observer Agreement for Categorical Data. *Biometrics* 33(1): 159–174.
12. Henson, R. M., Wyatt, S. W., and Lee, N. C. (1999). The National Breast and Cervical Cancer Early Detection Program. In *Community-based Prevention: Programs that Work*, R. C. Brownson, E. A. Baker, and L. F. Novick, eds. Gaithersburg, MD: Aspen (1999), pp. 122–139.
13. Sung, H. Y., Kearney, K. A., Miller, M., Kinney, W., Sawaya, G. F., and Hiatt, R. A. (2000). Papanicolaou Smear History and Diagnosis of Invasive Cervical Carcinoma Among Members of a Large Prepaid Health Plan. *Cancer* 88(10): 2283–2289.
14. Katz, S. J., Zemencuk, J. K., and Hofer, T. P. (2000). Breast Cancer Screening in the United States and Canada, 1994: Socioeconomic Gradients Persist. *American Journal of Public Health* 90(5): 799–803.
15. Hennekens, C. H., and Buring, J. E. (1987). *Epidemiology in Medicine*. Boston: Little, Brown and Company.
16. Streiner, D. L., Norman, G. R., and Blum, H. M. (1989). *PDQ Epidemiology*. Toronto: B. C. Decker.
17. Moody-Ayers, S. Y., Wells, C. K., and Feinstein, A. R. (2000). "Benign" Tumors and "Early Detection" in Mammography-screened Patients of a Natural Cohort with Breast Cancer. *Archives of Internal Medicine* 160(8): 1109–1115.

CHAPTER TEN

Analytic Ecological and Cross-Sectional Studies

Learning Objectives

▸ Describe the design and conduct of analytic ecological and cross-sectional studies.

▸ Summarize and give examples of the major strengths and weaknesses of the analytic ecological and cross-sectional study designs.

▸ Interpret the results of analytic ecological studies, including scatter plots, Pearson's correlation coefficient, coefficient of determination, and regression lines and equations.

▸ Analyze and interpret the results of analytic cross-sectional studies.

▸ Define crude prevalence rate, dependent and independent variables, exp, ln, and prevalence studies.

Overview

Analytic ecological and cross-sectional studies represent two relatively basic methods of confirming possible associations between exposures and outcomes. They are often employed when little is known about a potential relationship. Thus, they often precede more sophisticated epidemiologic studies. The analytic ecological study uses summary measures of exposure and outcome for each ecological unit being compared. These measures are usually obtained from secondary sources. The major weakness of the analytic ecological study is the possibility of making an ecological fallacy (i.e., assuming that an association at the group level also holds at the individual level). Analytic cross-sectional studies are conducted at a single point, or during a brief period, in time. Thus, exposure and outcome status are assessed simultaneously. Because of this one normally cannot tell whether the exposure preceded the outcome or vice versa. This is the major weakness of the cross-sectional study design. Because of the limitations of analytic ecological and cross-sectional studies it is not possible to use them to determine causal associations; they are suggestive only and are best thought of as preliminary studies.

Introduction

In chapter 4 it was established that ecological and cross-sectional studies could be classified as descriptive or analytic depending on their intent. Descriptive studies seek to *describe* patterns of exposure or outcome by person, place, or time variables. They do not test predetermined hypotheses, but they may be useful in initiating hypotheses for further investigation. Analytic studies, on the other hand, are concerned with *testing* predetermined hypotheses about the relationships between exposures and outcomes. Therefore, ecological and cross-sectional studies that only generate hypotheses belong to descriptive epidemiology, while those that actually test hypotheses are part of analytic epidemiology (see chapter 1).

This chapter discusses **analytic ecological studies** and **analytic cross-sectional studies**, which are designed to test predetermined hypotheses between exposure and outcome. The term "analytic" is used in this text simply to differentiate these studies from their descriptive counterparts. In common usage, no such differentiation in terminology is made, requiring the reader to infer from the context whether the study's intent is primarily descriptive or analytic. The basic design and types of ecological and cross-sectional studies were discussed in chapter 4. This chapter reiterates some of the key features of analytic ecological and cross-sectional studies, summarizes their major strengths and weaknesses, and discusses the more common methods of analysis and interpretation. Chapters 11–13 cover the other major analytic and experimental epidemiologic study designs.

Analytic Ecological Studies

Key Design Features

The most fundamental aspect of an ecological study is the *ecological unit*. As suggested in chapter 4, an ecological unit is typically a geographical area or time period that encompasses a defined population. For example, an ecological unit can be a city, county, state, or country or a particular day, month, year, or decade. For each ecological unit there is a summary measure of exposure and a summary measure of outcome, such as per capita salt consumption and the cause-specific mortality rate for stroke, respectively. It is important to understand that the summary measures are for the *entire* population encompassed by each ecological unit (i.e., they represent the experience of each population as a whole). This is because the *units of analysis* (defined in chapter 4) are the populations defined by each ecological unit and *not* the individuals within the populations.

It might be helpful at this point to describe briefly how one usually goes about conducting an analytic ecological study. These steps are illustrated in figure 10–1. First, one develops a hypothesis concerning the association between an exposure and outcome. Next, the ecological units to be compared are defined and selected. After this, summary measures of exposure and outcome are obtained for each ecological unit. Once the data on exposure and outcome have been obtained, the ecological units are usually plotted on a graph known as a *scatter plot*. A **scatter plot** is the pattern of points resulting when two variables are plotted on a graph, and each point represents one of the units of analysis formed by the intersection of the values of the two variables.[1] With regard to ecological studies, the intersections represent the ecological units with the x-axis representing the exposure levels and the y-axis representing the outcome levels. The data are then analyzed, and it is determined whether or not the hypothesized association exists. The analysis, which illustrates the use of a scatter plot, will be described shortly.

The exposure and outcome data for the ecological units are generally available from *secondary sources* that have been collected and recorded by someone else, usually for different reasons. Also, the information on exposure is typically from a different source than that on outcome (e.g., per capita salt consumption from a salt industry association and stroke mortality from a health organization, such as the World Health Organization).

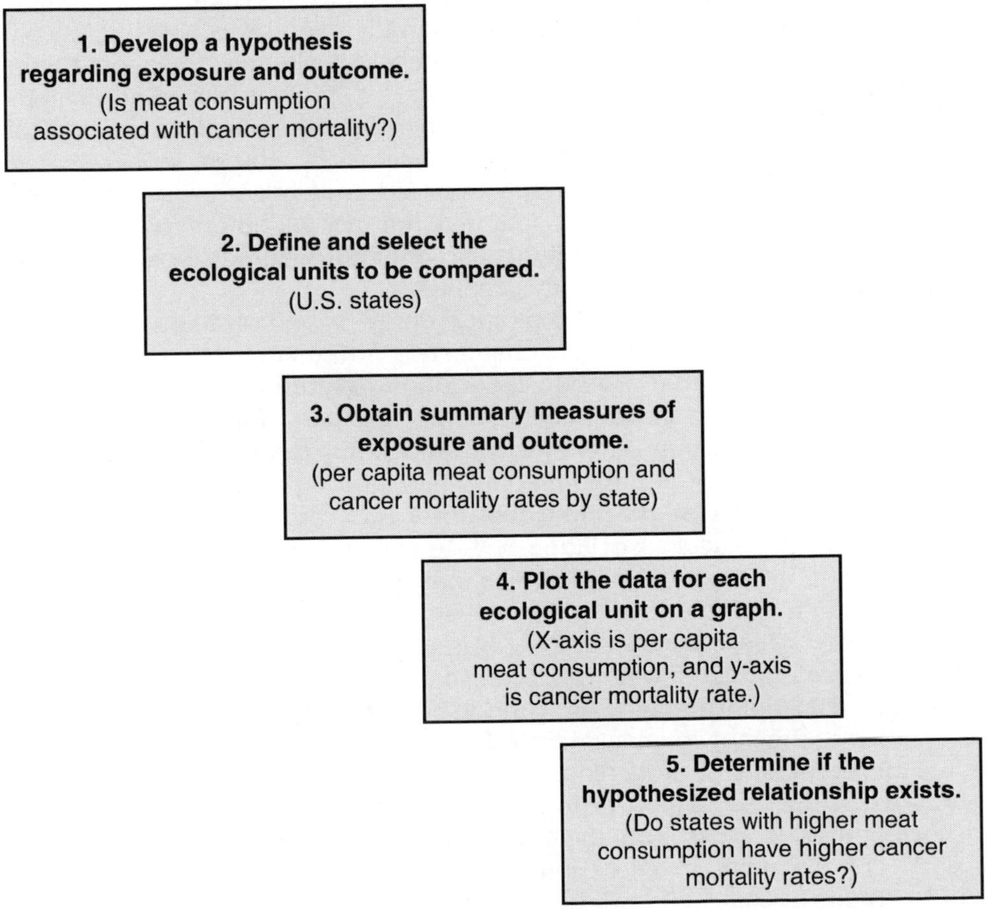

1. Develop a hypothesis regarding exposure and outcome.
(Is meat consumption associated with cancer mortality?)

2. Define and select the ecological units to be compared.
(U.S. states)

3. Obtain summary measures of exposure and outcome.
(per capita meat consumption and cancer mortality rates by state)

4. Plot the data for each ecological unit on a graph.
(X-axis is per capita meat consumption, and y-axis is cancer mortality rate.)

5. Determine if the hypothesized relationship exists.
(Do states with higher meat consumption have higher cancer mortality rates?)

Figure 10–1 Basic steps (with examples) in conducting an analytic ecological study

As indicated in chapter 4, there are several types of ecological studies. These include *multiple-group comparison studies*, which entail comparisons of many different populations in one study (e.g., multiple states or countries); *time-trend studies* in which one population is compared at different time periods (e.g., in 2000 and 2005); and *mixed studies*, which combine elements of both multiple-group and time-trend studies. All of these types can be classified as analytic or descriptive depending on whether or not there are predetermined hypotheses to be tested. *Exploratory studies* are always classified as descriptive studies, however, since there are no predetermined hypotheses to be tested due to their exploratory nature (see chapter 4).

Major Strengths and Weaknesses

The major strength of the analytic ecological study is that it can be used to test a preliminary hypothesis relatively quickly and at less expense than more sophisticated epidemiologic study designs. Before committing resources to undertake a case-control or prospective cohort study, for example, investigators might consider an ecological study when the hypothesis is still relatively undeveloped. Based on the findings of the ecological study, they could then decide if further study seems warranted. Thus, the findings of ecological studies may stimulate additional research by other investigators. When ecological studies in the 1970s revealed an inverse relationship between moderate levels of wine consumption and mortality from ischemic heart disease, the findings were intriguing enough to spawn a number of other epidemiologic studies involving different populations and different methods (see, for example, references 2–5 at the end of this chapter).

The major weakness of the ecological study is the possibility of making an *ecological fallacy* (defined in chapter 4). An *ecological fallacy* occurs when one concludes that a group association determined in an ecological study also holds at the individual level. Since the unit of analysis in an ecological study is the group versus the individual, any association between an exposure and outcome at the group level (i.e., among ecological units) does not necessarily exist at the individual level (i.e., among individuals). For example, the ecological association between wine consumption and mortality from ischemic heart disease implies that countries where moderate wine consumption is the rule tend to have lower levels of mortality from ischemic heart disease. This does not necessarily imply, however, that individuals who drink moderate levels of wine will lower their risk of mortality from ischemic heart disease. Unfortunately, we cannot be sure that a group association also holds at the individual level based on an ecological study alone. Therefore, the possibility of an ecological fallacy is a weakness of the ecological study when the association of interest is at the *individual* level. When the association of interest is at the *group* level, however, no such weakness exists. For example, if one wanted to know whether states with stricter enforcement of seat belt laws have lower rates of fatality from automobile crashes than those with less strict enforcement, an analytic ecological study would be an appropriate design. In this case, the phenomena of interest involve entire populations (i.e., states) instead of individuals, so an ecological fallacy is not a concern.*

Another potential weakness of analytic ecological studies is that the data on exposure and outcome generally come from secondary sources that have been collected by other persons for different purposes. Thus, the data may not be ideal for testing a given hypothesis. For example, per capita salt consumption may have to be approximated from data on sales of salt. Similarly, estimates of the proportion of smokers in different ecological units may come from data on the collection of tobacco taxes. In both cases, these surrogate measures may not accurately reflect the desired variables.

The use of summary measures poses other potential problems as well. Using summary data (e.g., average or per capita levels) for exposure or outcome may lead to imprecise or unstable associations if a high degree of variability exists within the ecological units being examined. Also, some exposure variables in ecological studies, especially social and environmental variables, tend to be more highly correlated with each other than they are on the individual level, making it difficult to isolate their independent effects on the outcome. For example, contaminated drinking water may be associated with cancer mortality based on an ecological study, but it may be difficult to separate the effects of specific contaminants on cancer mortality because of the strong intercorrelations between the contaminants.[7] When the Environmental Defense Fund released a report in 1974 showing a higher incidence of cancer mortality among white males who derived their drinking water from the Mississippi River compared to a similar group who relied on well water, it was believed that organic compounds in the water were responsible for the effect.[8] It would have been nearly impossible, however, to implicate specific organic contaminants with any degree of accuracy based on the ecological analysis due to the high intercorrelations among the myriad of organic compounds.

Other potential weaknesses of ecological studies include difficulty of controlling for potential confounders[9] and difficulty in establishing a correct temporal sequence between exposure and outcome.[7] Often data on potential confounders is either unavailable or of inconsistent quality among the ecological units being examined. Even if available, it may be difficult to incorporate the appropriate data into the analyses. This, of course, can limit the validity of the study findings.[9] In addition, because exposure and outcome are usually assessed simultaneously, the temporal sequence between exposure and outcome may not be clear. For example, an observed positive association between per capita alcohol consumption and unemployment levels across communities in the Midwest could be due to the fact that heavy drinkers are more likely to find themselves out of work or that loss of jobs is more likely to lead to heavy drinking. Table 10–1 summarizes the major strengths and weaknesses of analytic ecological studies.

---

* Due to the possibility of an ecological fallacy, group associations can only *suggest* associations at the individual level. This has led some epidemiologists to view all ecological studies as descriptive studies. This view, however, ignores those circumstances where the association of interest is at the group level and other considerations that are summarized by Szklo and Nieto, who support the classification of analytic ecological studies as distinct from descriptive ecological studies.[6]

Table 10–1 Major Strengths and Weaknesses of Analytic Ecological Studies

Strengths	Weaknesses
1. They are relatively quick and inexpensive to conduct.	1. Associations discovered may not hold at the individual level; thus, there is a possibility of making an ecological fallacy.
2. Significant findings may stimulate additional epidemiologic research at a relatively early stage of hypothesis development.	2. Available sources of exposure or outcome data may not be very accurate.
3. They may be the only practical design for uncovering associations at the group level.	3. Summary measures of exposure or outcome may hide wide variability in exposure or outcome leading to imprecise measures of association.
	4. It may be difficult to control for potential confounders.
	5. It may be impossible to establish a correct temporal sequence between exposure and outcome due to limited information.
	6. It may be impossible to isolate the independent effects of specific variables on

Analysis and Interpretation

The following discussion gives an idea of how the results of a *multiple-group comparison study*, one of the more common types of ecological studies, are analyzed and interpreted. It is assumed that the measures of exposure and outcome are continuous measures, which is typical in ecological studies. A detailed description of the variety of methods that can be used to analyze and interpret the various types of analytic ecological studies is beyond the scope of this text.

The results of multiple-group comparison studies are usually analyzed by first looking at the overall association between the exposure and outcome measures for the ecological units being compared. Typically, a scatter plot is constructed and an overall measure of correlation is calculated. The measure of correlation is often the **Pearson correlation coefficient** (r), which measures the degree of linear relationship between two continuous variables (i.e., exposure level and outcome level). *Pearson's r* ranges from -1 to $+1$, where $r = +1$ indicates a perfect positive linear relationship, and $r = -1$ indicates a perfect negative or inverse linear relationship. When $r = 0$ there is no relationship. Thus, the closer r is to the absolute value of one, the stronger the relationship. When one or both of the variables (exposure or outcome) cannot be considered continuous, other statistical procedures are available. Figure 10–2 illustrates three scatter plots and their respective correlation coefficients for different degrees of association between exposure and outcome. Note that while the r-values quantify the degree of association between the exposure and outcome, the scatter plots give one a visual sense of the degree of association. Also, each point on the scatter plot represents one unit of analysis (e.g., a state or a country).

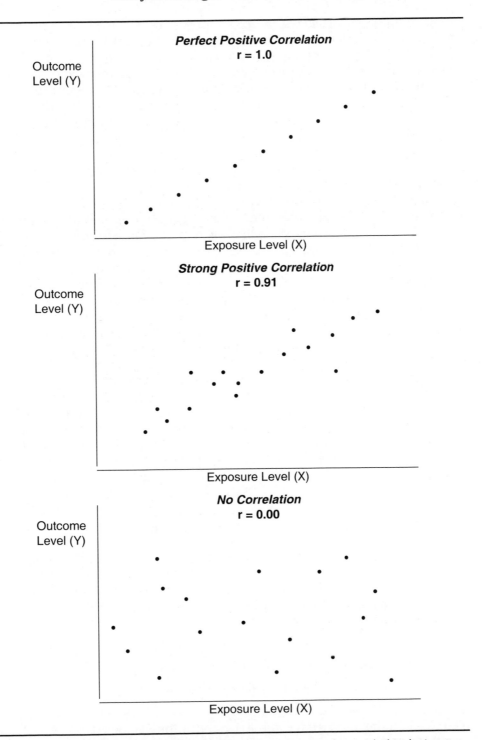

Figure 10–2 Scatter plots representing various degrees of association between exposure and outcome

In addition to producing a scatter plot and calculating the correlation coefficient, the relationship between exposure and outcome is commonly quantified using a form of regression analysis. When there is only one **dependent variable** (the hypothesized effect or outcome) and one **independent variable** (the hypothesized cause of the effect or exposure), *simple linear regression analysis* is used. When there is one dependent variable but more than one independent variable, *multiple linear regression analysis* is the appropriate method.[10, 11]

Let us assume that there is only one dependent and one independent variable represented by the measures of outcome and exposure, respectively. If the ecological units have been plotted on a scatter plot, *simple linear regression analysis* can be used to develop a **regression line** that best describes the relationship between the outcome and exposure values (i.e., a line that best fits the data). The regression line will have the basic formula: $Y = a + bX$, where Y is the outcome measure; X is the exposure measure; a is the intercept, the point where the regression line crosses the y-axis; and b is the slope of the regression line, which tells us the rate of change in Y for each unit change in X.[11] While we will not actually perform regression analysis here (it is described in most basic statistics textbooks), the important point to remember is that the formula for the regression line (the **regression equation**) represents a *model* that allows epidemiologists to predict the outcome level (Y) based on a knowledge of the exposure level (X), given the estimated intercept and slope of the regression line.[11] Depending on how the data points cluster or scatter, the prediction ability may range from perfect to none (see figure 10–3).

Hal Morgenstern has described how the regression equation ($Y = a + bX$) can also be used to estimate a relative risk (RR) for an ecological study.[7] This is done by calculating Y assuming everyone is exposed ($X = 1$) and then dividing that value by the value of Y assuming no one is exposed ($X = 0$). For simplicity, this can be expressed by the following formula:

(10.1)
$$RR \cong 1 + (b / a)$$

Note that in this formula a is the intercept, and b is the slope of the regression equation. As an example, assume that the following regression equation was produced by an analysis of results from an ecological multiple-group comparison study among 10 countries of the relationship between alcohol consumption and breast cancer:

$$Y = 1.2 + 0.6X$$

An RR for the study could be estimated as follows:

$$RR \cong 1 + (0.6 / 1.2) = 1 + 0.5 \cong 1.5$$

In other words, we would expect that those countries with high per capita alcohol consumption to have about 1.5 times the risk of breast cancer compared to those countries with low per capita alcohol consumption. This conclusion assumes that alcohol consumption preceded breast cancer, which might be a reasonable assumption if alcohol consumption data were determined for a time period that anteceded the determination of breast cancer rates by the approximate latency period for breast cancer. Using this method of estimating RR for continuous data depends on being able to dichotomize both exposure and outcome status in a meaningful way. In the example the exposure alcohol consumption was dichotomized as high and low, and the outcome breast cancer was dichotomized as present or absent.

An important related measure that is often cited when simple regression analysis is performed in an ecological multiple-group comparison study is r^2, which is known as the **coefficient of determination**. An analogous measure (R^2) is available when multiple regression is used. The coefficient of determination is a measure of the *magnitude of the effect* of the exposure on the outcome.[12] This measure reveals the proportion of the variance in the dependent variable (i.e., the outcome) that is explained by the independent variable (i.e., the exposure). Before one becomes overly impressed with seemingly high values of r, he or she should calculate r^2. For example, r = 0.80 produces r^2 = 0.64, which indicates that the exposure (independent variable) only explains 64% of the variance in the outcome (dependent variable). This means that 36% (1 − 0.64 = 0.36) of the variance must be due to other factors. An r of 0.50 explains only 25% of the variance in the outcome. That means that 75% (1 − 0.25 = 0.75) of the variance must be due to factors other than the exposure.

In summary, many analytic ecological studies involve production of a scatter plot, computation of a correlation coefficient, generation of a regression equation, and calculation of the coefficient of determination. Each of these reveals something about the linear relationship between the exposure and the outcome. When it is expected that the relationship is not linear or when a linear analysis reveals no relationship, other analytic procedures may be used. Finally, it should be noted that correlation and regression analysis are not restricted to the examination of results from ecological studies. These methods, in fact, are well suited to analyzing findings where the unit of analysis is the individual. In epidemiology, however, other methods are more commonly used when it comes to other analytic and experimental approaches. Figure 10–3 on page 190 shows the results of an ecological multiple-group comparison study.

Analytic Cross-Sectional Studies

Key Design Features

In cross-sectional studies one observes a sample of a population *at a single point* or *brief period in time*, that is, at a cross-section of the time continuum. Since exposure and outcome are assessed in the *same* time period, they are said to be determined simultaneously. The unit of analysis in cross-sectional studies is the individual. Therefore, relevant data on exposure and outcome are collected for each individual in the sample at the same time. Most

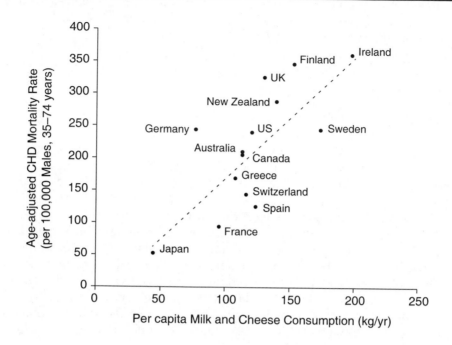

Analysis

r = 0.76

$r^2 = 57.8\%$

Regression Equation: Y = −13.6 + 1.9X

Explanation

The correlation between per capita milk and cheese consumption and the mortality rates in males from coronary heart disease is 0.76 for the 14 countries examined. Thus, those countries that consume higher per capita quantities of milk and cheese have higher rates of mortality from CHD in males than those that consume lower per capita quantities of milk and cheese, all other factors being equal. The regression model for this relationship explains 57.8% of the variability in the CHD mortality rates as indicated by r^2. The regression equation allows us to predict the rate of CHD mortality (Y) from a knowledge of per capita milk and cheese consumption (X). For Ireland, for example, X = 195; therefore, Y = −13.6 + 1.9 (195) = −13.6 + 370.5 = 356.9 deaths per 100,000 males, 35–74 years.

Sources: British Heart Foundation Health Promotion Research Group (1999). Coronary Heart Disease Statistics. Available: *http://www.dphpc.ox.ac.uk/bhfhprg/99stats* (Access date: February 15, 2000.); United States Department of Agriculture (1998). FAS Online: Fluid Milk and Cheese Consumption Per Capita, Selected Countries. Available: *http://ffas.usda.gov/dlp2/circular/1997/97-07-dairy/toc.htm* (Access date: February 15, 2000.)

Figure 10–3 Ecological correlation between milk and cheese consumption and mortality from coronary heart disease for 14 countries

cross-sectional studies employ population survey methods, such as face-to-face interviews, self-administered questionnaires, physical examinations, or telephone interviews.[13] Cross-sectional studies are sometimes referred to as **prevalence studies** (see chapter 5), since prevalence rates are the usual measures employed in the analysis stage. The major use of the analytic cross-sectional study is in testing preliminary hypotheses that may provide a basis for more definitive studies. Thus, the analytic cross-sectional study is most appropriately performed when relatively little is known about the potential causes of a particular health-related problem.

An investigation by C. A. Mancuso and colleagues illustrates the analytic cross-sectional study design.[14] The purpose of this study was to assess the effects of depressive symptoms on the functional status and health-related quality of life of asthma patients. Two hundred and thirty outpatients with moderate asthma, between 18 and 62 years of age, from a primary care internal medicine practice in New York City were interviewed using appropriate survey measures. An association between depressive symptoms and health-related quality of life was found with depressed patients being more likely to report lower health-related quality of life due to their asthma compared to those who were not depressed.

In the example above and other analytic cross-sectional studies four basic steps are usually apparent. First, one or more hypotheses about the relationship between exposure and outcome is formulated. Second, the target population is determined, and a sample of the population is selected, preferably a probability sample (see chapter 8). Third, appropriate measures of exposure and outcome are determined. Fourth, the data are collected and analyzed to determine if a valid association exists between exposure and outcome.

Major Strengths and Weaknesses

Like the analytic ecological study, the analytic cross-sectional study is generally quicker, more economical, and easier to undertake than more sophisticated epidemiologic designs. One reason for this is that no follow-up time is involved. Cross-sectional studies are essentially *one-time* surveys.* Another strength of the analytic cross-sectional study is that the sample may be more representative of the target population than in other analytic or experimental studies since it is easier to obtain a representative sample of the target population. In many case-control studies, for example, the sample may be quite unrepresentative of the desired target population because of a reliance on subjects seeking medical care.[15] A good example is a hospital-based case-control study, which depends on hospitalized patients for both the case and control groups. These subjects may not be very representative of any defined population, and the results therefore may be difficult to generalize. Another strength of the analytic cross-sectional study is that it may be the only appropriate design to use when the onset of disease is difficult to establish and when care is only sought in the advanced stages of the disease. Such is the case with osteoarthritis and some

---

* Exceptions are the panel study and repeated surveys, which are types of longitudinal cross-sectional studies (see chapter 4).

types of mental illness. In these circumstances it may be nearly impossible to determine incidence, and therefore prevalence, which can be determined in a cross-sectional study, may be the only useful measure of disease frequency.[15]

The major weakness of the analytic cross-sectional study design is that one cannot generally determine the *temporal sequence* between exposure and outcome, which is *necessary* to establish cause–effect relationships (see chapter 7). This problem is commonly illustrated by the association between poverty and mental illness. The so-called "Breeder Hypothesis" suggests that poverty causes mental illness, while the "Social Drift Hypothesis" suggests that mental illness causes poverty. A cross-sectional study that confirms the relationship between poverty and mental illness, however, usually cannot establish the direction of the relationship. Therefore, one needs to be cautious in interpreting the results of cross-sectional studies since, as was indicated in chapter 7, *association is not synonymous with causation*. This weakness disappears in those rare instances where the exposure is an inherent factor that does not change over time. For example, if a valid association was found between blood type and a certain disease based on a cross-sectional study, one could conclude confidently that blood type preceded the disease and not the other way around. Thus, it would be possible to establish a cause–effect relationship between blood type and the disease if other important criteria are also met (e.g., Hill's postulates).

There are other potential weaknesses of cross-sectional studies. First, there is the problem of possible *prevalence-incidence bias* (see chapter 8). Because cross-sectional studies normally measure prevalence versus incidence, samples tend to overrepresent disease cases of long duration, while underrepresenting those of short duration. This is due to the fact that cases that tend to recover or die soon after contracting the disease are less likely to be included in the sample. If the degree of association between exposure and disease differs for cases of short duration versus those of long duration, the results could be biased.

Another weakness is the unsuitability of cross-sectional studies for investigating rare diseases or other health-related problems. If the prevalence of a disease is only 2 cases per 100,000 population, then on average a sample of at least 500,000 subjects would be necessary to have a reasonable assurance that just 10 cases of the disease would be included in the sample. This certainly does not represent a cost-efficient method of testing a hypothesis!

Finally, it is possible that simultaneous assessments of *current* exposure and outcome could lead to erroneous results if exposure status has changed in a significant portion of the sample since the development of the outcome or if a significant portion of exposed persons no longer have the disease. This problem does not represent an inherent limitation of the cross-sectional study design but emphasizes the need for careful planning in designing this type of study. It may be necessary, for example, to ask subjects about when exposures occurred and their duration. Similarly, it may be necessary to test for evidence of past disease.[15] Table 10–2 summarizes the major strengths and weaknesses of analytic cross-sectional studies.

Table 10–2 Major Strengths and Weaknesses of Analytic Cross-Sectional Studies

Strengths	Weaknesses
1. They are relatively quick and inexpensive to conduct.	1. The correct temporal sequence between exposure and outcome cannot ordinarily be determined; thus, one cannot generally establish cause–effect relationships.
2. The findings may be more representative of the target population than in other studies because probability sampling is easier to implement.	2. There is a potential for prevalence-incidence bias because transitory or fatal cases are more likely to be missed.
3. They may be the only appropriate design when incidence cannot be established.	3. They are unsuitable for the study of rare outcomes.
	4. Associations based on current exposure or outcome status may not be representative of past exposure or outcome status.

Analysis and Interpretation

When exposure and outcome status are classified dichotomously, the results of a cross-sectional study can be analyzed using a simple 2×2 contingency table. If the exposure or outcome is measured on more than two levels (e.g., low exposure, moderate exposure, high exposure and/or no disease, moderate disease, severe disease), then a somewhat more complex table is used (e.g., 3×2, 3×3, etc.). For simplicity, the discussion of the analysis of cross-sectional studies will assume that exposure and outcome are each measured dichotomously.

The first step in analyzing the results of an analytic cross-sectional study is to place the frequencies of exposed and unexposed subjects in a contingency table according to whether the outcome is present or absent. The following table is a template for cross-sectional analysis.

	Outcome Status		
Exposure Status	**Present**	**Absent**	
Exposed	a	b	a + b
Unexposed	c	d	c + d
	a + c	b + d	n

The frequencies a, b, c, and d represent the number of exposed persons with the disease, the number of exposed persons without the disease, the number of unexposed persons with the disease, and the number of unexposed persons without the disease, respectively. The sums a + c and b + d represent the number of persons with and without the disease, respectively, without regard to exposure status. Similarly, a + b and c + d are the number of exposed and unexposed persons, respectively, without regard to outcome status. The total number of subjects in the sample is represented by n, which is the sum of a, b, c, and d.

These frequencies provide the data we need to calculate applicable prevalence rates and measures of association. The **crude prevalence rate** (i.e., overall prevalence rate) is calculated as follows: $PR = [(a + c) / n] \times 10^n$. If the data represent a *probability sample* (chapter 8), this is a *point estimate* (chapter 5) of the prevalence rate in the population. Two other prevalence rates that are important in cross-sectional studies are the prevalence rate among the *exposed* subjects ($PR_e = [a / (a + b)] \times 10^n$), and the prevalence rate among the *unexposed* subjects ($PR_{ue} = [c / (c + d)] \times 10^n$). These rates can be used to calculate relevant measures of association, namely, the **prevalence rate ratio** (PRR), commonly known as the **prevalence ratio**, and the **prevalence rate difference** (PRD), which are calculated as follows:

(10.2)

$$PRR = PR_e / PR_{ue}$$

(10.3)

$$PRD = PR_e - PR_{ue}$$

The PRR and PRD are analogous to the rate ratio and rate difference, which were discussed in chapter 6. The interpretation of the PRR and PRD differs, however, because they are based on prevalence rates instead of incidence rates. Because the prevalence ratio is more commonly used than the prevalence rate difference, it will be the focus of our discussion.

As with other *ratio* measures of association, the size of the PRR provides an indication of the *strength of an association* between an exposure and outcome. The PRR ranges from zero to infinity and has no units. A PRR of 1.0 indicates no association between exposure and outcome, while a PRR of 2.0 indicates that the outcome is two times *more common* in the exposed group versus the unexposed group. A PRR of 0.5 means that the outcome is only half *as common* in the exposed group compared to the unexposed group (i.e., it is actually twice as common in the *unexposed* group compared to the *exposed* group). In other words, the further the PRR departs from one, the greater the association between the exposure and outcome. This association can be positive (i.e., when the PRR is greater than one) or negative (e.g., when the PRR is less than one). Because the PRR is based on prevalence rates (point prevalence to be exact), the interpretation of the measure is restricted to statements about the *frequency or prevalence* of the outcome in the exposed group relative to the unexposed group. Unlike the risk ratio, statements about increased or decreased *risk* are inappropriate, since prevalence rates are generally poor estimates of risk (see chapter 6). The *percent relative effect* can be calculated for the PRR using Formula 6.3a or 6.3b. It represents the percent increased or decreased *prevalence* instead of risk, however.

The statistical significance of the PRR can be determined by the **chi-square test of independence** (χ^2), which for a 2 × 2 contingency table can be calculated as follows:[16]

(10.4)

$$\chi^2 = \frac{n\,(ad - bc)^2}{(a + b)\,(c + d)\,(a + c)\,(b + d)}$$

If the value of the chi-square is from 3.84 to 6.63, the association is considered statistically significant at the 0.05 level (i.e., $p \leq 0.05$). If the value is from 6.64 to 10.82, the association is significant at the 0.01 level (i.e., $p \leq 0.01$), and if the value is equal to or greater than 10.83, the association is significant at the 0.001 level ($p \leq 0.001$). These values appear in table 10–3.

Table 10–3 Common χ^2 Values and Their Associated P-Values*

χ^2	p	Example
0.00–3.83	> 0.05	($\chi^2 = 2.92$, p > 0.05)
3.84–6.63	≤ 0.05	($\chi^2 = 4.75$, p < 0.05)
6.64–10.82	≤ 0.01	($\chi^2 = 6.64$, p = 0.01)
10.83 or more	≤ 0.001	($\chi^2 = 12.91$, p < 0.001)

*Based on one degree of freedom, which applies to chi-square when calculated from a 2 × 2 contingency table

A 95% confidence interval for the PRR can be estimated using a formula developed by D. Katz and associates.[17] The values a–d are based on the 2 × 2 contingency table referred to earlier in this section.

(10.5)

$$95\%\ CI = \exp\left\{\ln(PRR) \pm 1.96\ \sqrt{[(b/a)/(a+b)] + [(d/c)/(c+d)]}\right\}$$

The term **ln** refers to the *natural logarithm*, so the expression ln (PRR) is the natural logarithm of PRR. The remainder of the expression is 1.96 times an estimate of the *standard error* of ln (PRR). The 1.96 corresponds to a 95% confidence interval based on a normal distribution. For a 99% confidence interval the multiplier is 2.58. The term **exp** refers to e, which is the base of the natural logarithm or the exponential. It has a value of about 2.7183, but like π, it is a universal constant whose exact value cannot be determined. In the formula exp is raised by the value of the expression. For further explanation of these terms see the glossary at the end of the text.

For those not so mathematically inclined, it may be comforting to know that most scientific calculators can readily compute ln and exp at the push of a button or two. Using the above equation, the 95% confidence interval for the PRR can be calculated in four simple steps:

1. Determine the natural logarithm of the PRR using a scientific calculator (this is usually accomplished by entering the PRR and pressing the ln button).

2. Calculate the value of the estimated standard error, i.e., $\sqrt{[(b / a) / (a + b)] + [(d / c) / (c + d)]}$, and multiply it by 1.96.

3. Subtract the value obtained in step 2 from that in step 1, and then raise exp to this power. Using a scientific calculator this is usually accomplished by pressing the exp or e^x button. On some calculators one has to press a second function button before pressing exp or e^x. The resulting value represents the *lower limit* of the confidence interval (i.e., the lower confidence limit).

4. Add the value obtained in step 2 to that obtained in step 1, and then raise exp to this power using a scientific calculator (see step 3). The resulting value represents *the upper limit* of the confidence interval (i.e., the upper confidence limit).

Example 10–1 illustrates the calculation and interpretation of the PRR, the chi-square test of independence, and the 95% confidence interval in an analytic cross-sectional study.

Example 10–1: Calculation and Interpretation of the Prevalence Ratio

Two epidemiologists wanted to know if cigarette smoking is associated with depression. To test their hypothesis, they randomly selected a sample of 149 adult males from Gilford County and initiated an analytic cross-sectional study. The results are shown in the following contingency table. Based on these data, calculate the crude prevalence rate of depression in the sample and the prevalence ratio (PRR). Determine if the PRR is statistically significant and calculate the 95% confidence interval for the PRR. Interpret your results.

Depression

Cigarette Smoking	Present	Absent
Exposed	27	34
Unexposed	26	62

Solution:

Earlier in this section a 2 × 2 template was developed using the letters a through d to represent the frequencies of specific combinations of exposure and outcome status. It is important to note the order in which these letters are used in the table since all the formulas in this section are based on that order. If a–d are ordered differently, the formulas provided in this section may no longer be valid.

Step 1: Calculate the *crude prevalence rate* based on the 2 × 2 template provided.

$$PR = [(a + c) / n] \times 10^n = [(27 + 26) / 149] \times 10^n = (53 / 149) \times 10^n = 0.356 \times 10^2 = 35.6 \text{ per } 100$$

Step 2: Calculate the *prevalence ratio* by dividing the prevalence rate among the exposed by the prevalence rate among the unexposed (i.e., $PRR = PR_e / PR_{ue}$).

$$PR_e = [a / (a + b)] \times 10^n = [27 / (27 + 34)] \times 10^n = (27 / 61) \times 10^n = 0.443 \times 10^2 = 44.3 \text{ per } 100$$
$$PR_{ue} = [c / (c + d)] \times 10^n = [26 / (26 + 62)] \times 10^n = (26 / 88) \times 10^n = 0.295 \times 10^2 = 29.5 \text{ per } 100$$
$$PRR = PR_e / PR_{ue} = (44.3 \text{ per } 100) / (29.5 \text{ per } 100) = 1.5$$

Step 3: Calculate the chi-square test of independence (χ^2) to determine if the PRR is statistically significant.

$$\chi^2 = \frac{n (ad - bc)^2}{(a + b)(c + d)(a + c)(b + d)}$$

$$= \frac{149 [(27 \times 62) - (34 \times 26)]^2}{(27 + 34)(26 + 62)(27 + 26)(34 + 62)}$$

$$= \frac{149 (1{,}674 - 884)^2}{(61)(88)(53)(96)}$$

$$= \frac{149 (790)^2}{27{,}312{,}384}$$

$$= \frac{149 (624{,}100)}{27{,}312{,}384}$$

$$= \frac{92{,}990{,}900}{27{,}312{,}384}$$

$$= 3.40$$

Step 4: Calculate the 95% confidence interval (CI) for the PRR.

$$95\% \text{ CI} = \exp \{\ln (PRR) \pm 1.96 \sqrt{[(b / a) / (a + b)] + [(d / c) / (c + d)]}\}$$

The *lower* confidence limit is:

$$\exp \{\ln (1.5) - 1.96 \sqrt{[(34 / 27) / (27 + 34)] + [(62 / 26) / (26 + 62)]}\} =$$

$$\exp \{0.41 - 1.96 \sqrt{[(1.3) / (61)] + [(2.4) / (88)]}\} = \exp (0.41 - 1.96 \sqrt{0.02 + 0.03}) =$$

$$\exp (0.41 - 1.96 \sqrt{0.05}) = \exp [0.41 - 1.96 (0.22)] = \exp (0.41 - 0.43) = \exp (-0.02) = 0.98^*$$

The *upper* confidence limit is:

$$\exp \{\ln (1.5) + 1.96 \sqrt{[(34 / 27) / (27 + 34)] + [(62 / 26) / (26 + 62)]}\} =$$

$$\exp \{0.41 + 1.96 \sqrt{[(1.3) / (61)] + [(2.4) / (88)]}\} = \exp (0.41 + 1.96 \sqrt{0.02 + 0.03}) =$$

$$\exp (0.41 + 1.96 \sqrt{0.05}) = \exp [0.41 + 1.96 (0.22)] = \exp (0.41 + 0.43) = \exp (0.84) = 2.3$$

Thus, the 95% CI is 0.98–2.3.

---

* Note that exp is being raised to a power representing a *negative* number. Thus, −0.02 must be entered into a calculator, not +0.02.

Answer: The crude prevalence rate of depression in Gilford County is estimated to be 35.6 cases per 100 adult males based on the sample. The prevalence ratio is 1.5, indicating that depression is 1.5 times more common among men who smoke cigarettes compared to those who do not. However, since the chi-square value of 3.40 is less than 3.84, the association between cigarette smoking and depression is *not* statistically significant ($p > 0.05$) (see table 10–3). This means that sampling error is a likely explanation for the finding. In other words, the variation of the PRR from a value of 1.0 (no association) was probably because of sampling error and not because of any true difference between prevalence rates in the exposed and unexposed groups. This assumes the study had adequate power to detect an association. The 95% confidence interval for the PRR was 0.98–2.3. This means that we are 95% confident that the population or true prevalence ratio ranges from 0.98 to 2.3. Because this confidence interval contains one, we know that the association is not statistically significant, which confirms the result of the chi-square test.

Comments:

1. Because this study used a probability sample, the crude prevalence rate is a point estimate of the population rate (see chapter 5 for an explanation of point estimate).

2. The PRR of 1.5 implies a weak association. The strength of an association represented by the PRR is interpreted in the same manner as that for other ratio measures of association (see figure 6–1). The PRR was not statistically significant, though, meaning that sampling error is a probable explanation for the finding. It should be noted, however, that the finding of no significance may also be due to a lack of *power*, which can result if the sample size is too small to detect a prevalence ratio of 1.5. The power of a study should be estimated before the study is initiated in order to minimize the chance of a type II error. Power and type II error (discussed in chapter 8) can be calculated using various software programs, including *Epi Info*, which can be downloaded free of charge from a Web site sponsored by the Centers for Disease Control and Prevention (see appendix B). In fact, the power of this study to detect a PRR of 1.5 is only 39% based on computerized power calculations. This is well below the 80% traditionally considered the minimally acceptable level. To reach 80% power, the sample size would need to be 371 versus 149. Once again, this reiterates the importance of estimating power prior to beginning a study.

3. It is important to realize that we do not know whether cigarette smoking preceded the development of depression or whether depression preceded cigarette smoking in this study. This is the major limitation of cross-sectional studies. Also, it would be improper to say that cigarette smoking increases the risk of depression even if the association was statistically significant since the prevalence ratio does not measure risk.

Other Issues in Analysis

The findings of analytic cross-sectional studies, like other epidemiologic studies, may be subject to various sources of selection and measurement bias, as well as confounding. In addition, there may be *interactions* (see chapter 11) between the exposure and other factors, such as age, sex, race/ethnicity, and so forth. These need to be examined and explained. To the extent possible, analytic cross-sectional studies should be designed to *prevent* sources of bias and confounding. Restriction and statistical control may be used to minimize confounding, as discussed in chapter 8. Matching, however, is rarely used in cross-sectional studies because there is usually no information on the subjects with regard to their status on potential confounders or exposure before the study is initiated.[15] The methods of controlling for confounding in the data analysis stage and for examining interactions are the same as those for other analytic studies. These are discussed in chapter 11 in the context of case-control studies and, therefore, are not explained here. Sampling error, which has been discussed in previous chapters, must also be considered in cross-sectional studies as is true for other epidemiologic studies as well.

Summary

- Analytic ecological studies generally are conducted by developing a hypothesis about the association between exposure and outcome and then selecting the ecological units to be compared. Next, summary measures of exposure and outcome are obtained for each ecological unit, and the data are then graphed on a scatter plot with the x-axis depicting exposure levels and the y-axis, outcome levels. Often one looks for a correlation between exposure and outcome and uses linear regression to predict outcome based on exposure.

- The major strength of analytic ecological studies is that they are relatively quick and inexpensive. Potential weaknesses include the ecological fallacy, inaccurate exposure and outcome data, difficulty in controlling confounding, difficulty in establishing the temporal sequence between exposure and outcome, and not being able to isolate independent effects of specific aspects of the exposure on the outcome.

- Analytic cross-sectional studies are conducted at a single point or brief period in time. After forming a hypothesis about the association between exposure and outcome, a sample of the target population is selected. The subjects are assessed simultaneously with regard to exposure and outcome status to determine if an association exists. A common measure of association is the prevalence ratio, and its significance is determined by a chi-square test.

- A strength of the analytic cross-sectional study is that it is relatively quick and inexpensive to perform. It may also represent the target population better than other analytic studies, and it may be the only analytic design to use when the onset of a given disease is difficult to establish. The major weakness is that one generally cannot establish the correct temporal sequence between exposure and outcome since they are measured simultaneously. Other potential weaknesses include prevalence-incidence bias, unsuitability for studying rare outcomes, and dealing with unknown changes in exposure or outcome status.

New Terms

analytic cross-sectional study	chi-square test	coefficient of
analytic ecological study	of independence	determination

crude prevalence rate	Pearson correlation	prevalence ratio
dependent variable	coefficient (r)	prevalence studies
exp	prevalence rate	regression equation
independent variable	difference	regression line
ln	prevalence rate ratio	scatter plot

Study Questions and Exercises

1. Describe how you would design an ecological study in the United States to examine the hypothesis that consumption of high levels of radium in drinking water are associated with bone cancer. Also, describe how you would design a cross-sectional study to test the same hypothesis. What are the strengths and limitations of your proposed designs?

2. An ecological study was performed among 12 countries to test the hypothesis that beef consumption is associated with gastrointestinal cancers. The following correlation was reported by the investigators: $r = 0.41$. The regression equation for the relationship was $Y = 3.3 + 0.2X$, where X is the per capita level of beef consumption in ounces per day, and Y is the age-adjusted mortality rate from gastrointestinal cancers per 100,000 population. Based on this information, how much of the variability in the gastrointestinal cancer mortality rates is explained by beef consumption? Is this a large amount, and why or why not? Also, if a country's estimated per capita beef consumption is 16 ounces per day, what is the estimated gastrointestinal cancer mortality rate in that country based on the study findings? Finally, what is the estimated relative risk of stomach cancer due to beef consumption, assuming a cause–effect relationship?

3. Two investigators were interested in testing the hypothesis that high educational attainment is associated with more frequent unintentional injuries in the home. To test their hypothesis the investigators selected a random sample of 5,000 men and women, 21 years of age and older, living in owner-occupied, single-family dwellings in Seattle, Washington, during February 2002. Data were also collected on potential confounders, such as age, sex, income level, and health status. The results of this cross-sectional study were as follows:

   • 10% of the sample had high educational attainment (defined as a college degree or higher) and unintentional injuries in the home in the previous 12 months

   • 10% of the sample had high educational attainment but no unintentional injuries in the home in the previous 12 months

   • 20% of the sample had low educational attainment (defined as having less than a college degree) and unintentional injuries in the home in the previous 12 months

   • 60% of the sample had low educational attainment but no unintentional injuries in the home in the previous 12 months

Based on this information, calculate and interpret the prevalence rate ratio and its 95% confidence interval. Assuming that the study was designed to minimize bias and confounding, was the investigators' hypothesis supported, and why or why not?

References

1. Vogt, W. P. (1993). *Dictionary of Statistics and Methodology*. Newbury Park, CA: Sage.
2. St. Leger, A. S., Cochrane, A. L., and Moore, F. (1979). Factors Associated with Cardiac Mortality in Developed Countries with Particular Reference to the Consumption of Wine. *Lancet* 1(8124): 1017–1020.
3. Nanji, A. A. (1985). Alcohol and Ischemic Heart Disease: Wine, Beer or Both? *International Journal of Cardiology* 8(4): 487–489.
4. Hennekens, C. H., Willett, W., Rosner, B., Cole, D. S., and Mayrent, S. L. (1979). Effects of Beer, Wine, Liquor in Coronary Deaths. *Journal of the American Medical Association* 242(18): 1973–1974.
5. Gronbaek, M., Deis, A., Sorensen, T. I., Becker, U., Schnohr, P., and Jensen, G. (1995). Mortality Associated with Moderate Intakes of Wine, Beer, or Spirits. *British Medical Journal* 310(6988): 1165–1169.
6. Szklo, M., and Nieto, F. J. (2000). *Epidemiology: Beyond the Basics*. Gaithersburg, MD: Aspen.
7. Morgenstern, H. (1982). Uses of Ecologic Analysis in Epidemiologic Research. *American Journal of Public Health* 72(12): 1336–1344.
8. Oleckno, W. A. (1982). The National Interim Primary Drinking Water Regulations: Part I—Historical Development. *Journal of Environmental Health* 44(5): 236–239.
9. Rothman, K. J. (1986). *Modern Epidemiology*. Boston: Little, Brown and Company.
10. Jekel, J. F., Elmore, J. G., and Katz, D. L. (1996). *Epidemiology, Biostatistics, and Preventive Medicine*. Philadelphia: W. B. Saunders Company.
11. Wassertheil-Smoller, S. (1990). *Biostatistics and Epidemiology: A Primer for Health Professionals*. New York: Springer-Verlag.
12. Norman, G. R., and Streiner, D. L. (1994). *Biostatistics: The Bare Essentials*. St. Louis: Mosby.
13. Last, J. M., ed. (1995). *A Dictionary of Epidemiology*. New York: Oxford University Press.
14. Mancuso, C. A., Peterson, M. G., and Charlson, M. E. (2000). Effects of Depressive Symptoms on Health-related Quality of Life in Asthma Patients. *Journal of General Internal Medicine* 15(5): 301–310.
15. Kelsey, J. L., Thompson, W. D., and Evans, A. S. (1986). *Methods in Observational Epidemiology*. New York: Oxford University Press.
16. Ferguson, G. A. (1976). *Statistical Analysis in Psychology and Education*, 4th ed. New York: McGraw-Hill.
17. Katz, D., Baptista, J., Azen, S. P., and Pike, M. C. (1978). Obtaining Confidence Intervals for the Risk Ratio in Cohort Studies. *Biometrics* 34: 469–474.

CHAPTER ELEVEN

Case-Control Studies

Learning Objectives

▸ Distinguish between exploratory and analytic case-control studies.

▸ Discuss the importance of exposure–outcome sequence, case definition, case and control selection, exposure assessment, and study power in the design of case-control studies.

▸ Compare and contrast the utility of population-based and hospital-based case-control studies.

▸ Calculate crude and Mantel-Haenszel odds ratios, their 95% confidence intervals, and the chi-square test of significance for the odds ratio.

▸ Interpret the results of unmatched case-control studies, including the results of stratification to uncover confounding and/or effect modification.

▸ Define population-based disease registry, source population, blinding, matched case-control studies, practical or clinical significance, stratification, multivariable methods, rare disease assumption, and test of heterogeneity.

Overview

Because case-control studies are subject to a number of potential sources of error, they must be carefully designed, conducted, analyzed, and interpreted. Some of the more important design considerations include establishing a proper temporal sequence between exposure and outcome, defining precisely what constitutes a case, selecting appropriate case and control groups, avoiding bias in determining exposure status, assuring adequate study power, and choosing the appropriate method of analysis. Potential sources of selection and measurement bias must be recognized and prevented to the extent possible. Potential confounding must be controlled, and effect modification, if present, should be identified and described. If properly designed and executed, case-control studies can further our understanding of disease etiology by establishing specific risk factors for disease. Analysis, which may be unmatched or matched, usually focuses on determining odds ratios, which can be interpreted as measures of association between the odds of exposure among cases versus controls.

Introduction

Case-control studies were discussed briefly in chapter 4. While the early origins of the case-control study can be traced back over a hundred years, it was not until the 1920s that the first modern case-control studies appeared in the literature.[1, 2] Today, this design is very common in epidemiology for reasons that will become apparent shortly. Case-control studies have been referred to as *retrospective studies*, although this term can be confusing since other types of epidemiologic studies may involve retrospective assessment. As discussed in chapter 4, the term is not recommended as a synonym for case-control studies.

Case-control studies can be *exploratory* or *analytic*. In **exploratory case-control studies** there is *no specific* a priori hypothesis about the relationship between exposure and outcome. Cases and controls are selected, and a variety of factors are examined to determine if any are related to the outcome. Exploratory case-control studies have been referred to in a disparaging manner as "fishing expeditions,"[2] but they can be valuable in identifying potential risk factors, especially when they concern an unfamiliar but serious or life-threatening disease. Exploratory studies are also useful in investigations of epidemics as a means of identifying possible causes of the outbreak (see chapter 14). *Analytic case-control studies*, which are the subject of this chapter, are designed to test *specific* a priori hypotheses about exposure and outcome.

In the classic case-control study individual subjects are selected on the basis of their outcome status *prior to* determining their exposure status. If the proportion of exposed subjects differs significantly between the case and control groups, and if there are no major sources of confounding or bias, an association between exposure and outcome is said to exist. It is important to recognize the sequence of inquiry in a case-control study. Outcome is *always* determined *before* exposure. Individual cases and controls are selected *first* and only then is exposure status determined for the cases and controls (see figure 11–1). Conceptually, this is the opposite of the cohort study (discussed in chapter 12) where exposure status is assessed first and outcome status is determined second. Because case-control studies are subject to a number of potential sources of error, they must be designed carefully if the findings are to be considered valid. The following sections discuss some of the more important design considerations for case-control studies followed by a discussion and illustration of how they are analyzed and interpreted. Major strengths and weaknesses of case-control studies are presented in table 11–1.

Design Considerations in Case-Control Studies

Establishing the Proper Temporal Sequence

Having the proper temporal sequence between exposure and outcome maximizes the value of case-control studies. In order to determine causal associations, the study exposure must precede the study outcome. The clearest way to accomplish this is to use *incident* (new) cases and assess *prior* exposure (i.e., exposure that occurred during a time period before the outcome devel-

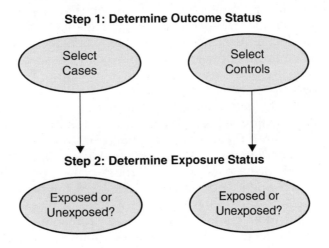

Figure 11–1 Sequence of determining exposure and outcome status in a case-control study

Table 11–1 Major Strengths and Weaknesses of Case-Control Studies

Strengths	Weaknesses
1. They are relatively quick and inexpensive to conduct.	1. Incidence rates in exposed and unexposed subjects ordinarily cannot be determined.
2. They are appropriate for studying rare outcomes.	2. They are not appropriate for studying rare exposures.
3. They can be conducted with moderate numbers of subjects.	3. Information on prior exposure or potential confounders may not be readily available, accurate, or of the same quality between cases and controls (e.g., due to differential recall).
4. They allow multiple potential risk factors to be examined in the same study.	
5. If properly executed, they can help in establishing cause–effect relationships.	4. It may be difficult to identify comparable case and control groups, and thus there is a greater potential for selection bias.

oped). Using prevalent (existing) cases or concurrent exposure does not invalidate a case-control study, but it limits the interpretation of the findings, because in these circumstances, one cannot be sure whether the exposure preceded the outcome, the outcome preceded the exposure, or the exposure and outcome occurred simultaneously. Thus, one cannot establish causal associations. This is one of the limitations of cross-sectional studies, which rely on prevalence data. Also, since prevalence is affected by both incidence and duration, when prevalent cases are employed in a case-control study one cannot always be sure of the extent to which an exposure is related more to disease prognosis than disease development.

Although desirable, determining incident cases for a case-control study is not as easy as it may first appear. For one thing, it is not always clear when new cases begin. Therefore, for pragmatic purposes, incident cases are usually defined as *newly diagnosed cases*, and the date of diagnosis is used as a proxy for when the disease began. With most acute conditions requiring prompt medical treatment (e.g., automobile-related injuries, botulism), the actual date of the outcome approximates the date of diagnosis quite well. This is not true for most chronic diseases (e.g., multiple sclerosis, emphysema), however. The date of diagnosis may be many years after the disease developed. Unfortunately, this fact can still lead to problems in ascertaining whether the study exposure preceded or followed disease initiation.

When diagnosis occurs long after disease initiation it may be important to assure that the exposure at least preceded the onset of *symptoms*, since in this situation it would be unlikely that one would have altered exposure because of the disease.[3] As illustrated in figure 11–2, the original exposure is

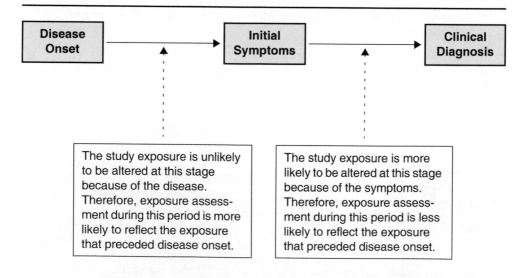

Figure 11–2 Problems in maintaining a correct temporal sequence between exposure and outcome in case-control studies when the period between disease onset and diagnosis is long

less likely to be changed before initial symptoms appear than after the symptoms, especially if they are bothersome. If exposure status is determined during the period between symptoms and diagnosis, and if this period is long, the true association between the study exposure and outcome might be missed. For example, changes in diet are less likely to be made by someone with stomach cancer prior to any symptoms than when early symptoms of heartburn and abdominal discomfort begin. By the time someone is diagnosed with stomach cancer, however, his or her dietary habits may be quite different than they were prior to cancer initiation. Furthermore, when prevalent cases are used in case-control studies there is a greater probability that exposure has been modified *after* disease diagnosis.[4] Patients with type 2 diabetes, for example, may have controlled their weight since their diagnosis, making it more likely that investigators would understate the role of obesity as a potential risk factor for diabetes when prevalent cases are examined sometime after diagnosis.

Defining and Selecting Appropriate Cases

If strict criteria are not employed to define precisely what constitutes a case in a case-control study, the case group may be diluted with noncases resulting in spurious associations (chapter 7). This can be a problem when different diseases have similar signs and symptoms but unrelated causes. Inadvertently including cases of a different disease with a different etiology in the case group can increase the probability of a type II error, that is, finding no association when one really exists. Using terminology we employed in the chapter on screening for disease detection (chapter 9), we can say that one needs to be careful to exclude *false positives* but to include *false negatives* in the case group. The best way to achieve this is to have reliable and widely accepted criteria for determining what constitutes a case and to use these criteria when selecting subjects for the case group.

The criteria for selecting subjects for the case group usually require evidence of the disease from clinical examination as well as appropriate diagnostic tests to confirm the clinical diagnosis. Sometimes this is relatively straightforward, and other times it can be more complicated. An English case-control study of the relationship between alcohol consumption and stroke used the World Health Organization (WHO) criteria for defining stroke cases.[5] If the authors had differentiated each of the various subcategories of stroke, the process of defining cases would have been more complicated. According to WHO, there are 10 types of strokes, not including transient ischemic attacks.[6] Having strict criteria for case inclusion sometimes may need to be tempered by practical considerations. For example, if there is missing information for a number of potential subjects, it may be necessary to relax the criteria somewhat. Sometimes investigators will classify cases as suspect, probable, and definite depending on how many of the criteria they satisfy. As additional information becomes available, classifications can be changed accordingly.

Cases for a case-control study generally come from patients admitted to clinical facilities (e.g., hospitals, clinics, nursing homes, rehabilitation centers) or from the general population. Studies that select cases from clinical facilities are commonly referred to as **hospital-based case-control studies**, even if sometimes the facilities are not hospitals per se. These cases are usually not representative of all possible cases in the general population because of differences in disease severity or socioeconomic factors related to hospitalization. This can affect external validity, but it will not affect internal validity if the controls are similar to the cases, especially with regard to their potential for past exposure. Likewise, *restriction* (chapter 8), when properly applied, does not invalidate epidemiologic studies as long as it is applied equally to the controls, and the controls are similar to the cases regarding potential confounders and potential exposure history.

Case-control studies where cases and controls are based on a total or representative sample of a defined population are known as **population-based case-control studies**. These studies are less common than hospital-based studies because of the time and expense involved in identifying eligible subjects and obtaining the required data. Cases obtained from these studies, however, should be representative of those in the target population. One way of identifying incident cases for population-based studies is to utilize a **population-based disease registry**, which is an ongoing system that collects relevant data and registers all cases of a particular disease or class of diseases as they develop in a defined population (e.g., a cancer registry). Not all registries are population-based, however, and thus some may only represent disease incidence within certain clinical facilities. Though not suitable for population-based studies, these registries may be used in connection with hospital-based studies.

Cases for a case-control study may be selected retrospectively or prospectively. In retrospective selection, for instance, one might identify all cases of leukemia at a medical center that were diagnosed for the first time between 1995 and 2000. In prospective selection one might identify new cases of leukemia as they are diagnosed during a forthcoming period. In both instances, controls would be selected during the same respective time periods. One advantage to selecting cases and controls retrospectively is that the investigator can go back as far as needed to get a sufficient number of subjects to maintain a desired level of power in the study. The usefulness of retrospective selection depends, however, on having an accurate database that also contains relevant information on exposure. Hospital records, for example, may have diagnoses on all admissions or discharges going back many years, but exposure data on intake forms may be incomplete or unreliable. Also, diagnostic methods or disease classifications may have changed during the specified time period. Selecting subjects prospectively may also be subject to problems. Better diagnostic procedures may be developed during the course of case selection, and the definition of the disease may change over time.

Selecting Appropriate Controls

Without controls there can be no case-control studies, but with the wrong controls there can only be regrettable case-control studies.

It is difficult to underestimate the importance of selecting appropriate controls in a case-control study. Put simply, failure to select proper controls can invalidate study results. The control group is important because it provides a basis for comparison by representing what is normal or expected. In fact, all analytic and experimental studies in epidemiology have a control or comparison group. In a cross-sectional study, for instance, those who are unexposed to the factor under investigation represent the control group.

Several factors need to be considered in selecting controls for a case-control study. First and foremost, controls should be *comparable* to cases except for the study disease and the frequency of the study exposure, which will vary between case and control groups depending on how strongly it is associated with the outcome. The *potential* for exposure, however, should be the same for cases and controls to avoid selection bias (chapter 8). Other characteristics that might confound a relationship, like age, sex, racial/ethnic background, socioeconomic level, occupational status, and certain lifestyle behaviors, should be similar between cases and controls. This usually can be achieved by restriction, matching, or statistical adjustment in the analysis stage of the study. The more investigators know about the study disease and previous research on the topic, the better they are able to identify those factors that should be measured in addition to the study exposure. For example, in a study of the relationship between tobacco use and oral cancer, one would want to be sure cases and controls are similar in regard to their drinking habits since alcohol consumption is a potential confounder for this association. In general, it is prudent to control for known or suspected risk factors for the outcome, since these could be confounders if they are also associated with the study exposure (see chapter 8).

To achieve comparability between cases and controls, the controls should come from the same population that generated the cases. This population is known as the **source population**. Ideally, controls should represent those who would have been cases had they developed the study disease.[7] If this is not possible, it is incumbent on the investigators to show that the controls are at least likely to be similar to hypothetical controls in the source population in terms of exposure frequency and other important characteristics. If not, selection bias or confounding may result. In general, to promote comparability, exclusions or restrictions placed on cases should also be applied to controls and vice versa. Thus, if cases consist of African-American males, 50–64 years of age, without a previous history of heart disease, who are admitted to St. Francis Hospital with a primary diagnosis of myocardial infarction, then the controls should consist of African-American males, 50–64 years of age, without a previous history of heart disease, who are admitted to St. Francis Hospital during the same time period but with other unrelated diagnoses. By selecting controls of the same race, sex, age group, medical history regarding heart disease, from the same hospital, and during the same time period, the investigators have provided some assurance that the case and control groups are alike on factors that could otherwise compromise the findings. Depending on the specific hypothesis being tested, there may be other factors that need to be controlled to minimize potential confounding or selection bias.

Controls from *population-based case-control studies* are usually selected randomly from the source population and are typically referred to as **population controls**. If selection is truly random, these controls should represent the actual exposure rate of subjects without the study disease in the source population and would therefore exemplify the ideal control group. Typical problems with control groups selected in this manner, however, include potential selection bias due to low rates of participation and possible measurement bias due to poor recall. Sometimes controls are selected from neighbors, family members, friends, or coworkers from the source population. These types of controls may improve participation and reduce recall bias, but they may also introduce a negative bias in the study results because the controls may be too similar to the cases with regard to exposure status; that is, they may not represent the true range of exposure that existed in the source population because of their similarity to the cases.

Hospital-based case-control studies generally use **hospital controls**, that is, patients admitted to same hospital(s) for reasons other than the study disease. Some, however, may employ population controls or neighbors, family members, or other associates of the cases. Using hospital controls is more convenient than selecting population controls and tends to result in greater participation with less recall bias since patients generally have had time to reflect about past exposures and events. Cases and controls from the same medical facilities are also more likely to resemble each other with regard to those selective factors that led to the use of the facilities (e.g., socioeconomic status). This may not hold for referral hospitals, however, where patients with a particular disease may be referred from a wider geographic area and be more affluent than patients without the disease.[8] Also, hospital controls may not represent the exposure distribution in the source population because they represent ill people who may be more likely to have an unfavorable risk profile than healthy people in the source population. Depending on what exposure is being studied, erroneous conclusions could result if the exposure is more *or* less common in hospital controls than it is in the source population.

A question that is frequently asked in selecting a hospital control group is, what diagnostic categories should be included? It is usually recommended that patients with a variety of diagnoses be chosen to comprise the control group with the important caveat that those patients with diagnoses that are known or likely to be related to the study exposure should *not be included*.[9] If they are, this could result in an over- or underestimation of the true association between the exposure and outcome depending on whether the diseases are positively or negatively related to the exposure. It would not be appropriate, for example, to include patients with emphysema or chronic bronchitis in the control group when testing the hypothesis that cigarette smoking causes lung cancer because we know that these diseases are also associated with cigarette smoking. Therefore, the magnitude of the relationship between smoking and lung cancer would be underestimated, since the controls would be expected to have a higher proportion of prior smokers than the source population. Choosing from a variety of diagnoses tends to minimize the impact of this error if any particular disease is unknowingly associated with the study exposure.

In summary, one must be careful when selecting a control group from hospitalized subjects. While there are some advantages in terms of convenience, better recall, and comparability between hospital cases and hospital controls, the chief disadvantage is that the exposure frequency may be different from that in the source population. This could lead to erroneous conclusions about the relationship between the study exposure and outcome in the target population, thus weakening the internal validity of the study. Table 11–2 lists some of the basic questions to ask when one selects a control group for a case-control study.

Table 11–2 Some Basic Questions to Ask When Selecting a Control Group for a Case-Control Study

- Do the controls come from the same source population as the cases?
- Are the controls similar to the cases with regard to their potential for past exposure?
- Are the controls similar to the cases with regard to potentially confounding factors?
- Have any restrictions or exclusions applied to cases also been applied to controls?
- Have hospital controls from diagnostic categories known to be associated with the study exposure been excluded from the control group?
- Have the controls been selected from the same time period as the cases?

Accurately Determining Exposure Status

Exposure status in case-control studies needs to be assessed carefully in order to minimize potential sources of measurement bias. Two common types of measurement bias that can result from the way exposure status is determined are interviewer bias and recall bias (see chapter 8).

Interviewer bias can result when an investigator interviews cases more thoroughly than controls to determine exposure status. Interviewer bias is a consequence of an interviewer being able to identify the cases and the exposure under study. Therefore, keeping the interviewer unaware of the subject's outcome status and the study hypothesis (i.e., **blinding** the interviewer) is a way of controlling this error. Unfortunately, blinding interviewers to outcome status usually is difficult because the interviewer can often recognize cases by overt signs or symptoms or because the subjects may share their outcome status with the interviewer before or during the interview. Interviewers, however, if different from the investigators, usually can be blinded to the specific hypothesis under investigation. This should reduce the usually unconscious tendency to search more thoroughly for a particular exposure among cases than controls during the interview. A similar bias can occur when medical records are being examined to determine exposure status. In this case, it is also best to blind the person gathering the information from the study hypothesis, and outcome status, if possible. The fundamental point to remember is that exposure status should be assessed in the same manner for cases and controls, even to the point of where the assessments take place. In addition, wherever feasible, data collected from subjects should be verified using other sources, such as laboratory tests, official records, and information from spouses, relatives, friends, or employers, in order to reduce further the probability of interviewer (or "data gatherer") bias.

Recall bias can occur because cases often remember past exposures better than controls, resulting in a positive bias for the association between exposure and outcome. This form of measurement bias results from a natural tendency among those with serious diseases or conditions to want to know why the outcome developed. The introspection that takes place makes cases more likely than controls to recall past exposures accurately, since controls generally have less, if any, vested interest in the findings. Recall bias can be reduced by blinding the subjects to the specific hypothesis and by consulting more reliable sources of data on subject exposure. Sometimes data on past exposures do not depend on subject memory, so recall bias is not a concern. Such is the case when *biomarkers* are used to determine exposure. **Biomarkers** are cellular or molecular indicators of exposure, such as elevated enzyme levels or toxic residues that may be found in the blood, saliva, urine, hair, or other body specimens.[1] A well-known biomarker for recent cigarette smoking, for example, is cotinine, a metabolite of nicotine. It can be found in the blood or other body specimens. Environmental and occupational studies frequently rely on biomarkers. Using carefully developed and tested study instruments, standardized procedures, and trained personnel are other ways of minimizing measurement bias.

Assuring Adequate Study Power

Even with the best efforts to minimize systematic errors, the results of a study may be inconclusive if there is insufficient study power. More than anything else, power is related to sample size. Therefore, a case-control study needs to have an adequate sample size to ensure a high degree of protection against type II error, which is more likely to occur when a study's power is low. Fortunately, software programs are available that can determine the sample size needed to obtain a desired level of power, given certain study parameters. One such program is available with *Epi Info* (see appendix B). There are also some Internet sites with applets that will calculate required sample size or power based on study parameters that you provide. *Epi Info* requires the following input to calculate required sample size for a case-control study:

- The confidence level desired (usually 95% corresponding to a p-value of 0.05)
- The level of power desired (usually between 80 and 95%)
- The ratio of controls to cases (may be 1:1, 2:1, 3:1, etc.)
- The expected frequency of the exposure in the control group (usually estimated from previous surveys in the source population);
- The smallest odds ratio one would like to be able to detect (based on *practical significance*)

As an example, assuming a 95% confidence level, 90% power, a control to case ratio of 1:1, and an expected exposure frequency of 10% in the control group, it would take 1,265 cases and 1,265 controls for a total sample size of 2,530 to detect an odds ratio as small as 1.50. The total sample size drops to 804 if one is content with detecting an odds ratio of 2.00, but jumps to 49,958 if one needs to detect an odds ratio as small as 1.10. The smallest detectable odds ratio needed should be based on **practical significance**, that is, what is meaningful from a public health or clinical point of view. This term is also referred to as **clinical significance**, and it is more crucial than statistical significance, which tells us nothing about the importance of an association.

Using multiple controls per case will lower sample size requirements for the *case group* but will increase the *total* sample size needed. For example, using three controls per case to detect an odds ratio of 1.50 for the parameters stated above will result in a 34.5% reduction in the number of cases required (from 1,265 to 829) but a 31.1% increase in the total sample size needed (2,530 to 3,316). This may be advantageous where the study outcome is relatively rare, and cases are more difficult to obtain than controls. The value added, however, begins to diminish after awhile. Using four instead of three controls per case in the above example reduces the number of required cases by only 6.6% (from 829 to 774), but increases the total sample size needed by 16.7% (from 3,316 to 3,870). Going from six to seven controls per case reduces the number of cases needed by only 2.2% but increases the total sample size required by 11.7%.

A rough estimate of the number of cases needed when multiple controls are used for any given set of parameters is provided by the following formula.[2]

(11.1)

$$\text{Number of cases} \cong [k\,(c + 1)] / 2c$$

Here, k = the original number of cases required based on a 1:1 control to case ratio, and c = the number of controls per case one plans to use. For example, if 1,265 cases are required based on a 1:1 ratio of controls to cases, and if one wants to see how many cases would be required if three controls were used per case, the estimate would be:

$$[1{,}265\,(3 + 1)] / (2 \times 3) = 1{,}265\,(4) / 6 = 5{,}060 / 6 = 843 \text{ cases}$$

This is close to the value of 829 calculated using *Epi Info*. The formula applies to both unmatched and matched analyses (see next section).

Analysis and Interpretation of Case-Control Studies

Analyzing Matched versus Unmatched Studies

The procedures for analyzing the results of case-control studies differ depending on whether the cases and controls are matched or unmatched. **Matched case-control studies** are those in which *pair matching* (chapter 8) has been used to increase the comparability of the cases and controls with regard to potentially confounding factors, such as age, sex, or race/ethnicity. In these studies every control is paired with a case so that case-control pairs are identical on the matched variables. Some of the advantages and disadvantages of pair matching in case-control studies are shown in table 11–3. The disadvantages tend to outweigh the advantages in most cases, and, therefore, frequency matching (chapter 8) with control for confounding in the analysis may be a viable alternative.[2] Procedures for analyzing matched case-control studies are described in exhibit 11–1.

Unmatched case-control studies are those in which controls are *not* pair matched with cases during the selection process. The results from unmatched case-control studies are analyzed differently from matched case-control studies as illustrated later in this chapter. It is important to note that matched analysis is only appropriate when pair matching has been used. If frequency matching has been used, an unmatched analysis should be employed since the cases and controls have not been paired as a new unit of analysis.

Table 11–3 Advantages and Disadvantages of Pair Matching in Case-Control Studies

Advantages	Disadvantages
1. Assures comparability between cases and controls on the selected variables	1. May be difficult or costly to find a sufficient number of controls that meet the criteria for matching if many variables are being matched
2. May simplify the selection of controls by eliminating the need to identify a random sample	2. Eliminates the possibility of examining the effects of the matched variables on the outcome
3. Useful in small studies where obtaining cases and controls that are similar on potentially confounding factors may otherwise be difficult	3. Can increase the difficulty or complexity of controlling for confounding by the remaining unmatched variables
4. Can assure adequate numbers of cases and controls with specified characteristics so as to permit statistical comparisons with regard to exposure and outcome	4. May produce case and control groups that are uncharacteristically similar with regard to the study exposure, especially if too many variables are matched (i.e., so-called "overmatching")
	5. Can result in a greater loss of data since a pair of subjects has to be eliminated even if only one subject is not responsive

Exhibit 11–1 Analysis and Interpretation of Matched Case-Control Studies

Introduction

Case-control studies where controls are *pair matched* to cases on various factors (e.g., age, sex, racial/ethnic background, smoking status, etc.) are known as *matched case-control studies*. Matching is used to increase the comparability of the cases and controls. Matching may be used in both population-based and hospital-based case-control studies where investigators want to control for potential differences in factors that might confound or bias an association. Matched case-control studies are analyzed differently than unmatched studies.

Analysis

Assuming dichotomous measures of exposure and outcome and a control to case ratio of 1:1, a matched case-control study can be analyzed using a 2 × 2 contingency table. This table, however, differs in important respects from that used to analyze unmatched studies. For one thing, the frequencies (a, b, c, and d) represent *case-control pairs*. The number of case-control pairs in which both cases and controls are exposed is represented by a, while the number of case-control pairs in which only the cases are exposed is b, and so on. The sum of the case-control pairs in the sample is indicated by n, which is *one-half* the total number of cases and controls in the study.

	Control		
Case	**Exposed**	**Unexposed**	
Exposed	a	b	**a + b**
Unexposed	c	d	**c + d**
	a + c	**b + d**	**n**

The odds ratio (OR) for a matched case-control study, which is interpreted the same as for an unmatched study, can be estimated by taking the ratio of the *discordant pairs*, that is, those case-control pairs where exposure status differs between cases and controls. Thus, the OR for matched analysis is:

$$OR = b / c$$

Significance of the OR can be calculated by a chi-square test for matched pairs (McNemar's test):

$$\chi^2 = (b - c)^2 / (b + c)$$

The χ^2 value is interpreted the same as in unmatched studies. Perhaps the easiest way of estimating the 95% confidence interval (CI) for a matched analysis is to use the following formula, which requires large values of b and c (say, at least 30 each).

$$95\% \text{ CI} = \exp [\ln (b / c) \pm 1.96 \sqrt{1 / b + 1 / c}]$$

Reference: Schlesselman, J. J. (1982). *Case-Control Studies: Design, Conduct, Analysis*. New York: Oxford University Press.

Using the Odds Ratio in Unmatched Analysis

If we use dichotomous measures of exposure and outcome, the results of an unmatched case-control study can be analyzed using the now familiar 2×2 contingency table as shown below.

	Outcome Status		
Exposure Status	**Cases**	**Controls**	
Exposed	a	b	a + b
Unexposed	c	d	c + d
	a + c	b + d	n

It is important to note that cumulative incidence rates in the exposed and unexposed groups, and hence the relative risk, cannot be derived from the above contingency table. This is because the ratio of cases (a + c) to controls (b + d) is seldom the same as the ratio of those with and without the study outcome in the source population. For example, when one selects 100 cases and 100 controls (a case to control ratio of 1:1) for a case-control study, this does not mean that there are an equal number of people with and without the study disease in the source population. More likely, the number of people in the source population with the study disease is far less than those without it (a ratio between 1:100 and 1:1,000 is more likely for most chronic diseases). Because the number of cases and controls is fixed at the beginning of a case-control study, a / (a + b) is not equivalent to the cumulative incidence rate among the exposed group, and c / (c + d) is not the same as the cumulative incidence rate among the unexposed group. Since the relative risk (RR) depends on these measures (i.e., RR = [a / (a + b)] / [c / (c + d)]), it cannot be calculated directly in a typical case-control study. Therefore, the usual measure of association in case-control studies is the *odds ratio* (OR), which does not depend on estimates of the incidence rates in the exposed and unexposed groups.

Though not always technically correct, many published case-control studies refer to the measure of association as the relative risk, and sometimes as the rate ratio. The OR approximates the *relative risk* and the *rate ratio* under the following conditions:[1, 3]

- incident cases are used,
- subject selection is unbiased, and
- the study outcome is rare.*

---

* Various suggestions have been offered in the literature for what constitutes a "rare" outcome. According to Last, an outcome with a cumulative incidence rate of less than 2 per 100 is a good rule of thumb to follow.[1]

Since most chronic diseases have relatively low incidence rates, it is not too difficult to meet these conditions when chronic diseases are being studied. The third condition, known as the **rare disease assumption**, is not necessary to approximate the relative risk when the controls are selected to represent the total population and not just those without the study disease. This is a very unusual way to select controls, however.[10] Also, the rare disease assumption is not necessary to approximate the rate ratio when:

- incident cases are used,
- subject selection is unbiased, and
- controls are selected from the same population as the cases and throughout the period during which the cases developed.

This latter requirement describes a method of sampling controls known as *density sampling*.[1]

Since the OR is a legitimate measure of association in itself, there is generally no need to depend on its approximation to other measures of association. However, when the OR can be used to estimate the relative risk, calculating *attributable risk percent* or *population attributable risk percent* (chapter 6) in a case-control study is greatly simplified.

The OR, which was discussed in chapter 6, is the usual measure of association in case-control studies. The OR can be calculated for unmatched studies using formula 6.5 in chapter 6. It is repeated here for convenience.

(Repeated 6.5)

$$OR = (a\ /\ c)\ /\ (b\ /\ d) = ad\ /\ bc$$

OR = 1 indicates no association between exposure and outcome. OR > 1 represents a positive association between exposure and outcome, and OR < 1 depicts an inverse association between exposure and outcome (i.e., the exposure is protective). The magnitude of the OR can be evaluated using the guidelines presented in figure 6–1.

Odds ratios can be interpreted in two ways. To illustrate, consider an association between smoking and heart disease where OR = 3.2. One could say that the odds of smoking are 3.2 times greater among those with heart disease compared to those without heart disease. This interpretation is based on a comparison of the *exposure odds* (i.e., the odds of exposure among cases and controls, respectively). Alternatively, one could say that the odds of heart disease are 3.2 times greater among smokers compared to nonsmokers. This interpretation is based on a comparison of the *disease odds* (i.e., the odds of the outcome among the exposed and unexposed, respectively). Since the derived formula for the OR (i.e., ad / bc) is the same whether the exposure odds or disease odds are used, either interpretation is acceptable.[2]

The statistical significance of the OR can be calculated using the chi-square test of independence shown in formula 10.4 and repeated here for convenience. The interpretation of the results of the chi-square can be found in table 10–3.

(Repeated 10.4)

$$\chi^2 = \frac{n\,(ad - bc)^2}{(a + b)\,(c + d)\,(a + c)\,(b + d)}$$

A 95% confidence interval for the OR can be estimated using the following method described by Barnet Woolf.[11] The letters a, b, c, and d refer to the frequencies in the contingency table shown at the beginning of this section.

(11.2)

$$95\% \text{ CI} = \exp\left[\ln(OR) \pm 1.96\,\sqrt{1/a + 1/b + 1/c + 1/d}\,\right]$$

Controlling Confounding

In general, potential confounding in a case-control study can be controlled by restriction or matching in the design stage or by statistical management in the analysis phase (see chapter 8). Control of potential confounding in the analysis phase is usually accomplished by stratification or multivariable methods. **Stratification** involves separating a sample into two or more subgroups according to specified levels of a third variable (e.g., the potentially confounding variable).[1] For example, to control for alcohol consumption in a study of the effect of cigarette smoking on automobile injuries, one might examine the association separately among drinkers and nondrinkers by calculating an odds ratio for each subgroup. These two subgroups represent two levels of stratification by drinking status, and the odds ratios represent the **stratum-specific odds ratios**. Since the stratum-specific odds ratios cannot be confounded by alcohol consumption (i.e., everyone in a subgroup has the same drinking status), they should be alike except for sampling error.* If confounding by alcohol consumption were present in the original relationship, we would expect the stratum-specific odds ratios to differ from the **crude odds ratio**, that is, the overall odds ratio prior to stratification. If there was no confounding, the odds ratios should all be similar. This is will be illustrated shortly.

The number of stratification levels may vary depending on the level of precision desired. The goal is to produce subgroups whose subjects are similar with regard to the potentially confounding factor. In the previous example, stratification on drinking status could have included several levels according to the number of drinks consumed per day if one thought that the degree of confounding varied depending on the amount of drinking. For example, drinking status might have been stratified by five levels (e.g., 0, 1–2, 3–4, 5–6, and more than 6 drinks per day). If stratification also included sex differences, then 10 categories would have been created (five categories for males plus five categories for females). If five age groups were also considered, then the number of stratification subgroups would rise to 50 ($10 \times 5 = 50$), producing 50 separate odds ratios to compare. It is easy to see that strat-

---

* Sampling error and small sample sizes can account for seemingly large differences in the stratum-specific odds ratios, which under ideal conditions would be the same if confounding were the only issue. Effect modification (described later) can also account for differences.

ification has it limits. As the number of subgroups increases, the analysis becomes more unwieldy, and the number of subjects in each subgroup decreases, which in turn reduces the power of the subgroup analyses, thereby increasing the potential for type II errors.

The increased potential for type II errors can be minimized by calculating the **Mantel-Haenszel odds ratio** (OR_{MH}), which is an overall combined measure of the stratum-specific odds ratios. In essence, it is a summary odds ratio *adjusted for* the stratification factor(s) and represents a weighted average of the stratum-specific odds ratios where the weights depend on the number of observations in each stratum.[12] For dichotomous levels of exposure and outcome, the OR_{MH} is calculated using the following formula described by Nathan Mantel and William Haenszel in 1959:[13]

(11.3)

$$OR_{MH} = \frac{\Sigma\,(a_i\,d_i\,/\,n_i)}{\Sigma\,(b_i\,c_i\,/\,n_i)}$$

To illustrate the use of this formula briefly, imagine two levels of stratification on a factor. For each level of the factor, a 2 x 2 contingency table is developed. The values in the cells of the first table are represented by a_1 through d_1 with a sum of n_1. The values in the cells of the second contingency table are represented by a_2 through d_2 with a sum of n_2. Therefore,

$$OR_{MH} = \frac{(a_1 d_1\,/\,n_1) + (a_2 d_2\,/\,n_2)}{(b_1 c_1\,/\,n_1) + (b_2 c_2\,/\,n_2)}$$

The OR_{MH} is an **adjusted odds ratio**. If it turns out that a given factor is not a confounder, the OR_{MH} will equal the crude odds ratio, but if the factor is a confounder, it will differ from the crude odds ratio to an extent depending on the degree and direction of confounding exhibited in the original relationship. Comparing the crude and adjusted odds ratios can be a more convenient way to determine if confounding is present than comparing the crude odds ratio to the stratum-specific odds ratios, especially if there are many of them.

The Mantel-Haenszel odds ratio should *not* be used to control for confounding when the stratum-specific odds ratios are not uniform; that is, when the differences in the stratum-specific odds ratios are not likely to be due only to sampling error. In these cases, a phenomenon known as *effect modification* may be occurring. This phenomenon should be described rather than controlled as discussed in the following section. A statistical test for significance of the OR_{MH} and an estimate of a 95% confidence interval are given in figure 11–3 on page 220. These measures may also be calculated using *Epi Info* (see appendix B).

Multivariable methods are efficient alternatives to stratification. These methods use specific mathematical models to analyze associations between exposure (an independent variable) and outcome (the dependent variable) while controlling simultaneously for potentially confounding factors. The most common type of multivariable analysis used in case-control studies is **multiple logistic regression**. Aside from its efficiency and convenience, this method is popular in analyzing data from case-control studies because the regression coefficients can be transformed easily into estimates of the odds ratios by calculating their exponentials.[14] For example, if a logistic regression coefficient is 0.724, the corresponding odds ratio would be 2.06 (exp (0.724) = 2.06). This is the odds ratio *adjusted* simultaneously for all the other independent variables in the model. Most output from computer application programs that provide logistic regression contains the logistic regression coefficients along with the adjusted odds ratios and their 95% confidence intervals. A detailed discussion of multivariable analysis is beyond the scope of this text. There are, however, many advanced epidemiology and biostatistics texts that discuss multivariable methods in more detail.

---

*Test of Significance**

$$\chi^2_{MH} = \frac{\{\Sigma a_i - \Sigma\,[(a_i + c_i)\,(a_i + b_i)\,/\,n_i]\}^2}{\Sigma\,(a_i + c_i)\,(b_i + d_i)\,(a_i + b_i)\,(c_i + d_i)\,/\,n_i^2\,(n_i - 1)}$$

95% Confidence Interval

$$95\% \text{ CI} = \exp\{\ln(OR_{MH})\,[1 \pm (1.96\,/\,\sqrt{\chi^2_{MH}})]\}$$

*Mantel-Haenszel chi-square test (χ^2_{MH}) with one degree of freedom based on contingency table analysis

Reference: Schlesselman, J. J. (1982). *Case-Control Studies: Design, Conduct, Analysis*. New York: Oxford University Press.

Figure 11–3 Test of significance and 95% confidence interval for the Mantel-Haenszel odds ratio (OR_{MH})

Identifying Effect Modification

Effect modification* occurs when the direction or magnitude of an association between the study exposure and outcome varies at different levels of a third factor.[8] This is perhaps most clearly seen in a stratified analysis. For example, assume the crude odds ratio for the relationship between exposure X and outcome Y is 3.0. When this relationship is stratified by sex, assume the stratum-specific odds ratios are 1.0 for females and 5.0 for males. This sug-

---

* Effect modification is a term popularized by Olli S. Miettinen in 1974.[15] Though widely used in epidemiology, some authors prefer to use the more common statistical term **interaction** (or statistical interaction). Although often used interchangeably, there is a subtle difference between these two terms. Effect modification refers to a real effect in the population, while interaction is a characteristic of the sample data, which only estimates what is occurring in the target population. For those interested in pursuing this topic see Kleinbaum, Kupper, and Morgenstern.[16] Effect modification or interaction can be additive or multiplicative and positive or negative as described by Szklo and Nieto.[14]

gests that sex is an *effect modifier*; that is, sex modifies the effect of X on Y differently depending the level of stratification. Among females, the odds of exposure to X is the same in cases and controls, but among males, the odds of exposure to X is five times greater in cases than controls. This implies that X is *not* a risk factor for Y among females but is a potentially significant risk factor among males. Thus, public health efforts to reduce Y by controlling X should target males over females.

Effect modification is distinct from confounding. Confounding is an annoyance that needs to be controlled so that we can get an accurate look at the relationship between an exposure and outcome. Effect modification, on the other hand, is a real effect that helps elucidate the relationship between an exposure and outcome in the presence of other factors. Therefore, it should always be described in a study.[8] When the subjects in a study are known to have risk factors for the outcome other than the study exposure, and these have not been controlled by restriction or pair matching, it is a good idea to perform a stratified analysis to evaluate whether these factors may be responsible for effect modification before attempting to control for potential confounding.

Although effect modification and confounding can occur together, effect modification should take priority in the sequence of analysis. The following steps should help determine if effect modification is likely:

- Observe the stratum-specific odds ratios to see if they differ materially in magnitude or direction, keeping in mind that odds ratios based on small sample sizes are more likely to be unstable.

- Consider whether effect modification makes biological sense based on other studies or evidence.

- Perform a **test of heterogeneity** to examine the probability that the stratum-specific odds ratios represent nonrandom differences. James J. Schlesselman illustrates the use of tests of heterogeneity.[2] Basically, these tests determine whether the stratum-specific odds ratios are significantly different.

If the evidence points to effect modification, the stratum-specific odds ratios and their 95% confidence intervals should be reported and discussed. It would not be appropriate to calculate a Mantel-Haenszel odds ratio, since this will mask the true variation in the stratum-specific odds ratios. If effect modification is unlikely, the Mantel-Haenszel odds ratio may be calculated. Effect modification also may be tested using multivariable methods, such as multiple logistic regression. Exhibit 11–2 on page 222 provides some hypothetical results from case-control studies employing stratification. Comparison of the crude odds ratio with the stratum-specific odds ratios provides a good indication of whether effect modification or confounding is present. When there are multiple levels of stratification and small numbers at each level, it may not be so clear whether effect modification or confounding is present without additional testing. Example 11–1 illustrates the use of stratification in a case-control study.

Exhibit 11–2 Examples of Confounding and Effect Modification in Case-Control Studies Using Stratification

Crude OR (OR$_C$)	Stratum-specific OR		Confounding	Effect Modification
	OR$_1$	OR$_2$		
4.00	4.00	4.00	None	Absent
3.50	1.05	1.04	Positive	Absent
1.00	2.50	2.48	Negative	Absent
2.75	1.10	6.35	None	Present
4.25	0.75	0.25	Positive	Present
2.00	1.00	1.10	Positive	Absent
3.75	0.75	2.85	Positive	Present
0.85	2.10	4.10	Negative	Present

In general, **confounding is present when** there is a difference between crude and adjusted odds ratios, that is, when:

$$OR_C \neq OR_1 = OR_2 \text{ or } OR_C \neq OR_{MH}$$

(Small differences in OR$_1$ and OR$_2$ are assumed to be due to random error.)

- If OR$_C$ > OR$_1$ = OR$_2$, the confounding is positive.
- If OR$_C$ < OR$_1$ = OR$_2$, the confounding is negative.

In general, **effect modification is present when** there is a difference between stratum-specific odds ratios, that is, when:

$$OR_1 \neq OR_2$$

(The difference should be more than random variation; differences in direction are most significant.)

In general, **confounding and effect modification are present when:**

$$OR_C < OR_1 \text{ and } OR_2, \text{ and } OR_1 \neq OR_2 \text{ or } OR_C > OR_1 \text{ and } OR_2, \text{ and } OR_1 \neq OR_2$$

Reference: Kleinbaum, D. G., Kupper, L. L., & Morgenstern, H. (1982). *Epidemiologic Research: Principles and Quantitative Methods.* Belmont, CA: Lifetime Learning Publications.

Example 11–1: Analysis of an Unmatched Case-Control Study

An epidemiologist wants to test the hypothesis that cigarette smoking increases the risk of fatal automobile injuries. To test his hypothesis, he selects 100 cases and 200 controls retrospectively from police and other official records in his county using random sampling procedures. Cases are county residents who died from injuries sustained in automobile crashes while driving with a valid driver's license. Controls are licensed drivers in the county, frequency matched to cases by age and sex. Interviews with spouses, friends, and co-workers of the cases and controls indicated that 68 of the cases and 104 of the controls were cigarette smokers. Based on this information, determine if the findings support the investigator's hypothesis.

During the study, data were also collected on the subjects' drinking habits. Of the 300 subjects studied, 192 (80 cases and 112 controls) were classified as drinkers. Of the cases who smoked, 58 were drinkers, and of the controls who smoked, 70 were drinkers. Based on this additional information, determine if drinking status is a confounder or effect modifier for this relationship.

Solution:

Step 1: Place the frequencies provided in the first part of the example in the appropriate cells of a 2 × 2 contingency table. Where there are missing values, calculate them from the data provided. For example, since there were 100 total cases, and 68 of these were cigarette smokers, the number of cases who did not smoke is 100 − 68 = 32. Likewise, the number of controls who did not smoke is 200 − 104 = 96.

Outcome Status

Exposure Status	Cases	Controls	
Smokers	68	104	172
Nonsmokers	32	96	128
	100	200	300

Step 2: Calculate the odds ratio from the contingency table using formula 6.5 repeated on page 217.

$$OR = ad / bc = (68 \times 96) / (104 \times 32) = 6{,}528 / 3{,}328 = 1.96$$

Step 3: Calculate the significance of the OR using the chi-square test of independence with one degree of freedom (formula 10.4).

$$\chi^2 = \frac{n\,(ad - bc)^2}{(a + b)\,(c + d)\,(a + c)\,(b + d)} =$$

$$300\,[(68 \times 96) - (104 \times 32)]^2 / (68 + 104)\,(32 + 96)\,(68 + 32)\,(104 + 96) =$$

$$300\,[(6{,}528) - (3{,}328)]^2 / (172)\,(128)\,(100)\,(200) =$$

$$300\,(3{,}200)^2 / 440{,}320{,}000 =$$

$$3{,}072{,}000{,}000 / 440{,}320{,}000 = 6.98$$

Since 6.98 is between 6.64 and 10.82, table 10–3 indicates that the chi-square is statistically significant at $p < 0.01$. Alternatively, we could have calculated the 95% confidence interval (CI) for the OR to determine the significance of the OR.

$$95\% \text{ CI} = \exp \left[\ln (\text{OR}) \pm 1.96 \sqrt{1/a + 1/b + 1/c + 1/d} \right] =$$
$$\exp \left[\ln (1.96) \pm 1.96 \sqrt{(1/68) + (1/104) + (1/32) + (1/96)} \right] =$$
$$\exp \left[0.67 \pm 1.96 \sqrt{(0.015) + (0.0096) + (0.031) + (0.010)} \right] =$$
$$\exp (0.67 \pm 1.96 \sqrt{0.066}) = \exp \left[0.67 \pm 1.96 (0.26) \right] = \exp (0.67 \pm 0.51) =$$
$$\exp (0.16), \exp (1.18) = 1.17, 3.25$$
$$95\% \text{ CI} = 1.17 - 3.25$$

Since the 95% confidence interval for the OR does not include the value one, the OR is statistically significant. At this point it appears that the hypothesis that cigarette smoking increases the risk of fatal automobile injuries is confirmed by the study. This is because the odds ratio shows a statistically significant relationship between cigarette smoking and fatal automobile injuries.

Step 4: To determine if drinking is a confounder or effect modifier for the association, one can stratify the analysis by drinking status as shown below.

	Outcome Status				Outcome Status	
Exposure Status	**Cases**	**Controls**		**Exposure Status**	**Cases**	**Controls**
Smokers	58	70		**Smokers**	10	34
Nonsmokers	22	42		**Nonsmokers**	10	54
	80	112	192		20	88	108

Stratum 1:	**Drinkers**	*Stratum 2:*	**Nondrinkers**

The values in the cells of the contingency tables are those provided in the problem or derived from those provided in the problem. For example, since the problem states that 68 of the cases are cigarette smokers and 58 of these are drinkers, it follows that the remaining 10 cases are nondrinkers (68 − 58 = 10). These cases are represented in the upper left-hand cell of the contingency table for nondrinkers. Also, since there are 100 cases and 80 are drinkers, there must be 20 nondrinkers among the cases (100 − 80 = 20), which is shown as the marginal total for the first column of the contingency table for nondrinkers.

Step 5: Calculate the odds ratio for each stratum using formula 6.5 (page 217) and compare them using the guidelines outlined in exhibit 11–2.

Drinkers:
OR = (58 × 42) / (70 × 22) = 2,436 / 1,540 = 1.58

Nondrinkers:
OR = (10 × 54) / (34 × 10) = 540 / 340 = 1.59

Since the stratum-specific odds ratios are nearly identical (1.58 and 1.59), but different from the crude odds ratio (1.96), confounding by drinking seems to be present (see exhibit 11–2). This is an example of positive confounding, since the crude odds ratio is apparently inflated because of a failure to account for confounding by drinking status. Based on the guidelines in exhibit 11–2, effect modification by drinking status does not appear to exist because the adjusted odds ratios are nearly identical.

Step 6: Since effect modification is not evident, a Mantel-Haenszel odds ratio (OR_{MH}) can be calculated using formula 11.3. The OR_{MH} is essentially a weighted average of the stratum-specific odds ratios that is influenced by sample size.

$$OR_{MH} = \Sigma\, (a_i\, d_i\, /\, n_i)\, /\, \Sigma\, (b_i\, c_i\, /\, n_i) =$$
$$\{[(58 \times 42)\, /\, 192] + [(10 \times 54)\, /\, 108]\}\, /\, \{[(70 \times 22)\, /\, 192] + [(34 \times 10)\, /\, 108]\} =$$
$$[(2{,}436\, /\, 192) + (540\, /\, 108)]\, /\, [(1{,}540\, /\, 192) + (340\, /\, 108)] =$$
$$(12.69 + 5.00)\, /\, (8.02 + 3.15) =$$
$$17.69\, /\, 11.17 = 1.58$$

Since there are more drinkers than nondrinkers in this problem, it is not surprising that the OR_{MH} is weighted toward the odds ratio among the drinkers (i.e., 1.58).

Answer: Based on the initial data, it appears that the hypothesis is supported by the study conducted in the county. That is, overall, cigarette smoking appears to be significantly associated with fatal automobile injuries (OR = 1.96, p < 0.01). Further analysis, however, reveals that the association is positively confounded by drinking status. That is, the overall OR is inflated due to a failure to adjust for drinking status. The adjusted OR of 1.58, therefore, provides a better estimate of the true association between cigarette smoking and fatal automobile injuries, assuming drinking status is the only confounder. Effect modification by drinking status is not apparent.

Comments:

1. An unmatched analysis is appropriate for this problem because pair matching was not employed. Frequency matching was used, but it does not require a matched analysis.

2. Since the outcome measure is death, we can be assured that the cases represent incident cases, which is desirable in a case-control study. Also, the exposure occurred prior to the outcome, which is the temporal sequence necessary to make statements about risk or causation.

3. This is a population-based case-control study since cases and controls were not selected from clinical facilities but directly from the county population. Since selection was random, it is reasonable to believe that the subjects are representative of licensed drivers in the county.

4. The crude odds ratio is 1.96. This is an estimate of the overall measure of association between exposure and outcome in the target population. Like a crude rate (chapter 6), the crude odds ratio (OR_C) may conceal confounding by other factors.

5. The stratum-specific odds ratios are calculated in the same manner as the crude odds ratio. The difference is that they represent odds ratios only for subgroups of a study population.

6. Because there was confounding in the association, the OR_{MH} of 1.58 is the appropriate measure of association to report. This says that odds of cigarette smoking are 1.58 times greater in drivers involved in fatal automobile injuries compared to those not involved in fatal automobile injuries *after adjusting for drinking status*. Alternatively, we could say, the odds of being involved in a fatal automobile injury is 1.58 times greater among cigarette smokers than non-cigarette smokers after adjusting for drinking status. Thus, the OR_{MH} is an adjusted odds ratio, and in this case it is the odds ratio adjusted for drinking status. Since the OR_{MH} is greater than one, it implies that there is still an association between cigarette smoking and fatal automobile injuries after accounting for drinking status, although it is not as strong as the OR_C indicated. In other words, the confounding by drinking status is only partial. If the overall association were entirely due to confounding by drinking status, the OR_{MH} would be one, implying no association between cigarette smoking and fatal automobile injuries.

7. Though not done in this problem, one would normally calculate whether the adjusted OR (i.e., the OR_{MH}) is itself statistically significant (or provide a 95% confidence interval). Formulas for doing this are provided in figure 11–3, but they can be rather cumbersome to use. It is easier to use a statistical package like *Epi Info* (see appendix B). Using *Epi Info*, it turns out that the OR_{MH} of 1.58 is not statistically significant (p > 0.05). The 95% confidence interval for the OR_{MH} is 0.91–2.77 based on exact confidence limits. Thus, it appears that the hypothesis that cigarette smoking is related to fatal automobile injuries is *not* supported by the study conducted in the county. While the crude odds ratio indicates a statistically significant relationship between cigarette smoking and fatal automobile injuries in the county, the association is not significant after adjustment for drinking status. This nonsignificant finding, however, is most likely due to low power. In the overall analysis, the power to detect a significant OR as low as 1.96 is 71.5% based on calculations using *Epi Info*. The power to detect a significant OR_{MH} as low as 1.58, however, is just 39.75%. This means that the probability of a type II error is a surprisingly high 60.25% or 0.6025 (i.e., $1 - 0.3975 = 0.6025$)! To increase the power to 90% power would require a sample size in excess of 900. One criticism of the study represented by this example is that power was apparently not determined before deciding on sample size.

Summary

- Case-control studies can be exploratory or analytic. Only analytic studies, however, test specific a priori hypotheses about associations between exposure and outcome. Case-control studies are conducted by determining outcome status (case and control groups) before determining exposure status.

- Many factors should be considered in designing case-control studies. There should be a proper temporal sequence between exposure and outcome; cases should be defined precisely to exclude noncases; controls should be comparable to cases, especially with regard to the potential for past exposure; exposure status should be assessed in the same manner for cases and controls; adequate power should be assured by determining the minimum sample size needed to detect clinically important differences; and the results should be properly analyzed and interpreted.

- One of the most crucial elements in the design of case-control studies is the selection of controls. Controls should come from the same source population as the cases to minimize the potential for selection bias. Exclusions or restrictions placed on cases should also be applied to controls. In population-based studies, controls are usually selected randomly from the source population. In hospital-based studies, controls are generally selected from patients with a variety of other diagnoses unrelated to the study exposure.

- Case-control studies can be analyzed using a matched or unmatched analysis depending on whether or not pair matching was used in the study design. Since incidence rates among exposed and unexposed groups generally cannot be determined in case-control studies, the odds ratio is the usual measure of association. When certain conditions hold, the odds ratio will approximate the relative risk or the rate ratio.

New Terms

adjusted odds ratio
biomarker
blinding
clinical significance
crude odds ratio
effect modification
exploratory case-
   control study
hospital controls
hospital-based
   case-control study

interaction
Mantel-Haenszel
   odds ratio
matched case-
   control study
multiple logistic
   regression
multivariable methods
population controls
population-based
   case-control study

population-based
   disease registry
practical significance
rare disease assumption
source population
stratification
stratum-specific odds ratio
test of heterogeneity
unmatched case-control
   study

Study Questions and Exercises

1. Obtain a copy of the following article: MacMahon, B., Yen, S., Trichopoulos, D., Warren, K., and Nardi, G. (1981). Coffee and Cancer of the Pancreas. *New England Journal of Medicine* 304 (11): 630–633. Critique the study in terms of the validity of its design, conduct, and analysis.

2. A case-control study using two controls per case was designed to test the hypothesis that lack of regular exercise (the exposure) increases the risk of bone fractures (the outcome) in elderly women. Of the 600 women studied (200 cases and 400 controls), 128 were regular exercisers (26 cases and 102 controls). Based on this information, determine if there is a statistical association between a lack of regular exercise and bone fractures in this group. Report the crude odds ratio, the value of the test of significance and its associated p-value, and the 95% confidence interval for the odds ratio. Also, interpret the odds ratio in words.

3. The investigators of the study described in the previous problem also collected data on the women's dietary habits, including average daily intake of calcium. Of those who did not exercise regularly, 50 of the cases and 112 of the controls had diets deficient in calcium. Of those who exercised regularly, 7 of the cases and 49 of the controls had diets deficient in calcium. The remainder of the subjects had diets adequate in calcium. Based on this information, use stratification to determine if calcium intake is a confounder or effect modifier for the relationship between lack of regular exercise and bone fractures, and explain why or why not. Also, report the odds ratio for each stratum along with the stratum-specific chi-square values and their associated p-values.

4. A case-control study was designed to see if body piercing by unlicensed merchants was associated with an increased risk of hepatitis B compared

to those receiving piercing from licensed merchants. Cases with clinically diagnosed hepatitis B were pair matched to controls without hepatitis B by age, sex, and number of previous body piercings. The results of the study appear in the contingency table below.

Control

Case	Exposed	Unexposed	
Exposed	96	23	119
Unexposed	14	87	101
	110	110	220

Based on this information, calculate the applicable odds ratio, the 95% confidence interval, and the significance of the odds ratio based on the applicable chi-square test. Be sure to use a matched analysis. Interpret your findings.

References

1. Last, J. M., ed. (1995). *A Dictionary of Epidemiology*. New York: Oxford University Press.
2. Schlesselman, J. J. (1982). *Case-control Studies: Design, Conduct, Analysis*. New York: Oxford University Press.
3. Kelsey, J. L., Thompson, W. D., and Evans, A. S. (1986). *Methods in Observational Epidemiology*. New York: Oxford University Press.
4. MacMahon, B., and Trichopoulos, D. (1996). *Epidemiology: Principles and Methods*. Boston: Little, Brown and Company.
5. Gill, J. S., Zezulka, A. V., Shipley, M. J., Gill, S. K., and Beevers, D. G. (1986). Stroke and Alcohol Consumption. *The New England Journal of Medicine* 315(17): 1041–1046.
6. World Health Organization (1992). *International Statistical Classification of Diseases and Related Health Problems, Tenth Revision*. Geneva: World Health Organization.
7. Wacholder, S., McLaughlin, J. K., Silverman, D. T., and Mandel, J. S. (1992). Selection of Controls in Case-Control Studies, I. Principles. *American Journal of Epidemiology* 135(9): 1019–1028.
8. Hennekens, C. H., and Buring, J. E. (1987). *Epidemiology in Medicine*. Boston: Little, Brown and Company.
9. Wacholder, S., Silverman, D. T., McLaughlin, J. K., and Mandel, J. S. (1992). Selection of Controls in Case-Control Studies, II. Types of Controls. *American Journal of Epidemiology* 135(9): 1029–1041.
10. Kahn, H. A., and Sempos, C. T. (1989). *Statistical Methods in Epidemiology*. New York: Oxford University Press.
11. Woolf, B. (1955). On Estimating the Relation Between Blood Group and Disease. *Annals of Human Genetics* 19: 251–253.
12. Elwood, J. M. (1988). *Causal Relationships in Medicine: A Practical System for Critical Appraisal*. New York: Oxford University Press.
13. Mantel, N., and Haenszel, W. (1959). Statistical Aspects of the Analysis of Data from Retrospective Studies of Disease. *Journal of the National Cancer Institute* 22: 719–748.
14. Szklo, M., and Nieto, F. J. (2000). *Epidemiology: Beyond the Basics*. Gaithersburg, MD: Aspen.
15. Miettinen, O. S. (1974). Confounding and Effect Modification. *American Journal of Epidemiology* 100:350–353.
16. Kleinbaum, D. G., Kupper, L. L., and Morgenstern, H. (1982). *Epidemiologic Research: Principles and Quantitative Methods*. Belmont, CA: Lifetime Learning Publications.

CHAPTER TWELVE

Prospective and Retrospective Cohort Studies

Learning Objectives

▸ Differentiate between prospective and retrospective cohort studies.

▸ Compare and contrast the advantages and disadvantages of cohort studies.

▸ Discuss the key design features of prospective and retrospective cohort studies as they relate to selection of the cohort and assessment of exposure and outcome status.

▸ Select, calculate, and interpret the appropriate measures of association, 95% confidence intervals, and the appropriate chi-square tests of significance in cohort studies using cumulative and person-time incidence rates, respectively.

▸ Explain the need for and basic approaches to estimating study power, controlling for potential confounding, and ascertaining effect modification in cohort studies.

▸ Define cohort, internal and external comparison groups, historical prospective cohort study, and Mantel-Haenszel relative risk.

Overview

There are two major types of cohort studies—prospective and retrospective. Both types follow a cohort over time to determine the incidence of the outcome among the exposed and unexposed groups. Prospective designs follow subjects from the study initiation to sometime in the future. Retrospective designs follow subjects from sometime in the past up to the present. Advantages of cohort studies include a clear temporal sequence between exposure and outcome, the possibility of studying multiple outcomes, and their usefulness in studying rare exposures. Disadvantages include the potential need for large sample sizes and losses to follow-up. If well designed, cohort studies provide strong support for causal associations. Analysis and interpretation of cohort studies depends on the type of incidence rates used.

Introduction

Cohort studies were introduced in chapter 4, and their basic design is illustrated in figures 4–4 and 4–5. One way these studies differ from other major analytic studies has to do with the sequence in which exposure and outcome status are determined. For example, in cross-sectional studies exposure and outcome are determined *simultaneously*, and in case-control studies outcome is determined *before* exposure. In cohort studies, however, exposure is determined *before* outcome. This is true for both major types of cohort studies—prospective cohort studies (PCSs) and retrospective (or historical) cohort studies (RCSs).*

While the sequence of exposure–outcome assessment is the same in RCSs and PCSs, there are some important differences between these two approaches. In a PCS the exposure status of the subjects is determined at the beginning of the study before any outcomes have occurred. Subjects' outcome status is then determined during follow-up into a future time period. The length of the study takes into account the outcome's incubation or latency period (see chapter 3). In an RCS, since outcomes have already occurred, the exposure status of the subjects is determined for a time period that existed in the past, and subjects' outcome status is determined during a subsequent time period up to the present. This strategy maintains the proper sequence of exposure–outcome assessment as illustrated in figures 4–4 and 4–5.

Both study types involve the formation of a **cohort**, which is a group of individuals who are followed over time. Thus, the cohort is comprised of the subjects of a cohort study. In a PCS the cohort is identified at the beginning of the study and followed into the future. In an RCS the cohort is historical; that is, it is constructed on paper, so to speak, as it once existed in the past. It is then traced from that time up to the present. Formation of a historical cohort depends on having access to appropriate historical records or documents that will allow the investigators to identify the subjects and their exposure status. Subjects' outcome status is then ascertained by consulting appropriate sources, such as death certificates, disease registries, and medical records.

Both types of cohort studies are *longitudinal studies* in that there is follow-up from an earlier to a later time period. When the exposure is considered a potential *risk factor* for the outcome, the expectation is that the exposed group will develop the study outcome at a greater rate than the unexposed group (i.e., there will be a positive association between exposure and outcome). On the other hand, when the exposure is suspected of being protective, it is hypothesized that the exposed group will develop the outcome at a lower rate than the unexposed group (i.e., there will be an inverse association between exposure and outcome). Cohort studies provide a good illustration of what is meant by an *observational study* (chapter 4) because

---

* Other names commonly applied to these types of studies can be found in table 4–1. Although not discussed here, another type of cohort study is the **historical prospective cohort study**, which is a combination of retrospective and prospective cohort designs. This type of study identifies a historical cohort and then follows it up into the future.

after identifying the exposed and unexposed groups, the investigators simply allow nature to take its course while recording outcomes as they occur. No intervention is applied, nor is there any attempt to manipulate the conditions of the study.

This chapter discusses the major advantages and disadvantages of cohort studies, outlines some of the important design considerations, and presents basic methods of analyzing and interpreting the study findings. In general, well-designed cohort studies provide the most definitive evidence possible from observational studies to support causal associations. They are only surpassed in this regard by experimental designs in epidemiology, which are the subject of chapter 13.

Advantages and Disadvantages of Cohort Studies

Advantages

Well-designed cohort studies offer a number of advantages. First, they clearly demonstrate an appropriate temporal sequence between exposure and outcome. Since exposure is determined *first* and in a time period *preceding* assessment of outcome, it is easier to ascribe the outcome to the exposure than it is in studies where the temporal sequence is more difficult to determine. You will recall that it is essential for exposure to precede outcome in order to demonstrate causal associations (see chapter 7). Of all the analytic studies discussed in this text, the cohort study best meets this criterion.

A second advantage of cohort studies is that they permit the direct calculation of incidence rates in both the exposed and unexposed groups. This makes it easy to calculate risk or rate ratios (or differences) as needed. Third, these studies permit multiple outcomes to be assessed in the same study. The Framingham Heart Study, for example, has been used to examine multiple outcomes in addition to heart disease, including seemingly unrelated conditions like gout and gallbladder disease.[1, 2] Fourth, they provide an indication of the incubation or latency period for communicable or noncommunicable diseases, respectively.[3] Fifth, they can be used to study exposures that are relatively uncommon. Because exposure status is determined first, cohort studies can be designed to assure that there are an adequate number of exposed and unexposed subjects at the study outset. This is not possible in case-control studies because exposure status is assessed after the subjects (cases and controls) have already been selected. Finally, since exposure status is determined *before* outcome, there is no opportunity for knowledge of a subject's outcome status to influence how exposure is assessed. In other words, one would not expect to encounter *exposure suspicion bias* (see chapter 8) in a properly designed cohort study.

Disadvantages

Some of the disadvantages of PCSs include potential large sample size requirements, long follow-up periods, and a need to reassess exposure on a frequent basis. Due to the relatively low incidence and long latency periods for many chronic diseases, sometimes thousands of subjects must be enrolled and followed for years or even decades in order to generate enough cases for valid statistical comparisons. In addition, where exposure status can change during the course of follow-up, periodic reassessments of exposure status are necessary. Also, outcomes must be determined as they develop. The Nurses' Health Study, for example, established a cohort in 1976 consisting of 121,700 female registered nurses from 11 states. Periodic follow-up to assess current exposure and outcome status has been conducted every two years since that time.[4] Because of these issues, the expense and resources necessary to conduct PCSs of chronic diseases can be substantial compared to other types of analytic studies. These disadvantages can be offset somewhat by employing RCSs, since the follow-up period has already occurred.[5] Retrospective cohort studies may not always be feasible, however, due to problems of identifying a suitable cohort or determining accurate exposure levels. These disadvantages may also be less of a problem in PCSs designed to study acute outcomes because of the shorter follow-up periods.

Another disadvantage of cohort studies is potential losses to follow-up. If a significant portion of the cohort is lost to follow-up, the study results could be biased. *Loss to follow-up bias*, a type of selection bias, was discussed in chapter 8. It can present a problem in both prospective and retrospective cohort studies. A further disadvantage is potential exposure misclassification, which can result in measurement bias (chapter 8). This can occur, for example, in PCSs when subjects change their exposure status during the follow-up period. If the investigators do not take the changes into account, the study results may be biased. Therefore, periodic reassessments of exposures that can change are important in PCSs. Exposure misclassification can also be an issue in determining exposure status in RCSs, since exposure is often determined from historical records that may be incomplete or inaccurate.

Another disadvantage of cohort studies is possible outcome misclassification. Advances in the ability to detect a particular disease during the course of follow-up may bring prior classifications of outcome status into question and lead to incorrect study results. Also, *diagnostic suspicion bias* (chapter 8) is possible in cohort studies to the extent that knowledge of a subject's exposure status influences the accuracy with which outcome status is determined. If the investigator is more likely to classify the exposed as having the study outcome than the unexposed, simply because he or she believes the exposure causes the outcome, diagnostic suspicion bias will result.[6] Table 12–1 summarizes the major advantages and disadvantages of cohort studies. While these advantages and disadvantages are meant to apply to cohort studies in general, some may be more applicable to PCSs and some to RCSs, respectively. Many also apply to other study types.

The remainder of this chapter deals with some important design considerations and the basic methods of analysis and interpretation of the findings from cohort studies. For simplicity, exposure status is treated as being dichotomous (i.e., exposed or unexposed). Some cohort studies may identify and compare various levels of exposure as opposed to just exposed and unexposed groups. The underlying principles, however, should be the same in either case. Because of some important differences in design considerations, prospective and retrospective cohort studies are discussed separately in the next few sections.

Table 12–1 Major Advantages and Disadvantages of Cohort Studies

Advantages	Disadvantages
1. They demonstrate a clear and appropriate temporal sequence between exposure and outcome.	1. Large sample sizes and long follow-up periods may be required to study diseases with long latency periods and low incidence (i.e., most chronic diseases), thereby increasing study complexity and cost.
2. They permit direct calculation of incidence rates in exposed and unexposed groups.	
3. They allow multiple outcomes to be evaluated in the same study.	2. There is a greater potential for loss to follow-up bias than in other analytic studies.
4. They provide an indication of the incubation or latency period for the outcome.	3. There is a potential for exposure misclassification due to changes in exposure during the follow-up period or because of inadequate information in retrospective designs.
5. They are suitable for studying rare exposures.	
6. Determination of outcome status is unlikely to bias the determination of exposure status.	4. There is a potential for outcome misclassification when advances in disease detection during the follow-up phase bring earlier classifications into question or when knowledge of exposure status biases the assessment of outcome status.
7. They can help in establishing cause–effect relationships if properly executed.	

Selecting the Cohort

Prospective Cohort Studies

Ordinarily, potential subjects for a PCS must meet at least two criteria in order to be eligible to participate: (a) they must be *free* from the study outcome, and (b) they must be *at risk* of developing the study outcome. To ensure these criteria are met, potential subjects need to be examined for current *and* prior outcome status before they are enrolled in the study. Because large numbers of individuals may need to be tested, only the most efficient screening or diagnostic methods should be used. Determining if potential subjects are at risk of the study outcome may be fairly straightforward for infectious diseases where serum antibody levels can be measured.[7] It can be more problematic with noninfectious diseases, however, since one may have to rely on individual recall or available medical records to determine disease history. Recall can be faulty, and medical records may be inaccurate or incomplete. Also, other factors may affect whether or not one is at risk of the study outcome. It is quite obvious, for example, that women should not be included as subjects in a study of the effects of diet on prostate cancer, since women do not have a prostate gland and cannot possibly be at risk. Likewise, women who have undergone a hysterectomy should not be included in a study of uterine cancer.

Possible sources of subjects for PCSs are numerous, and include general population samples, specific occupational groups, and members of prepaid health insurance plans or other large groups, such as the military, schools, unions, or church denominations. The Framingham Heart Study, for example, used a representative sample of adults residing in Framingham, Massachusetts, as its cohort.[8] Cohorts may be selected based on several factors, including how representative they are of the target population, expectations that they will participate for the entire length of the study, the quality or accessibility of exposure data, or simply convenience. Of course, findings from samples that are unrepresentative of the general population may be difficult to generalize.[7]

Sometimes a cohort is selected because it is known or suspected to be at high risk of the study outcome. If the study outcome is rare, selecting a high-risk group may be the only way of assuring that an adequate number of outcomes will develop for comparison purposes. For example, one might want to restrict a PCS of risk factors for cataracts to elderly individuals since this group is at higher risk of developing cataracts. Also, one might select a highly exposed group when exposure levels are relatively low in general population samples. Studies of the link between benzene and aplastic anemia, for example, have focused on occupational cohorts that work with the solvent since most individuals in the general population are not exposed to levels of benzene likely to be associated with this condition.

Generally, the *comparison group* in a PCS is represented by the unexposed portion of the cohort. This group is known as an **internal comparison group**, since it represents members of the original cohort. When the subjects are highly exposed individuals, however, it may not be possible to identify a suitable internal comparison group, since everyone is expected to have high levels of exposure to the factor being studied. In this and other instances, an **external comparison group** may be employed. An external comparison group is a group outside the original cohort that is used for comparison purposes. External comparison groups may include general population samples in the same geographic area with similar demographic characteristics as the exposed group, unexposed workers in the same industry as the exposed group (e.g., office workers in a pesticide manufacturing plant), and groups in similar but different occupations. An example of the latter might be hydroelectric plant workers when the exposed group is nuclear plant workers in a study of the effects of long-term, low-level radiation exposure on mortality rates.

> *The most critical point in selecting an external comparison group is that it must be as similar as possible to the exposed group in all regards except for the exposure(s) under study.*

Similarity between an external comparison group and the exposed group may sometimes be achieved by matching on relevant variables or controlling for potential confounders in the analysis. It is incumbent upon the investigators to have a good rationale for the comparison group selected, since selection bias may be an issue. A general population sample may not be a good comparison group to use, for instance, because it may include a portion who are exposed to the factor under investigation, thereby introducing a negative bias (chapter 8) in the results. Also, if a general population sample is compared to an occupational cohort, the healthy worker effect (chapter 8) may be operating. Sometimes PCSs utilize more than one external comparison group or a combination of internal and external comparison groups. This approach can increase the validity of the study if the results tend to be relatively consistent among the groups being compared.

Retrospective Cohort Studies

Selecting a cohort for an RCS proceeds in much the same fashion as that for a PCS. Because the cohort is historical, however, some unique issues must be considered. Jennifer L. Kelsey, W. Douglas Thompson, and Alfred S. Evans describe four important considerations.[7] First, the cohort must represent a group for which a large number of individuals have been exposed to the study factor. Second, a sufficient number of these individuals must have been exposed to high enough levels of the factor that an adequate number of outcomes are likely to have occurred. Third, there must be a sufficiently accurate source of existing data on exposure levels. Fourth, it must be possible to identify an appropriate comparison group. The comparison group is usually an external comparison group that is selected in a manner similar to that discussed for PCSs. In addition to the above considerations, it is important to have available sources from which to identify potentially confounding factors in the study and comparison groups, so that they can be controlled appropriately. Unfortunately, these sources are not always available, or if available, they are not always reliable.

Determining Exposure Status

Prospective Cohort Studies

With regard to determining *exposure status*, the sources or methods chosen in a particular study should be guided by considerations of accuracy, completeness, and practicality. Some of the more commonly used sources and methods to determine exposure are listed in table 12–2 on page 238. In general, because questionnaires and interviews rely on self-reported data, they may not always elicit accurate or complete responses, especially if the exposure relates to sensitive areas, such as illegal drug use or sexual behaviors. On the other hand, questionnaires or interviews may be the only possible ways to collect information that is not recorded elsewhere or that cannot be determined readily by testing. Also, questionnaires and interviews may provide a means of obtaining data on potential confounders that is not possible with other methods.[9]

The use of other modes of obtaining exposure data, such as existing records, physical examinations, body specimens, or environmental testing, will depend on the specific circumstances of the study. Body specimens, such as blood tests for elevated cholesterol levels, are highly objective means of determining exposure status but obviously cannot be used when the exposures of interest are variables like marital status, birth order, or seat belt use. Existing medical and other records may be convenient, but they may not always be complete or accurate for all members of the cohort, including the comparison group. Tests for environmental exposures, such as tests for radon gas concentrations in homes, may also be objective means of determining exposure status, but they may not give an accurate idea of the amount of exposure actually absorbed by the individual. The amount of radon absorption from a given concentration in the home, for example, may vary due to the behaviors of the subjects, such as how much time is spent in the home and the extent to which windows are opened for ventilation. In general, it is desirable to validate exposure status by using more than one data source whenever possible. Many studies of the effects of cigarette smoking, for instance, have queried subjects about smoking status using questionnaires or interviews, while taking blood measurements of cotinine, a *biomarker* (see chapter 11) for exposure to cigarette smoke.

Another issue relevant to exposure assessment in PCSs is change in exposure status during the follow-up period. In general, unless the exposure status is not subject to modification (e.g., blood type), it should be reassessed periodically to account for any changes. The frequency of reassessment will depend to some extent on the likelihood of change and the costs of reassessment. Where changes have occurred investigators can take this into consideration in the analysis of the data. For example, investigators at the University of Massachusetts, who studied the possible relationship between alcohol consumption and cataracts in female registered nurses, reassessed alcohol consumption status via questionnaires every two years during the 12 years of follow-up.[10] Because person-years (see chapter 5) constituted the denominators of the calculated incidence rates in the exposed and unexposed groups, it was possible to account for changes in exposure status during the study period. For example, if a subject was classified as a drinker for the first six years of the study and then gave up drinking for the remaining six years, that subject would have contributed only six person-years of risk to the exposed group, assuming she had not developed cataracts within the first six years. By the way, the investigators in this study found no general relationship between alcohol intake and the development of cataracts.[10]

Retrospective Cohort Studies

Determining exposure status in RCSs presents some unique problems, and, therefore, not all of the methods of exposure assessment listed in table 12–2 will be applicable in these studies. Questionnaires and interviews will have very limited use in RCSs due to the historical nature of the cohort. In some instances, close contacts who knew the subjects well may be questioned about the subjects' exposure. For many RCSs, however, past employment or company medical records will be the only available means by which to classify subjects on exposure status. These sources may not always be ideal, however, because of incomplete or inaccurate data that can increase the probability of exposure misclassification and, hence, measurement bias. In many cases, investigators may have to rely on job titles or other uncertain means of deduction to classify subjects on exposure status. A classic example is the study of the relationship of asbestos to lung cancer, which assumed that shipbuilders were exposed to the asbestos that was used to line the interior of the ship hulls. It is possible, however, that some of the shipbuilders actually had little or no contact with asbestos.

In some retrospective (and prospective) cohort studies, birth records are used as a source of information about exposure status. For example, an RCS conducted at Vanderbilt University in Nashville used birth certificates to classify the subjects on exposure status.[11] The study examined the relationship between certain maternal and child characteristics recorded on the birth certificates and mortality from community-acquired infections. The cohort for the study consisted of children who were less than five years old between 1985 and 1994. The authors found that children with three or more brothers and sisters and a birth weight of less than 1,500 grams had an approximate twentyfold increased risk of death from infection.

In some RCSs it may be impossible to estimate exposure status due to a lack of valid and reliable information. In these instances an RCS simply cannot be completed. In those rare circumstances where accurate data on past exposure have been collected for some reason, there should be few impediments to proceeding with an RCS.[7] One problem, however, that plagues many RCSs is the unavailability of specific data on potential confounders. This, of course, can lead to erroneous conclusions about the associations between exposure and outcome.

Determining Outcome Status

Prospective Cohort Studies

With regard to determining *outcome status*, accuracy, completeness, and practicality are again the major considerations. Outcome status should be determined using valid and reliable methods; the methods should be applied equally to exposed and unexposed subjects; and the methods should be acceptable to those being studied. Table 12–2 lists some of the more common methods of outcome assessment used in PCSs. When conclusive diagnostic tests are available and affordable, these may be the best methods to use. Depending on the outcome of interest, other methods may be suitable. For example, if the outcome of interest is a particular cancer, and a population-based cancer registry is available for that cancer, it would be a good source to consider for outcome assessment.

If the outcome is overall mortality, then death certificates may be an appropriate source from which to determine outcome status, since the

Table 12–2 Common Sources and Methods of Determining Exposure and Outcome Status in Cohort Studies

Exposure Status	Outcome Status
• Medical records	• Medical records
• Employment records	• Disease registries
• Birth records	• Death certificates
• Questionnaires	• Questionnaires
• Interviews	• Interviews
• Physical examinations	• Physical examinations
• Body specimens (blood tests, urine tests, etc.)	• Diagnostic tests
• Environmental tests	

reporting of deaths is nearly complete in the United States. Death certificates or databases derived from death certificates are generally less reliable for determining *specific* causes of death, however, because of possible recording errors or omissions. If the outcome has a high case-fatality rate, is rapidly fatal, and easily diagnosed, death certificates may be acceptable. Certain cancers fit these criteria (e.g., lung cancer), while many other chronic diseases (e.g., chronic bronchitis or diabetes) do not.[7] Thus, lung cancer is more likely to be reported on a death certificate as the *underlying cause of death* (see exhibit 2–1) than chronic bronchitis because it has a higher case fatality rate and is more rapidly fatal. Where possible, it is a good idea to use several sources of data for cross-validation purposes. As in case-control studies (chapter 11), it is also important to have strict criteria for diagnosis of the outcome that are determined *before* the study is initiated. These criteria should be widely accepted and verifiable.

Retrospective Cohort Studies

Assessment of outcome status for the subjects in an RCS usually relies on existing sources of data collected for other purposes. Some possible sources include death certificates, disease registries, and available medical records. The limitations of death certificates have already been discussed. Available medical records may vary in quality, completeness, or comparability. Interviews and questionnaires may be used if the survivors can be located and queried about their experiences relative to the study outcome. It will also be necessary, however, to find equally reliable data on those who have died or cannot be reached.

In general, investigators have a more difficult task identifying suitable sources of outcome data in RCSs compared to PCSs. In both types of studies, however, it is incumbent upon the investigators to use the same or equally accurate methods of assessing outcome for both the study and comparison groups if the results are to be valid. This is can be an issue when an external comparison group is used, since the data sources may be different for the two groups.

Analysis of Cohort Studies

The fundamental measure of disease outcome in a cohort study is the incidence rate. In fact, the type of incidence rate employed in a cohort study will determine the appropriate measure of association. If the *cumulative incidence rate* is used, the appropriate measure of association will be the relative risk (risk ratio) or the risk difference (or attributable risk). This is because these measures are calculated from the cumulative incidence rates in the exposed and unexposed groups (see chapter 6). Similarly, if the *person-time incidence rate* is used, the measure of association will be the rate ratio or the rate difference (or attributable rate). This is because these measures are calculated from the person-time incidence rates in the exposed and unexposed groups. The odds ratio is sometimes used as a measure of association in cohort studies when it is convenient to do so. Some multivariable methods of analysis, such as multiple logistic regression, generate odds ratios; therefore, odds ratios are more likely to be reported in these cases because of their ready availability. The use of the odds ratio was discussed in chapter 11 in relation to case-control studies where it is most commonly employed. It is not discussed further in this chapter. Since the two basic methods of analyzing cohort studies depend on the types of incidence rates used, they are discussed separately in the following two sections.

Analysis Based on Cumulative Incidence Rates

On the most basic level, cohort studies employing cumulative incidence rates can be analyzed using a standard 2 × 2 contingency table in a manner analogous to that used in cross-sectional studies (chapter 10).

	Outcome Status		
Exposure Status	**Present**	**Absent**	
Exposed	a	b	a + b
Unexposed	c	d	c + d
	a + c	b + d	n

If the results of a cohort study employing cumulative incidence rates are placed in a contingency table like the one shown above, it will be fairly simple to calculate measures of association based on risk (e.g., relative risk or risk difference). Unlike in case-control studies, in cohort studies cumulative incidence rates can be calculated directly from the data in the contingency table. This is possible because $a / (a + b)$ represents the actual proportion of cases that developed among the exposed group, and $c / (c + d)$ represents the actual proportion of cases that developed among the unexposed group. When multiplied by an appropriate rate base, these are the cumulative incidence rates in the exposed and unexposed groups. Thus, we can use them to calculate relative risk and risk difference (or attributable risk). These and other useful formulas are depicted in table 12–3.

Table 12–3 Common Measures Used in Cohort Studies Based on Cumulative Incidence Rates

---

Overall Cumulative Incidence Rate: $IR_C = [(a + c) / n] \times 10^n$

Cumulative Incidence Rate among the Exposed Group: $IR_{C\text{-}e} = [a / (a + b)] \times 10^n$

Cumulative Incidence Rate among the Unexposed Group: $IR_{C\text{-}ue} = [c / (c + d)] \times 10^n$

Relative Risk (or Risk Ratio): $RR = IR_{C\text{-}e} / IR_{C\text{-}ue} = \{[a / (a + b)] \times 10^n\} / \{[c / (c + d)] \times 10^n\}$

Attributable Risk (or Risk Difference): $AR = IR_{C\text{-}e} - IR_{C\text{-}ue} = \{[a / (a + b)] \times 10^n\} - \{[c / (c + d)] \times 10^n\}$

Attributable Risk Percent: $AR\% = [(IR_{C\text{-}e} - IR_{C\text{-}ue}) / IR_{C\text{-}e}] \times 100 = \quad \{[a / (a + b)] \times 10^n - [c / (c + d)] \times 10^n\} / \{[a / (a + b)] \times 10^n\}_{\|} \times 100$

Population Attributable Risk: $Pop\ AR = IR_C - IR_{C\text{-}ue} \{[(a + c) / n] \times 10^n\} - \{[c / (c + d)] \times 10^n\}$

Population Attributable Risk Percent: $Pop\ AR\% = [(IR_C - IR_{C\text{-}ue}) / IR_C] \times 100 = \{[(a + c) / n] \times 10^n - [c / (c + d)] \times 10^n\} / \{[(a + c) / n] \times 10^n\}_{\|} \times 100$

Chi-square Test of Independence: $\chi^2 = n (ad - bc)^2 / (a + b) (c + d) (a + c) (b + d)$

The statistical significance of the measure of association can be calculated using the chi-square test of independence (see formula 10.4 or table 12–3), and the results of the chi-square test can be interpreted based on information in table 10–3. A 95% confidence interval for the relative risk (RR) can be estimated using formula 12.1.[12] This formula is analogous to that for the 95% confidence interval for the prevalence ratio.

(12.1)

$$95\%\ CI\ for\ RR = \exp \{\ln (RR) \pm 1.96\sqrt{[(b / a) / (a + b)] + [(d / c) / (c + d)]}\}$$

The expression *exp* is the base e raised to the entire expression in braces. The expression ln (RR) is the natural logarithm of the relative risk, and the values a–d are derived from the standard 2×2 contingency table. A 95% confidence interval for the risk difference (RD) or attributable risk (AR) can be estimated using formula 12.2.[13]

(12.2)

$$95\% \text{ CI for RD} =$$
$$RD \pm 1.96 \sqrt{[IR_{C\text{-}e} (1 - IR_{C\text{-}e}) / (a + b)] + [IR_{C\text{-}ue} (1 - IR_{C\text{-}ue}) / (c + d)]}$$

$IR_{C\text{-}e}$ in formula 12.2 is the cumulative incidence rate in the exposed group and is calculated by $[a / (a + b)] \times 10^n$. Similarly, $IR_{C\text{-}ue}$ is the cumulative incidence rate in the unexposed group and is calculated by $[c / (c + d)] \times 10^n$. The letters a–d are those in the standard 2×2 contingency table. Before an example of the analysis of a cohort study based on cumulative incidence rates is provided, some other considerations should be noted. These include power analysis, confounding, and effect modification.

Power Analysis

As with other epidemiologic studies, the *power* of a cohort study should be considered before it is initiated in order to minimize the probability of a type II error. *Epi Info* (see appendix B) can be used to calculate the sample size needed to obtain a given level of power in a cohort study. To use *Epi Info* for this purpose, the following information is required:

- The confidence level desired (usually 95% corresponding to a p-value of 0.05)
- The level of power desired (usually between 80 and 95%)
- The ratio of unexposed subjects to exposed subjects
- The expected frequency of the outcome in the unexposed group (usually estimated from previous research)
- The smallest relative risk one would like to be able to detect, which should be based on practical significance

It is important to remember that the power of a study decreases as the sample size decreases. Therefore, cohort studies that experience large losses to follow-up or have significant missing data may have markedly less power than that determined at the initiation of the study. In addition, some subgroup analyses may be based on substantially smaller sample sizes and will have significantly less power than that in the overall analysis.

Confounding

Potential confounding in cohort studies can be controlled in the design stage by restriction or matching, or in the analysis stage by stratification or multivariable methods. The procedures are similar to those described in chapter 11. Instead of calculating the Mantel-Haenszel odds ratio in the stratification procedure, however, the **Mantel-Haenszel relative risk** (RR_{MH}) is calculated.[14] The formula for the RR_{MH} (see formula 12.3) is somewhat different from that for the OR_{MH}, but the logic of the derivation is similar (see formula 11.3 and the discussion in chapter 11 for details).

(12.3)

$$RR_{MH} = \Sigma [a_i (c_i + d_i) / n_i] / \Sigma [c_i (a_i + b_i) / n_i]$$

Effect Modification

Effect modification in cohort studies can be recognized by examining the stratum-specific relative risks in a manner similar to that for case-control studies (chapter 11). Exhibit 11–2, which shows how to recognize confounding and effect modification in case-control studies, can also be used with cohort studies by simply substituting "RR" for "OR" and "relative risk" for "odds ratio" wherever they occur in the exhibit. For example, if the relative risk in one stratum does not equal the relative risk in another stratum (i.e., $RR_1 \neq RR_2$), and the difference is unlikely due to random variation, then effect modification is probable. Example 12–1 provides an illustration of the analysis of a cohort study based on cumulative incidence rates.

Example 12–1: Analysis of a Cohort Study Based on Cumulative Incidence Rates

A prospective cohort study was conducted many years ago on a sample of young women in Omaha, Nebraska, to determine if there was an association between cigarette smoking during pregnancy and the incidence of miscarriages. Four hundred prospective mothers between 18 and 24 years of age were followed for the entire course of their pregnancies. Fifteen of the prospective mothers were lost to follow-up or died due to causes other than complications of pregnancy during the follow-up period. Thus, data were available for 385 mothers in the sample. Of the 385 mothers, 50 reported smoking cigarettes during pregnancy, and 10 of these had miscarriages. A total of 25 miscarriages occurred altogether. Assuming that the smoking and nonsmoking subgroups were similar with regard to potential confounders and that the study was not biased, calculate the relative risk (RR) of miscarriages in this population. Also determine if the RR was statistically significant and determine its 95% confidence interval. Interpret your results.

Solution:

Step 1: Place the frequencies provided in the example in the appropriate cells of a standard 2×2 contingency table. Missing cell or marginal values can be derived easily from the data provided. For example, a total of 50 women smoked cigarettes in the sample. Of these, only 10 had miscarriages. Therefore, the other 40 women who smoked cigarettes (50 – 10 = 40) did not have miscarriages. This number should be placed in the upper right-hand cell of the contingency table. Similarly, there were 25 women who had miscarriages. Of these women, 10 were cigarette smokers. Thus, 15 of the women who had miscarriages (25 – 10 = 15) must not have smoked cigarettes. This figure is placed in the lower left-hand cell of the contingency table.

	Outcome Status		
Exposure Status	**Present**	**Absent**	
Smokers	10	40	50
Nonsmokers	15	320	335
	25	360	385

Step 2: Calculate the cumulative incidence rates in the exposed and unexposed groups and the relative risk using the appropriate formulas in table 12–3.

$$IR_{C\text{-}e} = [a / (a + b)] \times 10^n = (10 / 50) \times 10^n = 0.200 \times 10^2 = 20.0 \text{ per } 100$$
$$IR_{C\text{-}ue} = [c / (c + d)] \times 10^n = (15 / 335) \times 10^n = 0.045 \times 10^2 = 4.5 \text{ per } 100$$
$$RR = IR_{C\text{-}e} / IR_{C\text{-}ue} = (20.0 \text{ per } 100) / (4.5 \text{ per } 100) = 4.4$$

Step 3: Calculate the statistical significance of the relative risk and its 95% confidence interval (CI) using the appropriate formula in table 12–3 and formula 12.1, respectively.

$$\chi^2 = n \, (ad - bc)^2 / (a + b) \, (c + d) \, (a + c) \, (b + d) =$$
$$385 \, [(10 \times 320) - (40 \times 15)]^2 / (50) \, (335) \, (25) \, (360) =$$
$$385 \, (3{,}200 - 600)^2 / 150{,}750{,}000 = 385 \, (2{,}600)^2 / 150{,}750{,}000 =$$
$$385 \, (6{,}760{,}000) / 150{,}750{,}000 =$$
$$2{,}602{,}600{,}000 / 150{,}750{,}000 = 17.26$$
$$95\% \text{ CI} = \exp \{\ln (RR) \pm 1.96 \, \sqrt{[(b / a) / (a + b)] + [(d / c) / (c + d)]}\}$$
$$\exp \{\ln (4.4) \pm 1.96 \, \sqrt{[(40 / 10) / 50] + [(320 / 15) / 335]}\} =$$
$$\exp [1.48 \pm 1.96 \, \sqrt{(4.0 / 50) + (21.3 / 335)}] =$$
$$\exp [1.48 \pm 1.96 \, \sqrt{(0.080 + 0.064)}] =$$
$$\exp (1.48 \pm 1.96 \, \sqrt{0.144}) = \exp [1.48 \pm 1.96 \, (0.38)] = \exp (1.48 \pm 0.74)$$

The *lower* confidence limit is: $\exp (1.48 - 0.74) = \exp (0.74) = 2.10$
The *upper* confidence limit is: $\exp (1.48 + 0.74) = \exp (2.22) = 9.21$
Therefore, the 95% confidence interval is 2.10–9.21.

Answer: The RR was 4.4, which is statistically significant as revealed by a chi-square value of 17.26. The significance of the chi-square value can be determined from information in table 10–3. Since 17.26 > 10.83, the association between cigarette smoking during pregnancy and birth defects in this population was statistically significant at $p < 0.001$. In other words, young women who smoked cigarettes during pregnancy were 4.4 times more likely to have children with birth defects than women who did not smoke cigarettes during pregnancy based on the Omaha, Nebraska, study. The 95% confidence interval for the RR is 2.10–9.21, indicating that we are 95% confident that the true RR of birth defects among children born to mothers who were pregnant at 18 to 24 years of age in this population was 2.10–9.21.

Comments:

1. The relative risk is a measure of association between the exposure (cigarette smoking during pregnancy) and the outcome (birth defects in the children of the pregnant women). The relative risk can be expressed as the number of times the outcome is more likely to occur in the exposed group compared to the unexposed group.

2. A statistical significance test (i.e., the chi-square test of independence) and its corresponding p-value are used to determine the probability that the population relative risk is one (a RR of one indicates no increased risk among the exposed group compared to the unexposed group). In this example, the probability that the population relative risk was one is less than 1 in 1,000 as indicated by the p-value of less than 0.001. This suggests that sampling error, which can account for differences between a sample RR and the population or true RR, was a very unlikely explanation for the findings, all other factors being equal.

3. The 95% confidence interval also indicates that the association between cigarette smoking during pregnancy and birth defects was statistically significant since the confidence

interval does not contain one. The confidence interval also tells us the likely range of the population relative risk. In this case we are 95% confident that the population relative risk lay between 2.14 and 9.39. We would expect it to be outside these limits only 5% of the time. Our best single estimate of the population relative risk in this population is 4.4. This is the *point estimate* of the relative risk.

Analysis Based on Person-Time Incidence Rates

Cohort studies using person-time incidence rates can be analyzed using the following tabular display:[14]

Exposure Status	Outcome	Person-time
Exposed	a	T_e
Unexposed	c	T_{ue}
	a + c	T

The value a represents the number of exposed subjects who developed the outcome, and the value c represents the number of unexposed subjects who developed the outcome. The values T_e and T_{ue} represent the total person-time units (e.g., person-years) generated by the exposed and unexposed groups, respectively. The value T is the sum of T_e and T_{ue}, and is thus the total number of person-time units generated by the study sample ($T = T_e + T_{ue}$). Notice that there are no row totals for the above tabular display. This is because the two columns represent different types of measures that cannot be added together.

Table 12–4 provides formulas for a number of measures that are commonly calculated when cohort studies are conducted using person-time incidence rates. The chi-square test of independence can be used to determine the statistical significance of the measure of association. Because it is calculated using person-time data, however, it is referred to as $\chi^2_{P\text{-}T}$, which is the **person-time chi-square**. It is interpreted in exactly the same manner as that for cohort studies using cumulative incidence rates (see table 10–3 for interpretation of the chi-square results). A 95% confidence interval for the rate ratio can be estimated using formula 12.4.[13]

(12.4)

$$\text{95\% CI for Rate Ratio} = \exp\left[\ln(\text{Rate Ratio}) \pm 1.96 \sqrt{1/a + 1/c}\right]$$

As in formula 12.1, the expression *exp* is the base e raised to the expression enclosed in brackets. The expression *ln (Rate Ratio)* is the natural logarithm of the rate ratio, and the values a and c are derived from the tabular display described at the beginning of this section. An approximate 95% confidence interval for the rate difference (or attributable rate) is given in formula 12.5.[13]

(12.5)

$$95\% \text{ CI for Rate Difference} = \text{Rate Difference} \pm 1.96 \sqrt{(a / T_e^2) + (c / T_{ue}^2)}$$

Here, the values T_e and T_{ue} and a and c are those defined in the tabular display shown at the beginning of this section.

Table 12–4 Common Measures Used in Cohort Studies Based on Person-Time Incidence Rates

---

Overall Person-Time Incidence Rate: $IR_{P\text{-}T} = [(a + c) / T] \times 10^n$

Person-Time Incidence Rate among the Exposed Group: $IR_{P\text{-}T\text{-}e} = (a / T_e) \times 10^n$

Person-Time Incidence Rate among the Unexposed Group: $IR_{P\text{-}T\text{-}ue} = (c / T_{ue}) \times 10^n$

Rate Ratio $= IR_{P\text{-}T\text{-}e} / IR_{P\text{-}T\text{-}ue} = [(a / T_e) \times 10^n] / [(c / T_{ue}) \times 10^n]$

Attributable Rate (or Rate Difference) $= IR_{P\text{-}T\text{-}e} - IR_{P\text{-}T\text{-}ue} = [(a / T_e) \times 10^n] - [(c / T_{ue}) \times 10^n]$

Attributable Rate Percent $= [(IR_{P\text{-}T\text{-}e} - IR_{P\text{-}T\text{-}ue}) / IR_{P\text{-}T\text{-}e}] \times 100 = \{[(a / T_e) \times 10^n] - [(c / T_{ue}) \times 10^n]\} / [(a / T_e) \times 10^n] \times 100$

Population Attributable Rate $= IR_{P\text{-}T} - IR_{P\text{-}T\text{-}ue} = \{[(a + c) / T] \times 10^n\} - [(c / T_{ue}) \times 10^n]$

Population Attributable Rate Percent $= [(IR_{P\text{-}T} - IR_{P\text{-}T\text{-}ue}) / IR_{P\text{-}T}] \times 100 = \{[(a + c) / T] \times 10^n - (c / T_{ue}) \times 10^n\} / \{[(a + c) / T] \times 10^n\} \times 100$

Person-Time Chi-Square Test of Independence: $\chi^2_{P\text{-}T} = \{a - [T_e (a + c)] / T\}^2 / \{T_e [T_{ue} (a + c)] / T^2\}$

Reference: Elmwood, J. M. (1988). *Causal Relationships in Medicine: A Practical System for Critical Appraisal.* New York: Oxford University Press.

As with cohort studies based on cumulative incidence rates, those based on person-time incidence rates should also consider the power of the study and potential confounding and effect modification. This can be done using procedures analogous to those for cohort studies based on cumulative incidence rates. The important difference is that the rate ratio is used instead of the relative risk. Example 12–2 provides an illustration of the basic analysis of a cohort study using person-time incidence rates.

Example 12–2: Analysis of a Cohort Study Based on Person-Time Incidence Rates

A 15-year PCS was carried out on 310 subjects to determine if there is an association between a family history of alcoholism and the development of problem drinking. It was hypothesized that those subjects with a family history of alcoholism would develop problem drinking at a significantly higher rate than those who had no family history of alcoholism. Of the 130 subjects with a documented family history of alcoholism, 30 became problem drinkers as defined in the study. Of the 180 subjects without a documented history of alcoholism, 20 became problem drinkers. The exposed group contributed a total of 1,954 person-years of observation during the study, while the unexposed group contributed 2,696 person-years of observation. Based on these findings and assuming the study provided adequate control for potential confounding and bias in the design or analysis, calculate the rate ratio for problem drinking, determine its 95% confidence interval, and calculate the χ^2_{P-T}. Interpret your findings.

Solution:

Step 1: Place the data provided in the example in the appropriate cells of a tabular display as follows:

Exposure Status	Outcome	Person-years
Exposed	30	1,954
Unexposed	20	2,696
	50	4,650

It is important to keep in mind that the values in the right column of the display are person-time units. In this example they are person-years.

Step 2: Calculate the person-time incidence rates in the exposed and unexposed groups and the rate ratio using the appropriate formulas in table 12–4.

$IR_{P-T-e} = (a / T_e) \times 10^n = (30 / 1,954) \times 10^n = 0.0154 \times 10^3 = 15.4$ per 1,000 person-years
$IR_{P-T-ue} = (c / T_{ue}) \times 10^n = (20 / 2,696) \times 10^n = 0.0074 \times 10^3 = 7.4$ per 1,000 person-years

Rate Ratio $= IR_{P-T-e} / IR_{P-T-ue} =$
(15.4 per 1,000 person-years) / (7.4 per 1,000 person-years) $= 2.1$

Step 3: Calculate the 95% confidence interval (CI) for the rate ratio and the person-time chi-square statistic (χ^2_{P-T}) using formula 12.4 and the appropriate formula in table 12–4.

95% CI $= \exp$ [ln (Rate Ratio) $\pm$ 1.96 $\sqrt{1 / a + 1 / c}$]
$\exp$ [ln (2.1) $\pm$ 1.96 $\sqrt{(1 / 30) + (1 / 20)}$] $=$
$\exp$ (0.74 $\pm$ 1.96 $\sqrt{0.03 + 0.05}$) $=$
$\exp$ (0.74 $\pm$ 1.96 $\sqrt{0.08}$) $= \exp$ (0.74 $\pm$ 0.55)
The *lower* confidence limit is: $\exp$ (0.74 $-$ 0.55) $= \exp$ (0.19) $= 1.21$
The *upper* confidence limit is: $\exp$ (0.74 $+$ 0.55) $= \exp$ (1.29) $= 3.63$
Therefore, the 95% CI $= 1.21$–3.63.
$\chi^2_{P-T} = \{a - [T_e (a + c)] / T\}^2 / \{T_e [T_{ue} (a + c)] / T^2\} =$
$\{30 - [1,954 (30 + 20)] / 4,650\}^2 / \{1,954 [2,696 (30 + 20)] / 4,650^2\} =$
$\{30 - [1,954 (50)] / 4,650\}^2 / \{1,954 [2,696 (50)] / 21,622,500\} =$
$[30 - (97,700 / 4,650)]^2 / [1,954 (134,800) / 21,622,500] =$
$(30 - 21.01)^2 / (12.18) =$
$80.82 / 12.18 = 6.64$

Answer: The rate ratio is 2.1 with a 95% CI of 1.21–3.63. This can be written: Rate Ratio = 2.1 (95% CI = 1.21–3.63). In this example, the rate ratio implies that the rate at which problem drinking develops is 2.1 times greater among those with a family history of alcoholism compared to those without a family history of alcoholism, all other factors being equal. The true (population) rate ratio is estimated to be 2.1 (point estimate), and we are 95% confident that the true rate ratio lies between 1.21 and 3.63. The rate ratio is statistically significant as revealed by a chi-square value of 6.64. Based on the data in table 10–3, the association is significant at $p = 0.01$. This means that a risk ratio as large as 2.1 is expected to occur by chance only 1 out of 100 times. Therefore, it is unlikely that the true rate ratio is one. This is the same as saying that the probability of a type I error in this problem is 1%.

Comments:

1. Not all of the data provided in the example were necessary to determine the rate ratio. The fact that 130 subjects had a family history of alcoholism and 180 did not was nonessential information, since the total number of person-years of observation was provided for both the exposed and unexposed groups. The number of person-years for each exposure group is required information, however, since person-years are the denominators for the person-time incidence rates upon which the rate ratio is calculated. If the number of person-years in the exposed and unexposed groups had not been provided, then it would have been necessary to provide additional information in the problem so that these measures could be calculated in the manner shown in example 5–2 (see chapter 5).

2. The rate ratio is a measure of association between the exposure (family history of alcoholism) and the outcome (problem drinking). Unlike the risk ratio, however, it does not measure the relative *risk* of developing problem drinking. Instead, it measures the relative *rate* at which problem drinking develops. Specifically, the risk ratio measures the probability of an outcome in the exposed compared to the unexposed subjects, while the rate ratio measures the pace at which the outcome develops in the exposed compared to the unexposed subjects. Under certain conditions (see chapter 11) the risk ratio can be used to approximate the rate ratio and vice versa.

Summary

- There are two major types of cohort studies—prospective cohort studies and retrospective (or historical) cohort studies. A distinguishing feature of both types of cohort studies vis-à-vis other major analytic studies is that the exposure status of the subjects is always assessed before their outcome status.

- Both prospective and retrospective cohort studies follow a cohort over time. In prospective designs the cohort is followed from the present (i.e., study initiation) into the future. In retrospective designs the cohort is followed from some time in the past up to the present.

- Well-designed cohort studies have a number of advantages, including maintaining a clear temporal sequence between exposure and outcome, allowing direct calculation of incidence rates, allowing multiple outcomes to be assessed, providing an indication of incubation or latency periods for diseases, allowing uncommon exposures to be assessed, and precluding exposure suspicion bias. Disadvantages include potentially large sample size requirements, long follow-up periods, losses to follow-up, exposure and outcome misclassification, and diagnostic suspicion bias.

- Important design considerations in cohort studies include selecting an appropriate cohort, including internal or external comparison groups; determining exposure and outcome status using valid and reliable sources; and reassessing exposure status during follow-up to account for any changes in exposure.

- Cohort studies are analyzed differently depending on the type of incidence rate employed. If cumulative incidence rates are used, the relative risk is the usual measure of association between exposure and outcome. If person-time incidence rates are used, the rate ratio is the typical measure of association.

New Terms

cohort	historical prospective	Mantel-Haenszel
external comparison	cohort study	relative risk
group	internal comparison group	person-time chi-square

Study Questions and Exercises

1. Describe how you would design a valid prospective cohort study to test the hypothesis that cigarette smoking during pregnancy increases the risk of Sudden Infant Death Syndrome (SIDS). Include in your description how you would select the cohort and the comparison group; how you would assess exposure and outcome status; how you would minimize potential sources of bias, confounding, and sampling error; and how you would analyze the data.

2. In January 2002, epidemiologists with the Frantrac Research Institute in Copenhagen were contracted by the Denmark Chemical Manufacturers Association to study the possible relationship between XG-47, an industrial solvent, and liver cancer. The epidemiologists collected the work records of all those who had been employed from 1975 to 1985 at the only plant using XG-47 to establish exposure levels and demographic profiles of the workers. Next, the epidemiologists conducted an extensive search to see what happened to the identified employees. This included an examination of the national cancer registry in Denmark to determine which workers had contracted liver cancer. There were a total of 345 workers, 145 of whom were exposed to XG-47. There were 12 cases of liver cancer among the exposed group, and 19 cases of liver cancer altogether. Based on this information, answer the following questions: (a) what type of study is represented here and why, (b) what is the applicable measure of association, (c) what is the value of the applicable measure of association, and (d) is the measure of association statistically significant? Based on your findings, what would you conclude about the relationship between XG-47 and liver cancer, assuming no significant bias or confounding in the study?

3. A prospective cohort study of the association between alcohol consumption and gall bladder disease was designed to follow a group of 400 healthy men over a five-year period. The men were tested for the presence of gall bladder disease at the end of each year during the follow-up period. Only new cases of gall bladder disease were recorded at each annual assessment. The results of the study were as follows:

    Among the 200 drinkers:
    10 subjects were positive for gall bladder disease in year three.
    15 subjects were positive for gall bladder disease in year five.

    Among the 200 nondrinkers:
    6 subjects were positive for gall bladder disease in year two.
    4 subjects were positive for gall bladder disease in year three.

    Based on these data, calculate the rate ratio for gall bladder disease in this group and its 95% confidence interval. Was there a significant association between alcohol consumption and gall bladder disease? Explain.

4. Indicate whether each of the following statements is true or false (T or F). For each false statement, indicate why it is false.

    ___ a. If the results of a cohort study showed a crude RR of 3.5 and an RR_{MH} of 6.3, one would be correct in concluding that effect modification was present.

    ___ b. Exposure suspicion bias is common in prospective cohort studies.

    ___ c. Death certificates tend to be relatively unreliable sources for determining specific causes of death in prospective cohort studies.

    ___ d. External comparison groups are always preferable to internal comparison groups in cohort studies.

    ___ e. A potential source of error in cohort studies is loss to follow-up bias.

References

1. Hall, A. P., Barry, P. E., Dawber, T. R., and McNamara, P. M. (1967). Epidemiology of Gout and Hyperuricemia: A Long-term Population Study. *American Journal of Medicine* 42(1): 27–37.
2. Friedman, G. D., Kannel, W. B., and Dawber, T. R. (1966). The Epidemiology of Gall Bladder Disease: Observations in the Framingham Study. *Journal of Chronic Diseases* 19(3): 273–292.
3. Friis, R. H., and Sellers, T. A. (1999). *Epidemiology for Public Health Practice*, 2nd ed. Gaithersburg, MD: Aspen.
4. Rim, E. B., Manson, J. E., Stampfer, M. J., Colditz, G. A., Willett, W. C., Rosner, B., Hennekens, C. H., and Speizer, F. E. (1993). Cigarette Smoking and the Risk of Diabetes in Women. *American Journal of Public Health* 83(2): 211–214.
5. Jekel, J. F., Elmore, J. G., and Katz, D. L. (1996). *Epidemiology, Biostatistics, and Preventive Medicine*. Philadelphia: W. B. Saunders Company.
6. Sackett, D. L. (1979). Bias in Analytic Research. *Journal of Chronic Diseases* 32: 51–63.
7. Kelsey, J. L., Thompson, W. D., and Evans, A. S. (1986). *Methods in Observational Epidemiology*. New York: Oxford University Press.
8. Brink, S. (1998). Unlocking the Heart's Secrets. *U.S. News & World Report* (On-Line). Available: http://www2.usnews.com/usnews/issue/980907/7fram.htm (Access date: January 15, 2000.)
9. Hennekens, C. H., and Buring, J. E. (1987). *Epidemiology in Medicine*. Boston: Little, Brown and Company.

10. Chasan-Taber, L., Willett, W. C., Seddon, J. M., Stampfer, M. J., Rosner, B., Colditz, G. A., Speizer, F. E., and Hankinson, S. E. (2000). A Prospective Study of Alcohol Consumption and Cataract Extraction Among U.S. Women. *Annals of Epidemiology* 10(6): 347–353.
11. Cooper, W. O., Hickson, G. B., Mitchel, E. F. Jr., Edwards, K. M., Thapa, P. B., and Ray, W. A. (1999). Early Childhood Mortality from Community-acquired Infections. *American Journal of Epidemiology* 150(5): 517–527.
12. Katz, D., Baptista, J., Azen, S. P., and Pike, M. C. (1978). Obtaining Confidence Intervals for the Risk Ratio in Cohort Studies. *Biometrics* 34: 469–474.
13. Ahlbom, A. (1993). *Biostatistics for Epidemiologists*. Boca Raton, FL: Lewis Publishers.
14. Elmwood, M. J. (1988). *Causal Relationships in Medicine: A Practical System for Critical Appraisal*. New York: Oxford University Press.

CHAPTER THIRTEEN

Experimental Studies in Epidemiology

Learning Objectives

▸ Differentiate between randomized controlled trials (RCTs), community trials, and natural experiments.

▸ Discuss the key design features of RCTs and community trials, respectively, in terms of sample selection, allocation to intervention and control groups, types of interventions, and assessment of outcomes.

▸ Describe the design and conduct of factorial and crossover designs of RCTs.

▸ Compare and contrast the strengths and potential weaknesses of RCTs and community trials, respectively.

▸ Calculate sample size requirements for RCTs using expected differences in proportions and analyze and interpret the findings of RCTs using person-time incidence rates.

▸ Describe and explain the use of eligibility criteria, randomization, and blinding in RCTs.

▸ Define carryover effects, crossover, effective sample size, effect size, end points, intention-to-treat analysis, meta-analysis, placebo, placebo-controlled trial, placebo effect, study protocol, survival analysis, washout period, and evaluation study.

Overview

Experimental studies in epidemiology include randomized controlled trials (RCTs), community trials, and natural experiments. RCTs randomly allocate individuals to experimental and control groups to test the effects of an intervention. Community trials are similar but allocate entire populations or communities. Natural experiments are unplanned situations in nature that resemble planned experiments. The major strength of experimental studies is their ability to substantiate causal relationships beyond that possible in observational studies. Major weaknesses of RCTs include their limited use and potential subject losses that can affect internal validity. The most serious problem in community trials is accounting for differences due to factors other than the intervention. Methods of analysis for experimental studies depend on the study objectives.

Introduction

Unlike observational studies, experimental studies are those in which the conditions of the study are controlled directly by the investigators.[1] Most important, the investigators control the degree of subject exposure. In the simplest case, some are intentionally exposed to a promising but unproven experimental agent, treatment, or procedure, and some are not. Experimental studies in epidemiology are often referred to as **intervention studies** because the investigators intervene into the lives of the subjects by manipulating the conditions of exposure. In observational studies, no such intervention occurs. Investigators simply observe and record the exposures that already exist or existed among the subjects.

As discussed in chapter 4, there are two major types of *planned* experimental studies in epidemiology. These are *randomized controlled trials* (also referred to as clinical trials) and *community trials* (also referred to as community intervention trials). One important distinguishing characteristic between these two types of studies is the unit of analysis. In randomized controlled trials the unit of analysis is the individual, while in community trials it is the group. A third, but unplanned, type of experimental study is the **natural experiment**. This represents a relatively rare situation in nature where the levels of exposure to a putative cause differ among a population in a way that is relatively unaffected by extraneous factors so that the situation resembles a planned experiment. This was the case in John Snow's nineteenth-century investigation of cholera deaths, due to the almost random fashion in which drinking water was supplied to area homes by two rival water companies. Another example is the conditions produced by the Chernobyl nuclear power plant disaster in the former Soviet Union. This created an unplanned opportunity to study the health effects of radiation exposure on populations according to the distance from the disaster site. Because they are relatively rare, natural experiments are not discussed further in this text. This chapter discusses some important design features of randomized controlled trials and community trials, their major strengths and weaknesses, and some of the basic approaches to analysis and interpretation of the findings from these studies.

Randomized Controlled Trials

A randomized controlled trial is an epidemiologic experiment where individual subjects are randomly assigned to either an experimental or control group to assess the effects of a preventive or therapeutic agent, treatment, procedure, or service.[1] In some randomized controlled trials there may be more than one experimental or control group. The control group is one where the subjects receive no intervention or one where they receive the standard or conventional intervention.

Randomized controlled trials (RCTs) are frequently referred to as the "gold standard" of epidemiologic studies.[2] This is because when they are well designed and conducted they provide the strongest possible evidence of causation that epidemiologic studies can deliver. This is due to the tightly controlled conditions of the experiment and randomization of the subjects, which tend to preclude other possible explanations for the findings, and because the results can be closely replicated by other investigators who use the same **study protocol** (i.e., study plan and procedures).

One of the first RCTs to be conducted was a study by Johannes Fibiger in a Copenhagen hospital in 1898.[2] In this study diphtheria patients were assigned to two groups based on their day of admission in order to test the efficacy of serum injection compared to traditional treatment for the disease. It was not until the middle of the twentieth century, however, that RCTs became established in the United States. A classic example is the large-scale polio vaccine field trials conducted in 1954. These studies demonstrated that the polio vaccine was highly effective in preventing poliomyelitis.[3] A more recent example is a study of the efficacy of pravastatin (a cholesterol-lowering drug) in reducing the risk of stroke.[4] As part of the findings, the authors reported that among heart patients pravastatin therapy reduced the risk of nonhemorrhagic stroke by 23% when compared to controls who were given a **placebo**, a similar appearing but inert substance.

As described in chapter 4, RCTs can be grouped into three categories—*preventive trials* (e.g., trials of vaccine efficacy on healthy volunteers), *intervention trials* (e.g., trials of lipid-lowering drugs in individuals at high risk of heart disease), and *therapeutic trials* (e.g., trials of the efficacy of various forms of therapy on survival of cancer patients). While each type of trial has a specific aim (primary, secondary, or tertiary prevention), the basic study design is the same. One of the first steps in designing an RCT is to develop the research hypothesis. This is followed by such steps as selecting the study sample, estimating sample size requirements, collecting baseline data on the subjects, allocating the subjects into experimental and control groups, applying the intervention, and assessing the outcomes during follow-up. These and other considerations should be a part of the overall study protocol.

Selecting the Sample

As noted in chapter 4, selecting a study sample for an RCT normally involves three steps (see figure 4–6). First, the *reference population* must be defined. This is the general population to which the investigators hope to generalize their findings. The reference population will depend on the particular problem or outcome being investigated. The reference population for a study of the efficacy of a new treatment for cervical cancer, for example, will be restricted at a minimum to women with cervical cancer, since men cannot contract the disease. Other restrictions, such as age, race, geographical location, and stage of cancer, may also be applied if they are believed to be important factors related to the outcome of the trial.[5] The reference population is generally more theoretical than practical, since it is usually impossible to identify and enumerate all of its members.

Once the reference population has been defined, the next step is to identify an *experimental population*. The experimental population is a practical representation of the reference population. It consists of a discrete subsample of the reference population that can be identified and counted (e.g., women with cervical cancer at three medical centers in Ohio between January and July 2002). The experimental population is more focused than the reference population, since it generally comes from a smaller geographic area during a finite time period. The most important consideration in identifying an experimental population, however, is its ability to produce valid results for the hypothesis being tested. Therefore, it must be large enough and likely to produce enough **end points** (study outcomes) to permit valid statistical comparisons between the experimental and control groups.[5]

In some cases, the experimental population may be more restrictive than the reference population to enhance compliance with the study protocol and improve the accuracy of the data collected. For example, restricting an adult female experimental population to registered nurses may increase compliance and reporting accuracy in a preventive trial of the benefits of calcium supplementation in maintaining bone density without seriously jeopardizing the generalizability of the findings to all adult women (the reference population). It is assumed here that registered nurses are more likely to comply with the study protocol and report results accurately because of their professional training in nursing. It is further assumed that if the calcium is efficacious for female nurses, it would also be efficacious in other females.

The final step in sample selection is choosing the *study sample* from the experimental population. The study sample includes fully informed, willing participants who meet the predetermined **eligibility criteria**. The eligibility criteria are based on the study objectives and should guide the identification of the reference and experimental populations, as well as the selection of the study sample. The eligibility criteria define who is to be included in the study (**inclusion criteria**) as well as who is to be excluded from the study (**exclusion criteria**). The goal of the eligibility criteria is to optimize the conditions for successful testing of the effects of an intervention. The inclusion criteria are usually based on demographic, geographic, medical, and/or temporal characteristics that may be relevant to the research question.[6] The exclusion criteria have to do with subject characteristics that may affect the validity of the study findings and with ethical issues related to questionable benefits or potential harm to subjects if they were included in the study. For example, a therapeutic drug trial may exclude severely ill patients who are unlikely to complete the study due to their illness and who could therefore threaten the validity of the findings. Similarly, the trial may exclude those taking medications known to interfere with the effectiveness of study drug, thereby decreasing any potential benefits to participation in the study.

In general, the eligibility criteria selected for an RCT should involve regard for the study objectives, the possible effects on internal and external validity of the study, the potential benefit or harm to the subjects, and issues related to convenience and efficiency. To illustrate the application of eligibility criteria, consider an RCT that was conducted at a hospital in Philadelphia.[7] The study was designed to evaluate the efficacy of lithium in treating aggressive behavior in children and adolescents. This study employed the following inclusion criteria: male and female patients with a history of severe aggressive behavior and a diagnosis of conduct disorder, who were 10–17 years of age and residing in an acute-care child and adolescent psychiatric inpatient ward of a teaching hospital. The exclusion criteria included mental retardation, pervasive developmental disorder, recent substance dependence, and a number of other psychiatric disorders, in addition to pregnancy, certain major medical problems, recent prescriptions for psychoactive drugs, and previous inclusion in a lithium trial. As you can see from this example, the eligibility criteria are very restrictive due to a number of considerations, including the research objective (e.g., includes only 10–17 year olds), convenience (e.g., includes only patients in a given hospital), threats to internal validity (e.g., excludes groups that may present compliance problems), and potential harm to the subjects (e.g., excludes pregnant adolescents and those with certain medical conditions). Table 13–1 summarizes some of the more common eligibility criteria employed in RCTs.

Table 13–1 Common Eligibility Criteria Used in Randomized Controlled Trials

Reasons for Inclusion	Reasons for Exclusion
• **Certain age, sex, or racial/ethnic characteristics** (e.g., African-American men, 60–79 years, for a study investigating an outcome of stroke—provides a high-risk group likely to produce sufficient end points for analysis)	• **Potential harm to participants** (e.g., patients with a previous history of hemorrhagic stroke for a study of a blood-thinning medication on memory improvement—may initiate another stroke)
• **Absence of certain diseases or conditions** (e.g., persons free of heart disease in a study of the efficacy of dietary management in preventing coronary heart disease—prevents erroneous results)	• **Intervention unlikely to be effective** (e.g., persons with a previous episode of mumps for a preventive trial of a new vaccine for mumps—mumps confers life-long immunity)
• **Not currently receiving the proposed intervention** (e.g., persons not currently taking vitamin C in a study of vitamin C and colds—prevents possible inflation of the magnitude of the effect)	• **Potential for poor compliance with the study protocol** (e.g., persons with drug or alcohol addiction—less likely to comply with the intervention in a study of the efficacy of meditation in treating anxiety)
• **Located in certain communities, hospitals, or clinics** (e.g., patients at ABC Community Hospital—convenient for investigators)	• **Practical difficulties with participation** (e.g., persons with certain mental disabilities—might result in inaccurate responses to study questions)
• **Meets eligibility criteria during certain time periods** (e.g., meets eligibility criteria between June 1 and December 31 of a given year—the period the study will commence)	• **Do not meet the inclusion criteria** (i.e., all who do not meet the inclusion criteria for a study are automatically excluded from the study)

Reference: Hulley, S. B., Cummings, S. R., Browner, W. S., Grady, D., Hearst, N., and Newman, T. B. (2001). *Designing Clinical Research*, 2nd ed. Philadelphia: Lippincott, Williams & Wilkins.

Determining Sample Size Requirements

Since many subjects in the experimental population of an RCT may be ineligible or unwilling to participate in the study, the size of the study sample is often substantially smaller than that of the experimental population. Small sample size can present serious concerns in RCTs because of the increased probability of sampling error. Inadequate sample size, for example, can mean that small, but clinically significant, differences go undetected.[*] The solution to this problem is to determine the sample size required to detect important differences *before* the study is initiated. In fact, this is critical. There have been too many irrelevant clinical trials where this advice has been ignored. Curtis L. Meinert, for example, states that some of these studies may even be "unethical in that they require patients to accept the risks of treatment, however small, without any chance of benefit to them or future patients."[8(p74)]

There are several ways to determine the sample size required to detect important differences *before* the study is initiated. Formula 13.1 provides one method of estimating the sample size requirements for RCTs when the measure of interest is the difference between two proportions.[9] This formula applies when there are only two groups (an experimental group and a control group) to be compared, when the groups are equal in size, and when the measure of interest is the difference between the proportions of some predetermined outcome (e.g., disease, death, recovery).

(13.1)

$$n = \frac{P_C(1 - P_C) + P_E(1 - P_E)}{(P_E - P_C)^2} \times 10.5$$

The n in the formula refers to the number of subjects required in *each* group. P_C is the proportion of outcomes *expected* in the control group, and P_E is the proportion of outcomes *expected* in the experimental group. $P_E - P_C$ is known as the **effect size**, which is the size of the difference one would like to be able to detect if it exists.[9] Formula 13.1 also assumes that the following parameters apply: p-value = 0.05, beta = 0.10, and power = 90%. Therefore, it should not be used if one is interested in other values of these parameters. To illustrate the use of formula 13.1 consider the following example. If one expected that those not receiving an experimental drug (the control group) to experience an overall survival rate of 25% (see formula 5.9) and those receiving the experimental drug (the experimental group) to experience an overall survival rate of 35%, then, given the parameters stated above, the sample size requirements for *each* group would be calculated as follows: {[(0.25 × 0.75) + (0.35 × 0.65)] / (0.35 – 0.25)^2} × 10.5 = (0.415 / 0.01) × 10.5 = 436. Thus, a total of 872 subjects (436 in each group) would be required for the study. If the expected survival rates were 25% and 30%, respectively, the sample size required in each group would be 1,670 or 3,340 total. As this

---

[*] One way of dealing with inconclusive results from small trials is to use **meta-analysis**, a method of statistically pooling the results of several studies on the same problem in order to identify overall trends and to form policy.[1]

illustrates, the smaller the effect size, the greater the sample size required. This is because it takes more power to detect small differences than it does to detect large differences.

Determining the required sample size at the beginning of a study is only part of the solution to minimizing sampling error in RCTs. Because of potential losses during the course of an investigation, the **effective sample size** (that remaining after losses) may be significantly below the original requirements. Some suggestions for assuring adequate sample size throughout a study include estimating the likely number of eligible volunteers through pilot testing, planning the study with an accessible population that is larger than required, and making contingency plans for obtaining additional subjects if necessary.[6] Many well designed RCTs are multicenter studies that pool resources to ensure that there are adequate numbers of subjects and end points for valid statistical comparisons. Also, sometimes groups at high risk of the outcome are targeted for study to increase the number of predicted end points and decrease sample size requirements. For example, since stroke incidence increases with age, one might restrict a study designed to test whether a particular intervention reduces the incidence of stroke to adults over 50 years of age, since this group is more likely to produce the number of end points needed than are younger age groups. A downside of this approach is that it may limit the generalizability of the findings. Lengthening the follow-up period of an RCT where feasible can have similar effects.[5]

Finally, it is important to note that the study sample may not be very representative of the experimental or reference population when many of the eligible subjects are unwilling to participate in the study. This will affect the external validity of the study, but it will not affect its internal validity.[5] Losses to follow-up and noncompliance, however, can affect internal validity.

Allocating Subjects into Experimental and Control Groups

Allocating subjects into experimental and control groups in RCTs involves *randomization*. **Randomization**, or random allocation, means that the assignment of subjects into experimental and control groups is by strictly random means. This assures that the subjects have the same probability of being assigned to either the experimental or control groups. Clinical trials that do not involve random allocation are not RCTs, and do not carry the same prestige in epidemiology as RCTs do. Randomization has the effect of increasing the comparability of the groups in terms of all factors other than the intervention being applied. Thus, selection bias has been essentially eliminated. Also, the randomized groups should be similar with regard to the distribution of anticipated, and even unanticipated, confounders. The key benefit of randomization is the similarity it should create between the experimental and control groups. Barring measurement errors, any differences in the groups, other than the intervention to be applied, should be due only to sampling error (chapter 8), which is always possible when random methods are used, but which fortunately can be estimated during the statistical analysis of the findings.

Randomization works best when the study sample is large. Chance differences between the groups due to sampling error are more likely to be a factor when the study sample is small (i.e., less than 100 subjects per group).[10] Consider, for example, a study sample of 10 subjects, five of whom are females. In the most favorable random distribution into an experimental and control group, two females would end up in one group and three in the other. The percentage of females in one group would be $(2 / 5) \times 100 = 40\%$. The percentage in the other group would be $(3 / 5) \times 100 = 60\%$. This represents a difference of 20% in the distribution of females between the two groups. If we got the most favorable random distribution with a study sample of 100 subjects, which had the same proportion of females as in the previous example (i.e., 50 females), then 25 (50%) would end up in each group. There would be no difference in the distribution of females between the groups. Thus, size is important when it comes to randomization. When the study sample in an RCT is small it may be helpful to employ a randomization technique that increases the probability that the experimental and control groups will be similar with regard to important, potentially confounding factors by decreasing the chances of sampling error. One such technique is **stratified randomization** (see figure 13–1). First, the researcher deliberately separates the subjects into

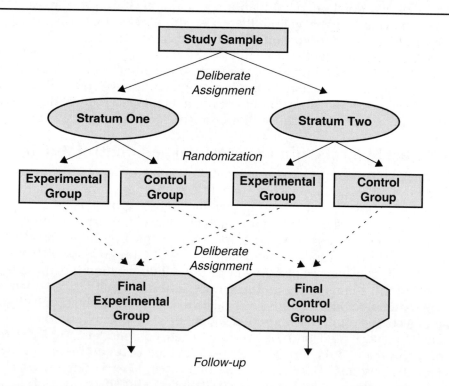

Source: Adapted from Fletcher, R. H., Fletcher, S. W., and Wagner, E. H. (1988). *Clinical Epidemiology: The Essentials,* 2nd ed. Baltimore: Williams and Wilkins.

Figure 13–1 Example of stratified randomization in a randomized controlled trial

different strata of the factor for which the technique is being employed (e.g., into groups of males and females). Next, the researcher randomly allocates the subjects from each stratum into experimental and control groups, which are then combined into the final experimental and control groups. The use of this technique should result in experimental and control groups that are nearly identical with regard to the stratification variables. This technique is best suited to studies with small sample sizes. It can also be used to detect *effect modification* in a study.[8] Stratified randomization becomes inefficient, however, when more than a few factors are stratified, so it should only be used for the potentially most important confounders. Finally, it is always a good idea to compare the randomized experimental and control groups, whether or not stratified methods have been used, to see if the resulting proportions of important potential confounders are similar in each group. If not, appropriate adjustments can be made in the analysis phase of the study.

Applying the Intervention and Assessing the Outcomes During Follow-up

In a typical RCT the experimental group is exposed to a promising, but unproven, agent, treatment, procedure, or service (i.e., intervention) in the hope that it will cure, ameliorate, or diminish a given problem without serious side effects, and the control group is exposed to either a placebo or the customary treatment for the problem. The subjects are followed up prospectively to determine if the intervention applied to the experimental group is efficacious when compared to the control group. This is accomplished by comparing some measure of the magnitude of the study outcome (e.g., incidence) in the experimental group with that in the control group.

Unfortunately, the assessment of outcomes during the follow-up period may be subject to measurement bias. One way this bias can occur is when the subjects are aware of which group they have been assigned to. This awareness can lead to differential rates in reporting outcomes between the experimental and control groups. It can also have a differential effect on compliance with the study protocol. For example, consider a **placebo-controlled trial** (an RCT in which the control group receives a placebo) to assess the efficacy of a new drug in the treatment of migraine headaches. If the subjects know which group they are in, those in the experimental group are more likely to report reduction in the severity and duration of their symptoms compared to those in the control group, even if the drug is not effective, simply because they expect the drug to be helpful. This is an example of the **placebo effect**, which is the tendency for those receiving a treatment to experience beneficial effects even when the treatment has no known therapeutic value. The members of the control group in this example would not be expected to report positive effects from the placebo due to their knowledge that it has no pharmacological value. They also are more likely to be noncompliant with the study protocol or withdraw from the trial than those in the experimental group for the same reason. Either way, bias could be introduced in assessing the outcomes of the study. If the subjects in the example do not know their group assignments, bias due to the placebo effect would be unlikely since the placebo effect would be expected to be operating independently of group assignment. Also, noncompliance with the study protocol or increased withdrawals among the control group might be less likely if the subjects think there is a chance they are in the experimental group.

One way of minimizing these problems is blinding (or masking)* the subjects to their own group assignment. In the parlance of epidemiology this is called a **single-blinded study**. This is a study in which the subjects are kept unaware of their group assignment, although the investigators are still aware. While a single-blinded study can minimize bias introduced by the subjects, it has no effect on bias on the part of the investigators. For example, by knowing the subjects' group assignments, the investigators may tend to record more positive outcomes in the experimental group than in the control group, if they believe the intervention is likely to be beneficial. A **double-blinded study**, in which *neither* the subjects nor the investigators are aware of the subjects' group assignments, helps to overcome both sources of bias. A double-blinded study generally is accomplished by using a sealed code for the assignments that is only broken at the conclusion of the study. Double-blinded studies are the standard for RCTs. A **triple-blinded study** also keeps those who are analyzing the data, if different from the investigators, unaware of the subjects' group assignments. This minimizes any data manipulation that might be attempted, consciously or unconsciously, to support the study hypothesis.

Blinding is also helpful in reducing confounding that occurs *during* the follow-up period. This can arise when the investigators pay more attention to the subjects in the experimental group than to those in the control group by perhaps suggesting, consciously or unconsciously, other ways that the experimental subjects can improve their condition. This can increase the probability that the intervention appears to be successful, due to unrecognized confounding by these other measures. Confounding also can occur among the subjects when, for example, those in the control group of a therapeutic trial seek other treatments more frequently than those in the experimental group because they learn they are taking a placebo. These so-called "cointerventions," which were not part of the original design, can confound the study results during the follow-up period.[6]

While blinding can help minimize measurement bias in ascertaining the study outcome or confounding during the follow-up period, it is not always feasible. Some studies, for example, cannot be blinded. A therapeutic trial to determine if back surgery is more efficacious than physical therapy in reducing chronic lower back pain can not be blinded since it would be obvious to patients and investigators as to who is receiving which treatment. In other cases, blinding may be difficult because of the problem of producing a suit-

---

* The terms blinding and masking and their derivatives (e.g., blinded and masked) are used interchangeably. Meinert and others prefer the use of masking over blinding, since the latter may be subject to confusion, especially when the outcome of interest is blindness (i.e., loss of vision).[8] The term *blinding*, however, is more commonly used in the literature and is probably more familiar to most people.

able placebo, especially where the intervention is likely to produce soon-to-be-discovered side effects like dry mouth, gastrointestinal upset, or fatigue. Blinding is most important when the outcome being assessed is subjective (e.g., pain, quality of life). When the outcome is truly objective (e.g., overall mortality, infection) blinding is less important since bias is unlikely to have any effect on reporting of the outcome.

In general, a well-designed placebo-controlled trial with randomization and double-blinding (or triple-blinding if necessary) is the ideal RCT. A placebo-controlled trial requires that the experimental intervention demonstrate a level of superiority that exceeds any placebo effect found in the control group. When a conventional treatment is used as the control, the experimental intervention must be shown to be superior to that treatment. Randomization has the potential of eliminating selection bias and confounding as alternate explanations for any association found between exposure and outcome. Double-blinding has the effect of minimizing measurement bias that can occur due to knowledge of subject assignments to experimental or control groups.

Variations in the Design of RCTs

Some of the more common variations in the design of the traditional RCT include factorial designs and crossover designs. A **factorial design** is intended to answer two or more research questions in one RCT. This can provide significant cost savings over separate trials. The simplest factorial design is the 2×2 design (see figure 13–2). In this design the study sample is randomized into an experimental and control group to test one hypothesis, and these groups are *each* randomized into an additional experimental and control group to test the second hypothesis. A potential limitation of this design is possible interactions between the interventions that can affect the magnitude of the outcomes. Therefore, unless one intends to test the effects of the interactions between the interventions, the design is best suited to interventions that operate independently of each other.[6]

A good example of a 2×2 factorial design is the Physicians' Health Study that involved over 20,000 male physicians, 40–84 years of age.[11] This was a preventive trial using a factorial design. It was planned to test two research hypotheses: (a) that aspirin reduces total cardiovascular mortality, and (b) that beta-carotene reduces cancer incidence. The first randomization produced an experimental group of physicians who took an aspirin every other day and a control group who took a placebo. The experimental group was further randomized into experimental and control groups that took beta-carotene or a placebo, respectively. The original control group was similarly divided into experimental and control groups that took beta-carotene or a placebo. Thus, the second hypothesis was tested among both the aspirin users and nonusers for a total sample size equivalent to that of the original study sample. In effect, two equally sized RCTs were conducted at the same time.

The **crossover design** is a variation in the RCT in which the intervention is applied at different times to each subject. In the most basic application of

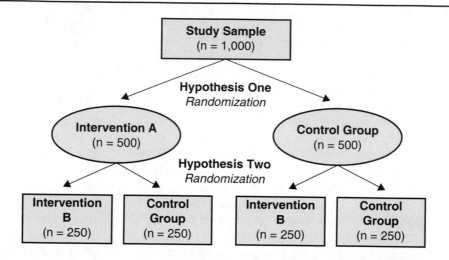

This study tests two hypotheses. The first hypothesis is that Intervention A will be efficacious in reducing a given outcome. The second hypothesis is that Intervention B will be efficacious in reducing another outcome. Note that the number of subjects being tested under Hypothesis One (n = 1,000) is the same as the number of subjects being tested under Hypothesis Two (n = 1,000). Therefore, the 2 × 2 factorial design is equivalent to two separate randomized controlled trials of the same size.

Figure 13–2 Example of a randomized controlled trial using a 2 × 2 factorial design

this design, the study sample is randomized into an experimental and control group as in a traditional RCT. After a specified period of time, however, the original experimental group becomes the control group, and the original control group becomes the experimental group (see figure 13–3). Only one hypothesis is being tested here, but the investigators can examine the effect of the intervention both within and between the two groups being compared.

The major advantages of the crossover design are reduced sample size requirements and decreased potential for confounding due to the fact that the subjects serve as their own controls.[6, 12] Comparing the same subjects in the experimental and control groups produces less statistical variance in the results, which in turn increases the power of the study, thereby reducing sample size requirements.[6] One of the disadvantages of this design is the longer time it takes to complete the study due to the need to follow the subjects twice (once with the intervention and once without the intervention). This can also increase the withdrawal rate due to subject fatigue. Another disadvantage is **carryover effects**, which are the residual effects of the intervention during the period after it has ended. A common way to deal with carryover effects is to introduce a **washout period**, a stage during which the effects of the intervention are believed to wear off. The assignment of the experimental group to the control group and vice versa begins only after the washout period has ended (see figure 13–3). Other disadvantages of crossover designs include their application only to interventions that provide temporary relief and the complexity of the analysis compared to that of traditional RCTs.[12]

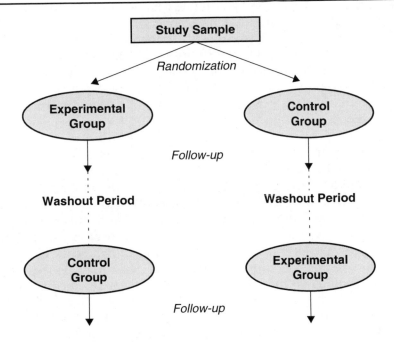

After the washout period, a time during which the subjects do not receive any intervention, those in the original experimental group become the control group, and those in the original control group become the experimental group. In a placebo-controlled trial, those receiving the intervention "cross over" to receive the placebo after a suitable washout period, and those receiving the placebo "cross over" to receive the intervention after the same washout period.

Figure 13–3 Example of a randomized controlled trial using a crossover design

Major Strengths and Weaknesses of RCTs

One of the most significant strengths of the RCT is its ability to demonstrate causal associations when appropriately designed. This strength stems from the use of controlled conditions and such powerful techniques as randomization and blinding that increase subject comparability and decrease potential bias and confounding. Another strength of the RCT is that the investigators control the level of exposure, which permits them to establish precise doses or procedures most appropriate to the experiment. Because of these strengths the RCT is widely accepted as the "gold standard" of epidemiologic studies, and it is the basis for many established medical and public health practices, including the use of cholesterol-lowering drugs in the prevention and management of heart disease and stroke, the use of segmental versus total mastectomy in the treatment of Stage 1 and 2 breast cancer,[13] the treatment of AIDS with azidothymidine (AZT), and immunization for various communicable diseases. Nevertheless, RCTs have a number of potential weaknesses that may make them unsuitable for studying many epidemiologic problems.

One of the chief weaknesses of the RCT has to do with its limited applicability. As suggested in chapter 4, ethical concerns limit the use of RCTs to circumstances of uncertainty. There must be enough confidence in the potential benefits of an intervention to expose some individuals to it, especially if it involves serious risks, but not so much confidence that it would be unethical not to offer it to others who might benefit from it. For example, say that a chemotherapy treatment using a prescription level of a drug previously approved by the U.S. Food and Drug Administration (FDA) for another use was being considered as a possible cure for Stage 3 pancreatic cancer. Evidence from extensive animal and preliminary human studies indicated that it produced a five-year survival rate of 80%, and the side effects of treatment were relatively mild. Would an RCT be appropriate to confirm that the treatment is efficacious compared to standard chemotherapy treatment? The answer is probably no because it would be unethical to deny some pancreatic cancer patients access to this medicine given that it has already been approved by the FDA and that the current five-year survival rate for treated Stage 3 pancreatic cancer is a dismal 3%.[14] Ethical considerations would also preclude an RCT to test the effects of cigarette smoking on the incidence of stomach cancer because it would be unethical to expose subjects to a known hazard with no clear benefits to the participants. This is why RCTs focus on interventions that have the potential to *reduce* rather than increase the risks of morbidity or mortality. In some cases, an RCT may need to be concluded early on ethical grounds because of cumulating evidence that the intervention may be highly beneficial or harmful.

Another potential weakness of RCTs is the bias that can result from differential rates of compliance, withdrawal, or losses to follow-up between the experimental and control groups. If any of these factors are significant, they can alter the magnitude or direction of the relationship between the intervention and the study outcome. To minimize bias resulting from these sources it is often helpful to: (a) exclude individuals who are likely to deviate from the study protocol at the outset of the study, (b) make the intervention as simple to comply with as possible, (c) maintain close contact with the subjects throughout the study, (d) encourage participation by emphasizing the scientific importance of the trial, and (e) follow up withdrawals or other losses or their family or friends to determine their outcomes wherever possible.[6]

Getting information on withdrawals and losses to follow-up is very important since it can be used to substantiate or refute the findings of a study. Sometimes where losses cannot be traced it is advisable to assume that none and all received the intervention and none and all had the desired outcome to determine the potential range of the study results. In general, withdrawals and losses to follow-up, even if equally distributed among the experimental and control groups, will diminish the power of the study, thereby increasing the probability of a type II error. The RCTs most likely to experience problems with noncompliance, withdrawals, or losses to follow-up are those that involve long, complex protocols; interventions with disagreeable side effects; or patients with severe or fatal diseases who fail to respond to the intervention. Many of the latter will seek other interventions during the course of the study.

Other weaknesses include the long-term commitment and considerable expenses that may be necessary to implement and complete a trial. Randomized controlled trials concerned with the reduction of chronic diseases, for example, may take years to complete at relatively high costs due to low incidence and long latency periods that consequently require long follow-up times and large sample sizes to detect small, but clinically significant, differences in the outcomes. Also, RCTs sometimes address narrowly focused questions in artificial settings, and their applicability to real-world situations may not always be clear. Finally, the reliance on volunteers and the use of strict exclusion criteria may make it difficult to recruit sufficient subjects for a study. These factors, as well as significant subject losses, can also limit the generalizability (external validity) of the findings from RCTs. Table 13–2 summarizes the major strengths and weaknesses of RCTs.

Table 13–2 Major Strengths and Weaknesses of Randomized Controlled Trials

Strengths	Weaknesses
1. They can demonstrate causal relationships with a high level of confidence, due to tightly controlled conditions not possible in observational studies. 2. They allow investigators to control the exposure levels as needed.	1. They have limited applicability due to ethical considerations and sometimes due to the artificial setting of the experiment. 2. There is potential for bias due to differential rates of noncompliance, withdrawals, and losses to follow-up among the study groups. 3. They are usually costly and time consuming to implement. 4. It may be difficult to achieve adequate sample size requirements due to reliance on volunteers and strict eligibility criteria. 5. They may have limited external validity due to the use of volunteers, eligibility criteria, and significant subject losses.

Analysis of RCTs

Planning the Analysis

Before beginning the analysis of an RCT one should examine if the experimental and control groups are similar with regard to important, potentially confounding factors. While randomization, especially with large samples, should equalize the experimental and control groups with regard to potential confounders, chance can still play a role, and therefore it is a good idea to see if the randomized groups are indeed comparable. The experimental and control groups should be similar with regard to factors like age, sex, race/ethnicity, or other potential risk factors that could confound the results. If there are significant differences on important variables, then methods of controlling confounding, such as stratification or multivariable methods (see chapter 11), need to be applied in the analysis.

In general, the results of an RCT should be examined using an **intention-to-treat analysis**. This means that the results should be analyzed based on the original subject assignments to the experimental and control groups at the time of randomization, whether or not all subjects in a group complied with the specified protocol. If there are significant numbers of subjects in the experimental group who did not complete the intervention or if there are subjects in the control group who sought the intervention, collectively known as **crossovers** (not to be confused with intentional crossover in a crossover design), an intention-to-treat analysis will *underestimate* the magnitude of the association between the study intervention and the outcome. Nevertheless, this is preferable to focusing only on compliant subjects, since this nullifies the benefits of randomization and can lead to erroneous conclusions about the effect of the intervention.[1, 6]

Removing those who did not comply with the study protocol may also limit one's ability to apply the findings to medical or public health practice, since it might not make sense to recommend interventions that result in high levels of noncompliance.[15] Also, some studies indicate that compliance itself may have positive effects independent of the intervention, regardless of whether or not one is in the experimental or control group (i.e., the placebo effect). In one study, those in the control group who complied by taking the placebo had a mortality rate of 15% compared to 28% among those who did not comply.[16] Sometimes investigators will analyze the results of an RCT in terms of compliance in order to compare the findings with the intention-to-treat analysis. If the findings are similar, this increases confidence in the results. If there are differences, however, the intention-to-treat analysis should prevail.[6]

Analytical Procedures

A number of techniques can be used to analyze the findings of RCTs. These range from relatively simple to complex. If there are two groups and the outcome variable is dichotomous, the results can be analyzed using procedures that have already been described in relation to observational studies. For example, one can calculate the person-time incidence rates in the experimental and control groups, respectively, and determine the rate ratio (table 12–4) and its 95% confidence interval (formula 12.4). Using formula 6.3b (repeated below), one can also calculate the *percent relative effect* of the intervention. Formula 6.3b is used because it is expected that the intervention will result in an improvement in the outcome (i.e., a decreased incidence rate). Thus, the relative effect measures the decreased *rate* of occurrence of the outcome when the rate ratio is the measure of association. A 95% confidence interval for the percent relative effect is calculated by applying formula 13.2 to the lower- and upper-confidence limits of the applicable rate ratio. *However, the upper confidence limit for the rate ratio is used to calculate the lower confidence limit for the relative effect, and the lower confidence limit for the rate ratio is used to calculate the upper confidence interval for the relative effect.* This is shown in formula 13.2 and illustrated in example 13–1.

(Repeated 6.3 b)

$$\% \text{ Decreased Change} = (1 - \text{Ratio}) \times 100$$

(13.2)

$$95\% \text{ CI for Decrease in the Rate Ratio} =$$
$$(1 - 95\% \text{ UCL of Rate Ratio}) \times 100 \text{ to } (1 - 95\% \text{ LCL of Rate Ratio}) \times 100$$

The CI in formula 13.2 refers to confidence interval, and 95% UCL and 95% LCL refer to the upper 95% confidence limit and the 95% lower confidence limit, respectively.

One could also analyze the findings of an RCT in a manner similar to that described in example 13–1 using cumulative incidence rates or proportions. If the outcome data are continuous (e.g., weekly blood pressure measurements over the course of a study), one might want to compare means between the experimental and control groups.

Example 13–1: Analysis of a Randomized Controlled Trial

A double-blinded randomized controlled trial was initiated to see if saw palmetto berry extract (an herbal remedy) is efficacious in reducing initial emergency urinary retention due to benign prostatic hyperplasia (BPH) in men. Initial emergency urinary retention was defined as the first episode during the study period of an inability to urinate due to BPH that required emergency medical attention. The study sample included a select group of adult men, 60–69 years of age, with diagnosed BPH, who were members of a large health maintenance organization (HMO). One thousand men who met the study selection criteria were randomized into two equally sized experimental and control groups. Those in the experimental group were instructed to take a standardized dose of 350 milligrams of saw palmetto berry extract each evening during dinner. The extract was provided in capsule form and free of charge by the HMO. Those in the control group were given the same instructions but were supplied with a placebo instead. The participants were given free prostate examinations by trained staff urologists every six months for the planned two-year study and were instructed to seek medical assistance if needed using a designated 24-hour telephone hotline. The end point of interest was initial emergency urinary retention, which typically requires immediate urinary catheterization.

At the conclusion of the study, the following data were reported:

- *Experimental group*: 40 incidents of initial emergency urinary retention during 960 person-years of follow-up
- *Control group*: 65 incidents of initial emergency urinary retention during 935 person-years of follow-up

Based on these data, was the treatment efficacious? Explain.

Solution:

Step 1: Place the data provided in the appropriate cells of a tabular display as follows:

Exposure Status	Outcome	Person-years
Exposed	a 40	T_e 960
Unexposed	c 65	T_{ue} 935
	105	1895

It is important to keep in mind that the values in the right-hand column of the display are person-years. Those in the left-hand column are frequencies (a = 40 and c = 65).

Step 2: Calculate the person-time incidence rates of initial emergency urinary retention in the experimental (exposed) and control (unexposed) groups and the rate ratio using the appropriate formulas in table 12–4.

$$IR_{P\text{-}T\text{-}e} = (a \, / \, T_e) \times 10^n = (40 \, / \, 960) \times 10^n = 0.042 \times 10^2 = 4.2 \text{ per 100 person-years}$$
$$IR_{P\text{-}T\text{-}ue} = (c \, / \, T_{ue}) \times 10^n = (65 \, / \, 935) \times 10^n = 0.070 \times 10^2 = 7.0 \text{ per 100 person-years}$$
$$\text{Rate Ratio} = IR_{P\text{-}T\text{-}e} \, / \, IR_{P\text{-}T\text{-}ue} = (4.2 \text{ per 100 person-years}) \, / \, (7.0 \text{ per 100 person-years}) = 0.6$$

Step 3: Calculate the 95% confidence interval (CI) using formula 12.4.

$$95\% \text{ CI} = \exp [\ln (\text{Rate Ratio}) \pm 1.96 \sqrt{1 \, / \, a + 1 \, / \, c}]$$
$$\exp [\ln (0.6) \pm 1.96 \sqrt{(1 \, / \, 40) + (1 \, / \, 65)}] =$$
$$\exp (-0.51 \pm 1.96 \sqrt{0.025 + 0.015}) =$$
$$\exp (-0.51 \pm 1.96 \sqrt{0.040}) = \exp (-0.51 \pm 0.39)$$

The *lower* confidence limit is: $\exp (-0.51 - 0.39) = \exp (-0.90) = 0.4$
The *upper* confidence limit is: $\exp (-0.51 + 0.39) = \exp (-0.12) = 0.9$
Therefore, the 95% confidence interval is 0.4–0.9.

Step 4: Calculate the *percent relative effect* using formula 6.3b and its 95% confidence interval. The 95% confidence interval can be calculated using formula 13.2, along with the 95% upper confidence limit (95% UCL) and the 95% lower confidence limit (95% LCL) already calculated for the rate ratio in step 3.

$$\% \text{ Decreased Change} = (1 - \text{Ratio}) \times 100 = (1 - 0.6) \times 100 = 0.4 \times 100 = 40\%$$
$$95\% \text{ CI for Decrease in the Rate Ratio} =$$
$$(1 - 95\% \text{ UCL of Rate Ratio}) \times 100 \text{ to } (1 - 95\% \text{ LCL of Rate Ratio}) \times 100 =$$
$$(1 - 0.9) \times 100 \text{ to } (1 - 0.4) \times 100 = 0.1 \times 100 \text{ to } 0.6 \times 100 = 10\%\text{–}60\%$$

Therefore, the 95% confidence interval for the percent relative effect is 10%–60%.

Answer: Based on the data, the treatment with saw palmetto berry extract is efficacious. Those in the experimental group had a 40% (95% CI = 10%–60%) reduction in initial episodes of emergency urinary retention due to BHP compared to those in the control group.

Comments:

1. Although not required, the tabular display provides a convenient way of exhibiting the data that are needed to calculate the rate ratio and its 95% confidence interval. The person-time units were provided in this example, but in some cases they may need to be calculated as described in chapter 5.

2. The rate ratio is a measure of association between the exposure (treatment with the saw palmetto berry extract) and the outcome of interest (initial emergency urinary retention due to BHP). Since RCTs are generally designed to see if an intervention improves an outcome, one would expect the rate ratio to be less than one if the intervention is efficacious. In this example the rate ratio was 0.6. Those in the experimental group developed initial emergency urinary retention at a rate of only 0.6 times as great as those in the control group.

3. A rate ratio of 0.6 indicates a moderate association between the exposure and outcome (see figure 6–1). Based on the 95% confidence interval for the rate ratio, we can say that we are 95% sure that the true rate ratio lies between 0.4 and 0.9. Since this interval does not contain one, we can also say that the rate ratio is statistically significant at $p \leq 0.05$. Statistical significance could also have been tested using the person-time chi-square test of independence (see table 12–4) and interpreting the results with the aid of table 10–3. Based on the information provided in the example, we can conclude that the findings of this study support the hypothesis that the saw palmetto berry extract is efficacious in reducing initial emergency urinary retention due to BHP. One could speculate, or demonstrate with additional clinical testing, that it reduces the size of enlarged prostate glands thereby improving urinary flow.

4. The *percent relative effect* is a convenient and simple way to communicate the efficacy of an experimental intervention. The percent relative effect ranges from 0 to 100%, and the closer it is to 100%, the more efficacious the intervention. In this example the percent relative effect was 40%. This indicates a 40% reduction in the outcome is due to the intervention, all other factors being equal. Since the rate ratio was statistically significant, and since the percent relative effect is based on the rate ratio, we can conclude that the percent relative effect is also statistically significant. It is more informative, however, to provide a 95% confidence interval for the percent relative effect. As illustrated in the solution to this problem, this can be derived from the confidence interval for the rate ratio. The 95% confidence interval for the percent relative effect also indicates statistical significance as long as it does not contain zero. Based on the calculated 95% confidence interval for the percent relative effect, we can be 95% sure that the true percent relative effect is between 10% and 60% in the sampled population.

A more complex way of analyzing data from RCTs involves **survival analysis**. This method can be useful when the follow-up periods vary widely for subjects or when the subjects enter a study at different times.[9] Basically, in survival analysis one plots the time for each subject from application of the intervention to a nonrecurrent event, such as death, disease, or another predetermined end point, on a *survival curve*. Survival curves can provide data on the percent survival (time until outcome) for any given time period, median survival time for a group, and other useful information.[17] The Cox Proportional Hazards model is an efficient method of multivariable survival analysis that allows one to control for several confounding factors.[9] A more detailed discussion of survival analysis is beyond the scope of this text. Those who are interested in the topic may want to consult the text of Mark Woodward[12] or other advanced textbooks of epidemiologic methods. Survival analysis may also be used in the analysis of the results of cohort studies.

Community Trials

Community trials were introduced in chapter 4. A community trial is an epidemiologic experiment where, unlike RCTs, the units of analysis are entire communities or groups of people. Most often the communities represent cities, towns, or villages, but they may also include other political subdivisions (counties, states) or other groupings of people such as schools, occupational settings, or nursing homes. Community trials generally have one of two major objectives: (a) to test etiologic hypotheses about health-related exposures and outcomes, or (b) to evaluate the impact of health-related programs, projects, or campaigns on communities. Community trials designed to meet the first objective are true epidemiologic studies; those designed to meet the second objective are **evaluation studies**. Technically, evaluation studies are *not* epidemiologic studies in the classical sense, although they may use the same epidemiologic methods. Because the methods are the same, many textbooks do not make this differentiation; nevertheless, it is important to know the difference.

As with RCTs, community trials involve a number of considerations that should be a part of an overall study protocol. Some of the important points are developing a research hypothesis, selecting the communities to be studied, collecting baseline data on the study outcomes, allocating the communities into experimental and control groups, applying the intervention, and assessing outcomes during the follow-up period. The following sections briefly discuss some of these issues.

Selecting the Communities

In the most basic community trial just two communities are compared. One serves as the experimental community, and the other serves as the control community. The Newburgh-Kingston study discussed in chapter 4 is an example of a two-community study.[18] Other well-known examples include the Pawtucket Heart Health Program conducted in Rhode Island[19] and the North Karelia Project conducted in Finland.[20] The Pawtucket program used a community-wide educational approach involving multilevel education, screening, and counseling to modify risks for cardiovascular disease. The North Karelia program also was aimed at reducing cardiovascular disease primarily through community-based educational and screening approaches. Both of these community trials were *evaluation studies*. The Newburgh-Kingston study, however, was an epidemiologic study. Community trials may also involve multiple intervention or control communities. An example is the Communities Mobilizing for Change on Alcohol study referred to in chapter 4.[21]

Whether two or more communities are involved in a community trial, selection of the experimental and control communities entails a number of considerations. First, the communities should be similar to each other. This is important for potential confounders, such as age, sex, and racial/ethnic distributions; income levels; population size; and access to relevant health care or public health resources. The communities should also exhibit relatively stable populations. If there is significant movement into or out of a community, it will be more difficult to detect changes due to an intervention. Another important issue is willingness of the communities to participate in an experimental study. This will involve discussions with those in positions of authority (e.g., city councils and mayoral staff), leaders in the communities, and others. It will also be important to inform community members of their participation via the media.[22] Finally, there should be sufficient evidence that the communities are experiencing high enough levels of the study exposures and outcomes to justify an experiment and to allow the investigators to detect any significant changes over time. As with RCTs, sample size must be estimated to ensure sufficient study power. The techniques for determining sample size are similar to those used for RCTs, although the subjects are groups.

Collecting Baseline Data on Study Outcomes

In order to determine if an intervention is effective, it is crucial to be able to measure changes in study outcomes over the course of the trial. This requires the collection of baseline data on study outcomes in each community, which can be compared with data collected during and after the conclusion of the study. Study outcomes may include reduction in the incidence or mortality of specific diseases, in the prevalence of known risk factors, or in changes in harmful behaviors or practices. For example, the Newburgh-Kingston study looked for a reduction in the incidence of dental caries resulting from fluoridation of the drinking water supply, and the Communities Mobilizing for Change on Alcohol study looked for a reduction in underage accessibility to alcohol due to changes in adolescent behaviors and the practices of establishments selling alcohol. The methods used to collect outcome data at baseline and throughout the study should be the same to reduce the possibility of measurement bias.[22]

Allocating Communities, Applying Interventions, and Assessing Outcomes

Ideally, the allocation of communities into experimental and control groups should be random as discussed in chapter 4. When this is not feasible, selection bias is a possibility, and its potential effects on the outcomes should be evaluated and discussed by the investigators. Random allocation to experimental and control groups requires that all of the participating communities are willing to support the intervention should they be chosen as an experimental group. Technically, community trials that use randomization to allocate communities to experimental and control groups are classified as true experiments, while those that do not are referred to as quasi-experimental studies (see chapter 4).

Once the communities have been allocated into experimental and control groups, the intervention is applied. This can take two basic forms depending on whether the purpose is to test an epidemiologic hypothesis about exposure and outcome (true epidemiologic study) or whether the study is designed to evaluate the impact of a program on community health status (an evaluation study). The intervention is considered effective to the extent that the experimental communities show a significantly greater reduction in the study outcomes compared to the control communities, all other factors being equal. Of course, the difference in outcomes between the communities should also be of *practical* significance.

It is important to realize that while community trials may involve collection, measurement, and analysis of data on individuals within the communities being compared, the ultimate interest is in comparing the results for the communities as a whole. Sometimes it can be confusing in deciding whether a trial is individual- or community-based. Key determining factors are that the control group represents an entirely different community from the one in which the intervention is applied and that the intervention is assigned at the community level. In RCTs we start with one group of individuals (the study sample) and split it into separate groups. Our interest is in individual responses to the intervention. Is the intervention more efficacious in those *individuals* who receive it than those who do not? In community trials we start with at least two different groups that remain intact during the investigation. Our interest is in community responses to the intervention. Is the intervention more effective in the *communities* receiving the intervention than those communities not receiving it? Project Northland, a community trial conducted in northeastern Minnesota, for example, used multilevel, community-wide approaches to preventing alcohol use among adolescents in 24 school districts and surrounding communities.[23] The investigators found that after three years of study, students *in the school districts* receiving the intervention reported significantly less alcohol use than those *in the school districts* that served as controls. It should be clear that the comparisons in this example are between the overall experiences of the separate school districts and not between exposed and unexposed individuals in the sample. This community trial, by the way, was an evaluation study.

Major Strengths and Weaknesses of Community Trials

Community trials have a number of potential strengths and weaknesses. In terms of strengths, well-designed and controlled community trials can provide strong evidence to support causal associations. In the general hierarchy of epidemiologic studies with regard to their ability to establish causation, community trials generally are listed ahead of prospective cohort studies and just behind RCTs. Community trials may also be more appropriate than RCTs when community intervention is considered important. Thomas D. Koepsell discusses some instances where community interventions may be appropriate.[24] At least two of these suggest circumstances where community trials may be preferable to RCTs:

1. *When the intent of the intervention is to prevent more cases of disease than could be achieved by targeting only selected individuals.* A community trial can be an effective way of determining whether a

given strategy can reach a broad group of individuals with varying levels of risk for the outcome of interest. An intervention aimed at an entire community has the potential of preventing more cases of the disease than intervention trials aimed only at high-risk individuals. This is particularly true when the risk factors are very common in a population, such as those for heart disease (e.g., obesity, high cholesterol, hypertension, sedentary lifestyle).

2. *Where the outcome is influenced by the social context.* It is generally more desirable to study an intervention in the context of its social setting if one believes the social milieu influences compliance with the intervention (e.g., studies of the management of problem drinking). Conversely, interventions in RCTs that are found to be promising in the controlled conditions of a clinical environment may not work well in more natural social settings. Community trials provide an opportunity to test interventions in "real-life" situations, whereas some RCTs may involve more artificial surroundings.

Also, it might be more advantageous to conduct a community trial when the intervention being tested would be less costly than a clinical intervention applied to a given population. For example, treating individuals with AIDS would be more expensive to implement in a large population than public service announcements aimed at helping individuals recognize the risk factors for the disease, assuming this method works.

Community trials have a number of potential weaknesses. Some of the more important are:

1. *Changes in the study outcomes may be due to causes other than the intervention.* These can occur because of differences in the makeup of the communities being compared (e.g., due to inherent differences in resident attitudes, behaviors, or norms), changes in the composition of one or more of the communities due to significant population growth or decline during the trial period, different secular trends operating in different communities, and other events occurring in one or more of the communities. The two-community study is most susceptible to this problem. Studies with multiple intervention and control groups provide a basis for recognizing and possibly accounting for inconsistent findings among the experimental or control communities.[24] Changes in study outcomes due to causes other than the intervention can produce erroneous results.

2. *Depending on the types of interventions, community trials can be expensive and time consuming.* Trials involving multiple, complex interventions and numerous communities are especially subject to these limitations. Those that hope to demonstrate declines in the incidence of chronic diseases will also take longer to complete as will those studies that rely more heavily on primary versus secondary data collection.

3. *Randomization of communities into experimental and control groups may not always be feasible.* This can affect the comparability of the

communities in unrecognized ways and can lead to selection bias. As mentioned previously, community trials that do not involve random- ization are technically quasi-experimental studies. They lack some of the rigor of experimental studies and, hence, some of the credibility.

4. *Because the findings of community trials are based on group data, it is possible to commit an ecological fallacy.* Just as in ecological stud- ies, drawing inferences about individuals based on a community trial may lead to incorrect conclusions since the associations are based on aggregate data.

Table 13–3 summarizes the major strengths and weaknesses of community trials.

Table 13–3 Major Strengths and Weaknesses of Community Trials

Strengths	Weaknesses
1. They can provide strong evidence in support of cause–effect relationships. 2. They may be the most appropriate epi- demiologic design in certain situations (e.g., when risk factors for the outcome are very common and when the social context influences compliance with the intervention).	1. Differences in the study outcomes may be due to causes other than the inter- vention (this is especially true for studies that involve only one intervention and control group). 2. They may be expensive and time con- suming to conduct. 3. Selection bias may occur when random- ization of the intervention is not feasible. 4. An ecological fallacy can occur if infer- ences based on group data are made about individuals in the communities.

Analysis of Community Trials

One way of analyzing the findings of community trials is to test for differences on the outcome variables based on the aggregate experiences of each of the communities being compared. These differences between the experimental and control communities may be calculated in terms of proportions, rates, or means and tested for statistical significance using the appropriate methods (e.g., chi-square tests, t-tests). Tests of means assume that the populations being tested have equal variances on the outcome measures, which are usu- ally met when the populations being compared are of similar size. A problem arises, however, when the results are based on a two-community study. As mentioned in the previous section, these studies may be subject to changes in outcomes caused by factors other than the intervention. This can confound the results of a community trial in possibly unaccountable ways. For a more detailed discussion of the approaches to the analysis of community trials, including the problem with two-community comparisons, see Koepsell.[24]

Summary

- In experimental studies, the investigators directly control the study conditions. There are two main types of planned experimental studies—randomized controlled trials (RCTs) and community trials. A third, unplanned type of experimental study is the natural experiment, a situation in nature resembling the conditions of a planned experiment.

- An RCT is an epidemiologic experiment where individual subjects are randomly assigned to experimental and control groups to assess the efficacy of an intervention. Important design considerations involve sample selection, randomization of subjects, application of the intervention, and outcome assessment during follow-up.

- The major strength of RCTs is their ability to demonstrate causal associations. Weaknesses include limited use due to ethical concerns, potential errors of inference due to noncompliance and subject losses, time and cost commitments, and possibly limited external validity.

- Community trials are epidemiologic experiments where the units of analysis are groups, usually cities or towns. They may be designed to test etiologic hypotheses about exposure and outcome (true epidemiologic studies) or to evaluate the impact of programs, projects, or campaigns on community health status (evaluation studies). Important design elements include community selection, collection of baseline data, allocation of communities to experimental and control groups, application of the intervention, and outcome assessment.

- Strengths of community trials include support for causal associations and usefulness when community intervention is considered important. Weaknesses include difficulty in attributing changes to the intervention, especially in two-community comparisons; time and cost commitments; and potential problems using randomization.

- Analysis of experimental studies may involve comparisons of incidence rates, proportions, means, and other advanced measures. Special considerations may apply for community trials.

New Terms

carryover effects	exclusion criteria	placebo effect
crossover	factorial design	placebo-controlled trial
crossover design	inclusion criteria	randomization
double-blinded study	intention-to-treat	single-blinded study
effect size	analysis	stratified randomization
effective sample size	intervention study	study protocol
eligibility criteria	meta-analysis	survival analysis
end point	natural experiment	triple-blinded study
evaluation study	placebo	washout period

Study Questions and Exercises

1. Describe how you would design a valid randomized controlled trial to test the hypothesis that Low-Chol, a new oral medication to lower serum cholesterol, decreases the risk of death from coronary heart disease in healthy men, 40–54 years of age, at high risk for the disease. Include in your description how you would select the study sample, determine the subject eligibility criteria, ascertain the appropriate sample size, allocate the subjects into experimental and control groups, apply the intervention, and assess the outcomes during follow-up.

2. Assume the randomized controlled trial you designed in item 1 was implemented with the following results:

Exposure Status	CHD deaths	Person-years
Taking Low-Chol	29	16,500
Not Taking Low-Chol	62	19,350
	91	35,850

Assuming that the study was designed to minimize bias and confounding, determine if Low-Chol is efficacious in reducing deaths due to coronary heart disease based on the study findings. To support your conclusion provide the percent relative effect and its 95% confidence interval. Interpret these measures.

3. Describe how you would design a valid community trial to test the hypothesis that air pollution abatement in large cities reduces childhood asthma. Include in your description how you would select the communities to study, allocate them to experimental and control groups, apply the intervention, collect the appropriate data to evaluate, and assess the effectiveness of the intervention.

4. Indicate whether each of the following statements is true or false (T or F). For each false statement, indicate why it is false.

____ a. There are three major types of unplanned experimental epidemiologic studies—randomized controlled trials, community trials, and natural experiments.

____ b. Randomized controlled trials are subject to ecological fallacies.

____ c. Stratified randomization is most useful in a randomized controlled trial when the sample size is large.

____ d. The study sample for a randomized controlled trial is selected from the experimental population.

____ e. Intention-to-treat analysis tends to overestimate the magnitude of the association between a study intervention and outcome in a randomized controlled trial if the number of crossovers is large.

___ f. Technically, evaluation studies are not true epidemiologic studies.

___ g. Blinding in a randomized controlled trial tends to minimize the capacity of the placebo effect to bias the study results.

___ h. The smaller the effect size, the smaller the sample size required in a randomized controlled trial.

___ i. The internal validity of a randomized controlled trial is not affected by a study sample that is not representative of the experimental population.

___ j. Two-community studies are more subject to errors due to confounding than multiple-community studies.

___ k. In a factorial design of a randomized controlled trial each subject is assigned to the experimental group at one time or another.

___ l. Loss to follow-up in randomized controlled trials can increase the probability of a type II error.

References

1. Last, J. M., ed. (1995). *A Dictionary of Epidemiology*. New York: Oxford University Press.
2. Meldrum, M. L. (2000). A Brief History of the Randomized Controlled Trial: From Oranges to the Gold Standard. *Hematology/Oncology Clinics of North America*: 14(4): 745–760.
3. Francis, T., Jr., Napier, J. A., Voight, R. B., Hemphill, F. M., Wenner, H. A., Korns, R. F., Boisen, M., Tolchinsky, E., and Diamond, E. L. (1955). Evaluation of 1954 Field Trials of Poliomyelitis Vaccine. In *The Challenge of Epidemiology: Issues and Selected Readings*, C. Buck, A. Llopis, E. Najera, and M. Terris, eds. Washington, DC: Pan American Health Organization, 1988, pp. 838–854.
4. White, H. D., Simes, R. J., Anderson, N. E., Hankey, G. J., Watson, J. D., Hunt, D., Colquhoun, D. M., Glasziou, P., MacMahon, S., Kirby, A. C., West, M. J., and Tonkin, A. M. (2000). Pravastatin Therapy and the Risk of Stroke. *New England Journal of Medicine* 343(5): 317–326.
5. Hennekens, C. H., and Buring, J. E. (1987). *Epidemiology in Medicine*. Boston: Little, Brown and Company.
6. Hulley, S. B., Cummings, S. R., Browner, W. S., Grady, D., Hearst, N., and Newman, T. B. (2001). *Designing Clinical Research: An Epidemiologic Approach*, 2nd ed. Philadelphia: Lippincott Williams & Wilkins.
7. Malone, R. P., Delaney, M. A., Luebbert, J. F., Cater, J., and Campbell, M. (2000). A Double-Blind Placebo-Controlled Study of Lithium in Hospitalized Aggressive Children and Adolescents with Conduct Disorder. *Archives of General Psychiatry* 57(7): 649–654.
8. Meinert, C. L. (1986). *Clinical Trials: Design, Conduct, and Analysis*. New York: Oxford University Press.
9. Wassertheil-Smoller, S. (1990). *Biostatistics and Epidemiology: A Primer for Health Professionals*. New York: Springer-Verlag.
10. Elwood, J. M. (1988). *Causal Relationships in Medicine: A Practical System for Critical Appraisal*. New York: Oxford University Press.
11. Hennekens, C., and Eberlein, K. (1985). A Randomized Trial of Aspirin and Beta-carotene Among U.S. Physicians. *Preventive Medicine* 14(2): 165–168.
12. Woodward, M. (1999). *Epidemiology: Study Design and Data Analysis*. Boca Raton, FL: Chapman and Hall/CRC.
13. Fisher, B., Bauer, M., Margolese, R., Poisson, R., Pilch, Y., Redmond, C., Fisher, E., Wolmark, N., Deutsch, M., Montague, E. et al. (1985). Five-year Results of a Randomized Clinical Trial Comparing Total Mastectomy and Segmental Mastectomy With or Without Radiation in the Treatment of Breast Cancer. *New England Journal of Medicine* 312(11): 665–673.
14. Cooper, G. M. (1992). *Elements of Human Cancer*. Boston: Jones and Bartlett Publishers.
15. Greenberg, R. S., Daniels, S. R., Flanders, W. D., Eley, J. W., and Boring, J. R. (1996). *Medical Epidemiology*, 2nd ed. Norwalk, CT: Appleton and Lange.
16. Coronary Drug Project Research Group (1980). Influence of Adherence to Treatment and Response of Cholesterol on Mortality in the Coronary Drug Project. *New England Journal of Medicine* 303(18): 1038–1041.

17. Motulsky, H. (1995). *Intuitive Biostatistics*. New York: Oxford University Press.
18. Ast, D. B., and Schlesinger, E. R. (1956). The Conclusion of a Ten-year Study of Water Fluoridation. *American Journal of Public Health* 46(3): 265–271.
19. Carleton, R. A., Lasater, T. M., Assaf, A. R., Feldman, H. A., and McKinlay, S. (1995). The Pawtucket Heart Health Program: Community Changes in Cardiovascular Risk Factors and Projected Disease Risk. *American Journal of Public Health* 85(6): 777–785.
20. Puska, P., Salonen, J. T., Nissinen, A., Tuomilehto, J., Vartiainen, E., Korhonen, H., Tanskanen, A., Ronnqvist, P., Koskela, K., Huttunen, J. (1983). Change in Risk Factors for Coronary Heart Disease During 10 Years of a Community Intervention Programme (North Karelia Project). *British Medical Journal* 287(6408): 1840–1844.
21. Wagenaar, A. C., Murray, D. M., Gehan, J. P., Wolfson, M., Forster, J. L., Toomey, T. L., Perry, C. L., and Jones-Webb, R. (2000). Communities Mobilizing for Change on Alcohol: Outcomes from a Randomized Community Trial. *Journal of Studies on Alcohol:* 61(1): 85–94.
22. Lilienfeld, D. E., and Stolley, P. D. (1994). *Foundations of Epidemiology*, 3rd ed. New York: Oxford University Press.
23. Komro, K. A., Perry, C. L., Williams, C. L., Stigler, M. H., Farbakhsh, K., and Veblen-Mortenson (2001). How Did Project Northland Reduce Alcohol Use Among Young Adolescents? *Health Education Research* 16(1): 59–70.
24. Koepsell, T. D. (1998). Epidemiologic Issues in the Design of Community Intervention Trials. In *Applied Epidemiology: Theory to Practice*, R. C. Brownson and D. B. Petitti, eds., pp. 177–211. New York: Oxford University Press.

CHAPTER FOURTEEN

Applications of Epidemiology
Disease Outbreaks, Disease Clusters, and Public Health Surveillance

Learning Objectives

▶ Explain the meaning and the differences among the terms epidemic, endemic, disease outbreak, and disease cluster.

▶ Describe the primary and secondary purposes of disease outbreak investigation.

▶ Discuss the steps involved in disease outbreak investigations.

▶ Interpret epidemic curves as to the probable type of epidemic, and for common source epidemics, the probable time of exposure.

▶ Construct and interpret attack rate tables using the appropriate statistical measures.

▶ Discuss the problems of investigating disease clusters.

▶ Describe the objectives, major uses, and sources of data for public health surveillance systems.

▶ Describe the ideal characteristics of an effective public health surveillance system.

▶ Define public health surveillance, active surveillance, passive surveillance, sentinel surveillance, cancer cluster, emerging and reemerging infectious diseases, index case, sentinel event, vector, and vehicle.

Overview

Disease outbreaks are localized epidemics that usually involve communicable diseases or acute poisonings. Outbreaks are investigated primarily to prevent further cases and similar outbreaks in the future. The steps in outbreak investigation are well established and should guide the investigation to a conclusion about the cause of the outbreak. Major types of outbreaks are common source and propagated outbreaks. Disease clusters are said to occur when cases of a relatively uncommon disease are grouped in space or time. Identifying the causes of nonrandom clustering can be a difficult task. Public health surveillance is the ongoing collection, analysis, interpretation, and dissemination of health-related data for public health purposes. Surveillance is important in detecting disease outbreaks, identifying trends in health problems, and establishing program priorities.

Introduction

This chapter addresses three common applications of epidemiology—the investigation of disease outbreaks, the detection of disease clusters, and public health surveillance. Public health authorities frequently become aware of potential disease outbreaks through observations and reporting by physicians, nurses, or laboratory workers who notice abnormal numbers of cases of a disease or unusual symptoms or clinical findings.[1] Disease clusters are usually reported by members of the public who become aware of the grouping of generally uncommon diseases believed to have common environmental causes. Public health surveillance is a key element of public health practice and the means by which diseases and other conditions are recorded, tracked, and monitored to detect potential disease outbreaks or clusters and, ultimately, to protect and improve public health.

Purpose of Investigating Disease Outbreaks

Although the terms epidemic and endemic were defined in chapter 1, it should be helpful to reiterate and elaborate on the meaning of these terms before discussing the purpose of disease outbreak investigations. An epidemic is the occurrence of a specific disease at a frequency that is *clearly in excess* of normal expectations for a given population, time, and place. It may involve a communicable or noncommunicable disease or other health-related event (e.g., lead poisoning). The *usual* frequency of the disease is referred to as the endemic level. Therefore, in order to determine if a disease is epidemic, we compare its frequency in a given population, time, and place to the endemic level of the disease to ascertain if its occurrence is clearly in excess.

A commonly raised question is what constitutes "clearly in excess"? While there is no definitive answer to this question, one must realize that even the frequency of an endemic disease fluctuates, and *expected* increases based on past experience do not constitute epidemics. The presence of an epidemic implies that something *unusual* is happening in a population and that there is a certain cause for the sudden increase in the incidence of the disease. An investigation is the usual way of determining the cause and its appropriate management. Sometimes a suspected epidemic will turn out to be due to sporadic, unrelated cases of the disease, a different disease with similar symptoms, changes in reporting procedures, new diagnostic criteria for the disease, population changes that affect the incidence rate, or other factors.[2] These situations do not represent epidemics. For example, we expect influenza rates in the Midwest to rise substantially in the late fall and early winter and to be at relatively low levels at other times of the year. Influenza is not, however, epidemic in the fall and winter months unless the incidence rate is substantially higher than anticipated for that time of year. Instead, influenza is following an *expected* cyclic (seasonal) pattern (see chapter 1). Finally, it is worth mentioning that "clearly in excess" does not necessarily mean statistically different from expected levels. Even one case of smallpox in a population would be considered epidemic, since the World Health Organization has certified this disease to be globally eradicated.[3]

The term **disease outbreak** is often used synonymously with epidemic, but technically it refers to an epidemic confined to a localized area, such a town or within an institutional setting like a day-care center. Epidemics, on the other hand, are not limited to localized areas, and very large epidemics (those that generally traverse international borders and affect large numbers of people) are known as pandemics.[4] Disease outbreak investigations, therefore, may be more limited in their scope than some epidemic investigations. In addition, they usually involve communicable diseases or acute poisonings. Also, a disease outbreak should be differentiated from a **disease cluster**, which is the occurrence of a group of cases, usually of a relatively uncommon disease (e.g., leukemia), in space or time whose distribution is *believed not to be due to chance.*[4] Members of the public are often the first to report suspected disease clusters and to demand that public health authorities investigate. These investigations usually reveal that the cluster is either a random variation from an expected pattern or a collection of diseases with different etiologies. More will be said about disease clusters later in this chapter.

The primary purpose of investigating a disease outbreak is to identify the cause of the outbreak so that effective controls can be initiated to prevent further spread of the disease and to prevent similar outbreaks from occurring in the future. Outbreak investigation also provides opportunities for research, training, and program improvement.[2] Disease outbreaks can present opportunities to learn more about the natural history of a disease, to identify important risk factors, and to test control procedures. The investigation of outbreaks also provides opportunities to train new and aspiring epidemiologists. The Centers for Disease Control and Prevention (CDC), for example, operates a number of training programs. Furthermore, local and state public health departments can benefit from outbreak investigations by identifying program weaknesses or gaps that may have led to an outbreak. Sometimes outbreak investigations are initiated because of public demands or political pressure even when the existence of an outbreak is highly doubtful. This chapter focuses on the primary purpose of disease outbreak investigation, which is the protection of public health.

Framework for Investigating Disease Outbreaks

General Guidelines

The investigation of a disease outbreak can be a time-intensive and laborious process depending on the nature of the disease, its distribution, and the need for answers. Michael B. Gregg and others have outlined the major tasks that should be completed in investigating a disease outbreak.[5] The most basic steps are described briefly in exhibit 14–1. These steps are not always followed sequentially and some may be completed simultaneously; therefore, they are best perceived as guidelines. The investigation of a disease outbreak rarely proceeds in an orderly fashion from step one to step two and so on. In many cases the next step begins before the previous step has been completed. This is due to the fact that data are continually being collected or evaluated during the investigative process. Just as a homicide detective may revisit the scene of the crime several times during an investigation or interview suspects and witnesses on more than one occasion, the epidemiologist performing an investigation of a disease outbreak may go back and forth among the steps as new information comes to light.

Exhibit 14–1 Basic Steps in Investigating a Disease Outbreak

1. Verify the Existence of an Outbreak

It is important to be reasonably sure that one is dealing with an outbreak before committing valuable resources. The existence of an outbreak is established by determining if the rate of reported cases of the disease exceeds expected levels. Most local or state health departments should have ongoing surveillance systems that track reportable diseases over time and that can be used to verify an outbreak. The cases may be unconfirmed at this point, and one should also be aware of factors that might artificially increase the rate of reported cases (e.g., recent changes in reporting procedures). Verifying the existence of an outbreak may involve telephone surveys of physicians, hospitals, or clinics and examination of absentee records from schools or places of work.

2. Confirm the Diagnosis of the Disease

Some outbreaks may be due to familiar diseases, and others may be due to unrecognized diseases. In either case, it is important to confirm the diagnosis of the disease early in the investigation. Sometimes this can be done in step one. Confirming the diagnosis should keep the investigation on track and help in identifying the cause of the outbreak. Diagnosis should be established by standard laboratory procedures wherever possible, although it is not necessary, nor always possible, to confirm every case of the disease by laboratory means. Clinical diagnosis may be the norm.

3. Prepare a Case Definition and Count Cases

Once the diagnosis has been established, it is important to develop a working case definition using accepted criteria. The criteria will include signs and symptoms of the disease and any restrictions by person, place, or time variables. The purpose of the criteria is to differentiate cases from noncases, and the criteria should be kept as simple and objective as possible (e.g., presence of fever, bloody diarrhea, elevated white blood cell counts). For convenience, cases can be classified as *suspect* (those meeting some of the criteria), *probable* (those meeting most of the criteria), and *definite* (those with laboratory confirmation). Cases can be moved along the suspect-to-definite spectrum as additional evidence becomes available. This helps to minimize false positives. Once the case definition has been prepared, one needs to find and record the number of cases. This may involve contacting or visiting health care providers, laboratories, institutions, and businesses or conducting community surveys. In addition, one should collect as much information on the cases as possible (demographic information, time of onset, clinical features, possible exposures, contacts, etc.).

4. Characterize the Data by Person, Place, and Time Variables

Characterizing the data that were collected in step three by person, place, and time variables is equivalent to performing a descriptive epidemiologic study. The purpose is to provide a comprehensive profile of the cases that will suggest hypotheses as to the cause of the outbreak. The profile can be updated during the course of the investigation as necessary. Person variables include personal characteristics, like age, sex, race, and occupation, as well as personal behaviors that may be related to exposure (e.g., eating raw shellfish). Place variables can reveal the geographic distribution of cases and clustering around potentially important factors (e.g., water supplies, wooded areas). Time factors usually refer to time of onset of the disease. When plotted against the number of cases, the graphic display that results (i.e., the epidemic curve) can reveal the likely mode of transmission of the disease and other clues that may be helpful in identifying the cause of the outbreak.

5. Formulate and Test Hypotheses

The results of the previous steps generally should be sufficient to develop specific hypotheses about the causes of the outbreak. Testing hypotheses may be as simple as comparing the hypotheses with the known facts or may involve case-control or retrospective cohort studies to confirm the suspected causes.

6. Prepare a Written Report and Conduct Control and Prevention Measures

The report of an outbreak investigation should be definitive. If it is not possible to come to definitive conclusions following the previous steps, it may be necessary to extend the investigation. Generally, one wants to reach conclusions that eliminate alternative explanations. Definitive conclusions should facilitate cooperation in implementing control and prevention efforts, which should be aimed at curtailing the current outbreak, if it is still in progress, and preventing future outbreaks due to insights gained from the investigation. Some level of control should also be possible in earlier steps.

References: Gregg, M. B. (1996). Conducting a Field Investigation. In *Field Epidemiology*, M. B. Gregg, ed. New York: Oxford University Press, pp. 44–59; Centers for Disease Control and Prevention (1992). *Principles of Epidemiology: An Introduction to Applied Epidemiology and Biostatistics*, 2nd ed. Atlanta: The Centers.

Person, Place, and Time

One of the most revealing steps in the investigation of a disease outbreak comes when one characterizes the data by person, place, and time variables (the fourth step in exhibit 14–1). This step can provide specific information about potential risk factors that is helpful in generating hypotheses about the nature and causes of the outbreak. This information is enhanced when it can be presented in graphic form. For example, when cases are plotted on a spot map (chapter 2) by *place* of occurrence or residence, along with other geographic features, one may get visual clues that suggest the possible source of the outbreak. Figure 14–1 is a spot map showing a hypothetical distribution of cases of histoplasmosis.* The grouping of the cases near an abandoned amusement park strongly suggests that the park may have been the source of the infection. As mentioned in chapter 2, one must be careful in interpreting

---

* Histoplasmosis is a respiratory disease caused by inhalation of dusts contaminated by the droppings of infected pigeons and other birds.

spot maps if the population is not evenly distributed over the mapped area.[4] In these instances area-specific disease rates should be used instead of the number of cases to account for differences in population density among the areas being compared.[2] As indicated in chapter 1, unless the denominators (e.g., the populations at risk) are the same, we should always confine our comparisons to rates and not to numerators alone (i.e., raw numbers).

The appropriate rates to use in investigating disease outbreaks are **attack rates**, which are cumulative incidence rates applied to a narrowly but well-defined population being observed over a limited time period.[5] The calculation of attack rates proceeds in the same manner as cumulative incidence rates (see formula 14.1), but they are often reported as percentages (i.e., using a rate base of 10^2 or 100). Attack rates are usually calculated by age, sex, race, occupation, and other relevant *person* variables to reveal potentially high-risk groups.

(14.1)

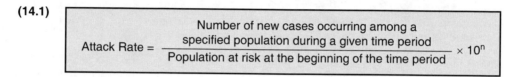

$$\text{Attack Rate} = \frac{\begin{array}{c}\text{Number of new cases occurring among a}\\\text{specified population during a given time period}\end{array}}{\text{Population at risk at the beginning of the time period}} \times 10^n$$

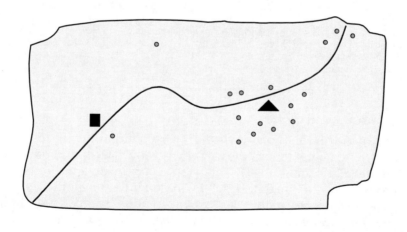

■ **Elementary School**   ▲ **Abandoned Amusement Park**   ○ **Histoplasmosis Case**

(Based on an actual outbreak that occurred in the Midwest in the 1970s)

Figure 14–1 Spot map showing a grouping of cases of histoplasmosis near an abandoned amusement park along a river

When the distribution of cases is plotted by *time* of disease onset, a wealth of information is revealed about a disease outbreak, including its magnitude, its likely source and mode of transmission, its possible duration, and the nature of the disease, including its probable etiological agent and incubation period.[5] This information is useful in generating hypotheses about the cause of the disease outbreak. A graphic representation of the case distribution by time of onset in the form of a histogram is known as an **epidemic curve**. Usually, epidemic curves are constructed for the outbreak as a whole, but they can also be constructed for specific person or place variables to determine how these variables influence the time of disease onset or exposure.[5] The use of epidemic curves in generating hypotheses about the types of disease outbreaks is discussed in the following section.

Epidemic Curves and Types of Outbreaks

The shape and characteristics of an epidemic curve can aid in the identification of the probable type of outbreak, which in turn may suggest possible causes for an outbreak as discussed in the previous section. There are several factors other than the type of outbreak, however, that can influence the shape and characteristics of epidemic curves. These include the size of the time intervals used in graphing an epidemic curve (in general, the x-axis should be in time units about one-fourth of the length of the incubation period of the disease or less),[2, 5] the thoroughness of case finding, the certainty of the diagnosis, the length of the incubation period of the disease, the number of susceptible individuals, and the point one is at in the outbreak. Because of these factors, epidemic curves should not be used in isolation to draw conclusions about the type of outbreak. The accumulated data should always be viewed as a whole.

There are three basic types of disease outbreaks or epidemics: *common source, propagated,* and *mixed.* Each of these exhibits a characteristic epidemic curve as described below.

Common Source Outbreaks

A **common source outbreak** is an outbreak that results from the exposure of a susceptible group of people to a common agent of disease (e.g., pathogenic organism, toxic substance). An outbreak of salmonellosis resulting from the consumption of contaminated egg salad during a church-sponsored buffet luncheon is an example of a common source outbreak. In this example, the egg salad is considered the **vehicle*** that supported the growth and transmission of the salmonella organism, which is the common agent of the disease. Common source outbreaks can be further classified as *point source outbreaks, continuing source outbreaks,* or *intermittent source outbreaks.*[5]

---

* In the context of epidemiology, a *vehicle* is an inanimate substance or object, such as food, water, bedding, or surgical equipment, that is capable of transmitting an agent of disease to a susceptible host. The vehicle serves as an intermediary in disease transmission, and the mechanism of transmission is considered indirect. A vehicle may or may not support the growth of the agent.[2, 3]

A **point source outbreak** is a type of common source outbreak where the duration of exposure to the common agent of disease is relatively brief and virtually simultaneous among those exposed. The epidemic curve typically shows a rapid rise in the number of cases to a peak level followed by a more gradual decline as illustrated in figure 14–2. Point source outbreaks are relatively short-lived and normally conclude within a time frame equal to the range of the incubation period of the disease.

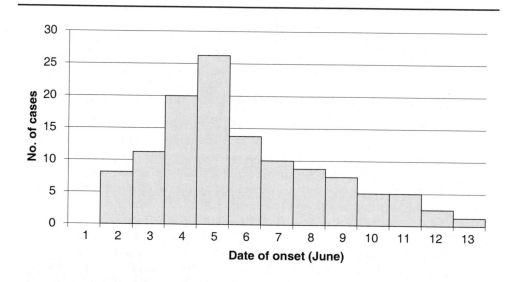

Hypothetical outbreak of cryptosporidiosis, a waterborne parasitic disease, with an approximate incubation period of 1–12 days. Notice that the outbreak shows a rapid rise in the number of cases to a peak level followed by a more gradual decline, and that it lasts for a duration equal to the range of the incubation period of the disease (i.e., 12 days).

Reference: Chin, J., ed. (2000). *Control of Communicable Diseases Manual,* 17th ed. Washington, DC: American Public Health Association.

Figure 14–2 Example of an epidemic curve representing a point source outbreak

A **continuing source outbreak** is a common source outbreak where the exposure to the common agent of disease is prolonged beyond a brief period, and the exposure is not simultaneous among those exposed. For example, a continuing source outbreak might occur when visitors at a park consume contaminated water over a period of several days. The epidemic curve usually shows a rapid rise in the number of cases to a plateau followed by a gradual decline. Continuing source outbreaks are expected to last longer than the time range of the incubation period of the disease because the exposure period is protracted, and not all are exposed at the same time. Figure 14–3 shows an example of a continuing source outbreak.

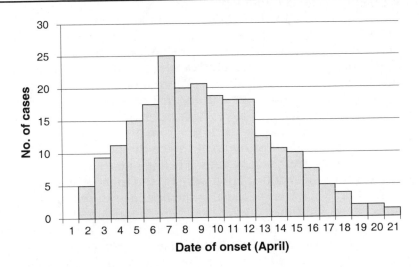

Hypothetical outbreak of cryptosporidiosis, a waterborne parasitic disease, with an approximate incubation period of 1–12 days. Notice that the outbreak shows a rapid rise in the number of cases to a plateau followed by a gradual decline, and that it lasts for a duration longer than the range of the incubation period of the disease (i.e., greater than 12 days).

Reference: Chin, J. ed. (2000). *Control of Communicable Diseases Manual,* 17th ed. Washington, DC: American Public Health Association.

Figure 14–3 Example of an epidemic curve representing a continuing
source outbreak

An **intermittent source outbreak** is a common source outbreak where the exposure to the common source of disease is irregular. An epidemic curve for this type of outbreak may show small clusters or individual cases spread out over a relatively protracted time period.[5] An intermittent source outbreak might occur, for example, in a cafeteria when contaminated roast beef is served as an entree on Monday, in sandwiches on Wednesday, and as a component of soup on Friday. The intermittent exposure should leave gaps in the epidemic curve. Because of the variety of epidemic curves that might be produced by intermittent source outbreaks, this type of outbreak is not illustrated here.

If one knows the specific disease responsible for a common source outbreak, it is easy to estimate the probable time of exposure to the common source that may have caused the outbreak. Using the epidemic curve, and assuming the outbreak is already over, one simply goes to the first case of the disease in the outbreak and counts backwards the minimum length of the incubation period of the disease. Then one goes to the last case of the disease in the outbreak and counts backwards the maximum length of the incubation period of the disease. The time range created by this process is the probable time of exposure to the common source. For example, if the disease has an incubation period of four to eight days, one would go to the first case of the disease represented on the epidemic curve and count backwards four days (i.e., the minimum incubation period). He or she would then go to the last case of the disease on the curve and count backwards eight days (i.e., the maximum incubation period). If the first case occurred on November 6, one would count back four days to November 2. If the last case occurred on November 18, one would count back eight days to November 10. Thus, one would expect that the common source exposure occurred from November 2–10. This would likely imply a continuing source outbreak, since the presumed exposure was not brief but prolonged over several days. If counting backwards from the minimum and maximum incubation period were to lead to the same date, it would imply a point source outbreak because of the brief exposure time.

The procedure described above is illustrated using two examples in exhibit 14–2. The incubation periods for most communicable diseases are available in the *Control of Communicable Diseases Manual* from the American Public Health Association[3] or from other sources. If you know the probable time of exposure, but not the disease, and hence not the incubation period, you can reverse the process by counting forward from the first point of exposure to the first case of the disease on the epidemic curve and from the last point of exposure to the last case of the disease on the epidemic curve to determine the probable incubation period of the disease and perhaps from this and other information determine the identity of the disease.

Propagated Outbreaks

A **propagated outbreak** is a progressive outbreak that usually is due to direct person-to-person transmission of the disease (e.g., via touching, sneezing, coughing, or sexual relations) or by indirect transmission through a **vector**, which in the context of epidemiology is an animate source, such as a fly, mosquito, or rodent, which is capable of transmitting an agent of disease to a susceptible host.* The epidemic curve for a propagated outbreak due to person-to-person spread is typically characterized by a relatively gradual rise in case numbers and a steeper decline,[5] such as that illustrated in figure 14–4 on page 290. In some instances there may be more than one peak separated by distances approximately equal in length to the average incubation period of the disease. These additional peaks represent secondary and tertiary spread of the disease.[2]

The epidemic curve for a vector-borne disease may be difficult to distinguish from that for person-to-person spread. It has been described as beginning slowly, showing irregular peaks, and slowly tailing off.[5] In general, the epidemic curves for propagated outbreaks tend to show a longer duration than those for common source outbreaks, although, as stated previously, several other factors can affect the shape of epidemic curves.

---

* The vector serves as an intermediary in disease transmission, and the mechanism of transmission is considered indirect. The vector may be infected with the disease organism or may be simply a mechanical carrier.[2, 3]

Exhibit 14–2 Estimating the Probable Time of Exposure in Common Source Outbreaks

Step 1: Go to the first case on the epidemic curve and count backwards the length of the minimum incubation period of the disease from, but not including, the first case.

Step 2: Go to the last case on the epidemic curve and count backwards the length of the maximum incubation period of the disease from, but not including, the last case.

Step 3: Record the probable time of exposure, which is the resulting time interval.

Examples: Common Source Outbreaks Each with an Incubation Period of 1–12 days

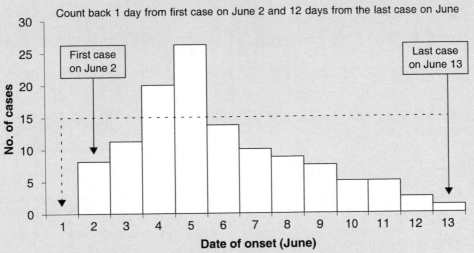

Count back 1 day from first case on June 2 and 12 days from the last case on June

Probable time of exposure in the above example is June 1

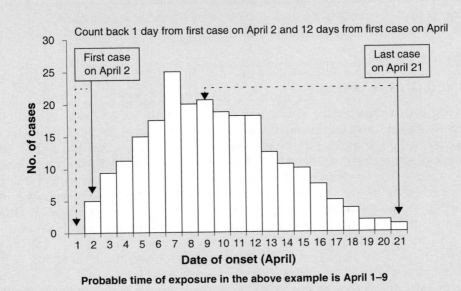

Count back 1 day from first case on April 2 and 12 days from first case on April

Probable time of exposure in the above example is April 1–9

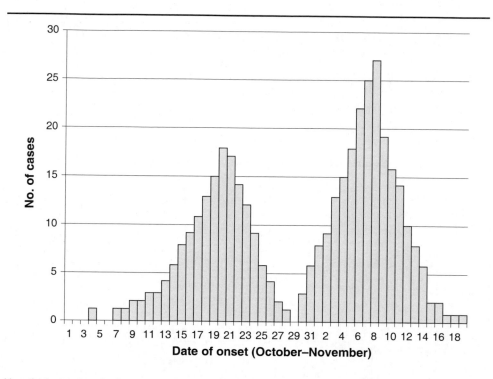

Hypothetical outbreak of an unspecified viral disease causing fever, malaise, and rash with an incubation period of 15–23 days. Notice that the outbreak shows a relatively gradual rise in case numbers and a steeper decline. Also note that there are two peaks separated by a distance approximately equal to the average incubation period of the disease (i.e., 19 days). The average incubation period can be estimated as follows: $(15 + 23) / 2 = (38 / 2) = 19$.

Figure 14–4 Example of an epidemic curve representing a propagated (person-to-person) outbreak

Mixed Outbreaks

Mixed outbreaks are a combination of common source and propagated outbreaks. Often these begin with a common source exposure that is followed by person-to-person spread of the disease. An example is a common source outbreak of shigellosis, an acute bacterial disease causing diarrhea and fever, that results from a contaminated water supply and proceeds to spread among the residents by direct person-to-person contact. The epidemic curve frequently shows a single large peak and subsequent smaller peaks.[6] Other combinations of common source and propagated outbreaks are also possible.

A concept that can be useful in disease outbreaks of all types is the **index case**, which is the first case in a defined group to come to the attention of the investigators.[4] Often the index case is the one who introduced the causative agent (e.g., an infected food handler, an elementary school student with streptococcal sore throat, an employee with hepatitis A). Discovering and interviewing the index case may be helpful in discovering how and why the outbreak began.

Testing Hypotheses Using Analytic Studies

As indicated in step five of exhibit 14–1, it is sometimes necessary to carry out additional studies to substantiate a given hypothesis about the cause of an outbreak. Often these investigations involve case-control studies (chapter 11) or retrospective cohort studies (chapter 12). These designs are very useful because they can be performed "after the fact" (i.e., both designs are retrospective in nature) and because they involve controlled comparisons.

In case-control studies, cases with the disease are compared to a similar group of individuals without the disease to test the hypothesis that the disease is linked to a specific exposure. This same basic hypothesis can be tested in retrospective cohort studies where individuals in the cohort who were exposed to a given factor are compared to those in the cohort who were not exposed to the factor to determine if the factor is linked to the disease. The use of these studies in regard to disease outbreak investigations is discussed briefly in the following sections.

Case-Control Studies

Case-control studies are most useful in the investigation of disease outbreaks when a specific cohort cannot be easily defined. This may occur, for example, when the cases are widely dispersed. Since cases have already been identified in a previous step of the investigation (step 3), the central issue is defining an appropriate control group. The control group should be as similar as possible to the case group but without the disease. Problems in identifying a suitable control group were discussed in detail in chapter 11. In general, randomly selected individuals from the source population matched by age and sex, and sometimes other important variables, constitute the preferred control group. Practical matters, however, such as achieving adequate participation and cooperation from a sufficient number of controls, may need to be considered. In practice, typical members of control groups in disease outbreak investigations include neighbors, friends, coworkers, and family members. Investigators need to be cautious, however, in choosing controls based on convenience since they may introduce selection bias into the study.[2]

Once the case and control groups have been defined, it is necessary to solicit information about exposures suspected of causing the disease. Common methods of collecting appropriate data include questionnaires, interviews, and examinations. The methods used should be identical for both case and control groups to avoid potential measurement bias. Because case-control studies cannot normally produce attack rates, the usual measure of association is the odds ratio (formula 6.5), which can be calculated using a contingency table for each exposure to be examined. The statistical significance of an association can be measured using the chi-square test of independence (see formula 10.4 and table 10–3).

Retrospective Cohort Studies

The retrospective cohort design works well when a specific cohort can be easily defined. For example, in the common source outbreak of salmonellosis referred to earlier in this chapter, the cohort would be all those who attended the church-sponsored buffet luncheon. This cohort could be enumerated easily and followed up to determine who ate what foods.

Typically, in a retrospective cohort analysis of a disease outbreak several exposures are examined simultaneously using an **attack rate table**. This is very common in outbreaks due to foodborne illness. Specifically, the attack rate table is used to determine which food(s) is likely to be responsible for the outbreak. The use of a food attack rate table is illustrated in example 14–1. The attack rate table divides the cohort into the exposed group (i.e., those who ate the designated foods) and the unexposed group (i.e., those who did not eat the designated foods). Attack rates are then calculated in each group by dividing the number ill by the total ill and well for each item being examined.

To determine which food is most likely to have served as a vehicle for the outbreak, one could calculate the relative risk of the disease for each suspected food item by dividing the attack rate among those who ate a specified food by the attack rate among those who did not eat the food. The food with the highest relative risk that is statistically significant will be suspect. Statistical significance of the relative risk can be computed using the chi-square test of independence (see formula 10.4 and table 10.3). As an alternative, one could determine the attributable risk for each suspected food by subtracting the attack rate among those who did not eat the food from the attack rate for those who did eat the food. In this case one would be looking for the food with the greatest, statistically significant, attributable risk. Statistical significance of the attributable risk can be calculated using the same chi-square test as for the relative risk.

In either case, it is also beneficial to calculate the attributable risk percent (formula 6.7, but using attack rates instead of incidence rates, or formula 6.8). This will reveal the percent of the risk of the disease in the exposed group that is due to the exposure. The closer this measure is to 100%, the more likely a suspected food accounted for the outbreak. An attributable risk percent of 85%, for example, says that 85% of the risk of the disease among those who ate the suspected food was due to eating the food. The other 15% of the risk must have been due to reasons other than eating the food, assuming the reporting is accurate. An attributable risk of less than 100% will always result when some of those who report not eating the suspected food contract the disease. This can be due to cross-contamination between foods, the presence of other contaminated foods, or other sources related or unrelated to the outbreak. It can also be due to faulty recall, as when one reports not eating a particular food when in fact he or she did. A low attributable risk percent for a particular food suggests that the food may not be the source of the outbreak.

Example 14–1: Analysis of a Foodborne Outbreak Using an Attack Rate Table

An investigation of an outbreak of staphylococcal food poisoning occurred during the second week of January, 2002. The case definition produced by the investigators was acute onset of nausea, cramps, and vomiting between 9:00 P.M. and 4:00 A.M. January 6–7, among members and spouses of the Order of the Elephant Lodge who attended an annual banquet at the Hungry Horse restaurant in Fremont City, Texas, on the evening of January 6. As part of a retrospective cohort study to test their hypotheses about which foods were involved in the outbreak, the investigators began developing an attack rate table. A partially completed table showing the number of individuals who came down with food poisoning as defined above and the number who did not is provided for each food investigated. Complete the attack rate table, including the attack rates for each suspected food, and determine the most likely food responsible for the outbreak. Justify your response.

	Attack Rate Table							
	Exposed Persons *Those Who Ate Suspected Foods*				**Unexposed Persons** *Those Who Did Not Eat Suspected Foods*			
Suspected Food	**Ill**	**Well**	**Total**	**Attack Rate (%)**	**Ill**	**Well**	**Total**	**Attack Rate (%)**
Ham	36	5			2	11		
Potato Salad	40	4			9	6		
Peas	16	15			10	13		

Solution:

Step 1: For each food in each exposure category (those who ate the suspected foods and those who did not eat the suspected foods) add the number of ill and well persons together to obtain the total or population at risk. Then calculate each food-specific attack rate by dividing the number of ill persons by the specific population at risk. Place this information in the attack rate table.

Food-specific Attack Rates for the Exposed Group:
Ham: $[36 / (36 + 5)] \times 100 = (36 / 41) \times 100 = 87.8\%$
Potato salad: $[40 / (40 + 4)] \times 100 = (40 / 44) \times 100 = 90.9\%$
Peas: $[16 / (16 + 15)] \times 100 = (16 / 31) \times 100 = 51.6\%$

Food-specific Attack Rates for the Unexposed Group:
Ham: $[2 / (2 + 11) \times 100 = (2 / 13) \times 100 = 15.4\%$
Potato salad: $[9 / (9 + 6)] \times 100 = (9 / 15) \times 100 = 60.0\%$
Peas $= [10 / (10 + 13)] \times 100 = (10 / 23) \times 100 = 43.5\%$

The completed attack rate table appears on the next page. The figures added to the table are in italics.

Attack Rate Table							
	Exposed Persons *Those Who Ate Suspected Foods*				Unexposed Persons *Those Who Did Not Eat Suspected Foods*			
Suspected Food	Ill	Well	Total	Attack Rate (%)	Ill	Well	Total	Attack Rate (%)
Ham	36	5	*41*	*87.8*	2	11	*13*	*15.4*
Potato Salad	40	4	*44*	*90.9*	9	6	*15*	*60.0*
Peas	16	15	*31*	*51.6*	10	13	*23*	*43.5*

Step 2: The next step in determining the most likely food responsible for the outbreak of staphylococcal food poisoning is to calculate the relative risk (RR) of food poisoning, or the attributable risk (AR), for each suspected food.

Ham: RR = 87.8% / 15.4% = 5.7 or AR = 87.8% − 15.4% = 72.4%
Potato salad: RR = 90.9% / 60.0% = 1.5 or AR = 90.9% − 60.0% = 30.9%
Peas: RR = 51.6% / 43.5% = 1.2 or AR = 51.6% − 43.5% = 8.1%

Based on the high RR or the large AR, the ham appears to be the most likely food involved in the outbreak.

Step 3: We should next determine the attributable risk percent (AR%) in each case using either formula 6.7 (using attack rates) or 6.8. We will use formula 6.8, which is [(RR − 1) / RR] × 100. Both formulas should yield the same results.

Ham: AR% = [(5.7 − 1) / 5.7] × 100 = 82.5%
Potato salad: AR% = [(1.5. − 1) / 1.5] × 100 = 33.3%
Peas: AR% = [(1.2 − 1) / 1.2] × 100 = 16.7%

These results support the suspicion that the ham is responsible for the outbreak. A high percentage of the risk of staphylococcal food poisoning among those consuming the ham was actually due to eating the ham (82.5%) and not to other factors.

Step 4: Although the findings appear to confirm that the ham is the most likely responsible for the outbreak, we should still perform a chi-square test to see if the apparent association between ham and the food poisoning is statistically significant. If it is not, it suggests that the findings are likely to be due to sampling error (i.e., chance). The formula for the chi-square test is: χ^2 = n (ad − bc)^2 / (a + b) (c + d) (a + c) (b + d) based on a standard 2 × 2 contingency table. Using the figures in the attack rate table, we can produce a 2 × 2 contingency table from which we can calculate a chi-square value and interpret it using table 10–3.

Food Poisoning

Exposure Status	Present	Absent	
Ate the Ham	**a** = 36	**b** = 5	41
Did Not Eat the Ham	**c** = 2	**d** = 11	13
	38	16	54

$$\chi^2 = n \, (ad - bc)^2 / (a + b) \, (c + d) \, (a + c) \, (b + d) =$$
$$54 \, [(36 \times 11) - (5 \times 2)]^2 / (41) \, (13) \, (38) \, (16) =$$
$$54 \, (396 - 10)^2 / 324{,}064 = 54 \, (386)^2 / 324{,}064 = 54 \, (148{,}996) / 324{,}064$$
$$= 8{,}045{,}784 / 324{,}064 = 24.8$$

According to table 10–3, a chi-square value of 24.8 is statistically significant at $p < 0.001$.

Answer: Contaminated ham eaten at the Hungry Horse restaurant on the evening of January 6, 2002, is the most likely explanation for the staphylococcal food poisoning outbreak that occurred among the members of the Order of the Elephant Lodge and their spouses in Fremont City, Texas on January 6 and 7. Those individuals who ate the ham were 5.7 times more likely to get staphylococcal food poisoning than those who did not eat the ham. Also, 82.5% of the risk of food poisoning among those who ate the ham was due to eating the ham. The difference in attack rates between those who ate and did not eat the ham at the dinner was statistically significant at $p < 0.001$, indicating that chance was an unlikely explanation for the findings.

Comments:

1. An attack rate table is a convenient method of determining which exposures are likely to be responsible for an outbreak. Though frequently used in point source outbreaks involving vehicles, such as food, beverages, or water supplies, attack rate tables may be used in any retrospective cohort analysis of an outbreak, including propagated outbreaks. In propagated outbreaks involving person-to-person spread of disease, for example, one may develop an attack rate table based on the characteristics of the individuals involved in the outbreak (e.g., by age, sex, or racial/ethnic group). Also, the factors examined in an attack rate table do not need to be dichotomous. One could look at the amount of food eaten, for example.

2. While the relative risk or the attributable risk is the most important measure in identifying the probable "cause" of an outbreak, the attributable risk percent provides an important perspective. The relatively high attributable risk percent found in this example helps to confirm that the ham is the likely source of the outbreak. It indicates that among those who ate the ham, only 17.5% (100% − 82.5% = 17.5%) of the risk of food poisoning could not be explained by eating the ham. It is possible that some of the cases that occurred in the unexposed group were due to faulty memory (e.g., forgetting that one tasted the ham) or eating foods that contained or were contaminated by the ham. In general, when the attributable risk percent is low, say less than 50%, one would want to search for other factors that might explain the outbreak.

3. Another measure that can be useful in assessing the role of a factor in an outbreak is the population attributable risk percent (formula 6.10a, but using attack rates). This measure would tell us how many of the cases might not have occurred had the ham not been contaminated at the banquet. The population attributable risk percent (Pop AR%) for ham is calculated as follows: [(Overall attack rate − attack rate in those who did not eat the ham) / overall attack rate] × 100. Based on the data in the attack rate table, the overall attack rate for the ham is: [(36 + 2) / (41 + 13)] × 100 = 70.4%. Therefore, the Pop AR% = [(70.4% − 15.4%) / 70.4%] × 100 = 78.1%. This implies that about 78% of the cases of staphylococcal food poisoning in this outbreak could have been prevented if the ham were not contaminated. To the extent that other cases were due to cross-contamination by the ham, the use of ham in other foods, etc., the percent of cases that could not be explained by eating the ham would be even less.

4. To support a conclusion that contaminated ham was responsible for the outbreak, it would be helpful to have laboratory confirmation that the ham was indeed contaminated

with staphylococcal toxin and that those who developed food poisoning were affected by the same toxin. This may not always be possible, however (e.g., the ham may have been completely consumed or the leftovers may have been discarded, and the cases may have already recovered).

5. While it has been implied that the ham was responsible for, or the "cause" of, the outbreak, it is really only a *proxy* for the real cause, which is the staphylococcal organisms that produced the enterotoxin that causes staphylococcal food poisoning. This distinction is critical to preventing similar outbreaks in the future. After all, suggesting that ham not be served at future banquets will not be sufficient to prevent additional outbreaks of staphylococcal food poisoning at the Hungry Horse restaurant. What epidemiologists need to know is how the ham became contaminated, and what might be done to prevent a similar occurrence in the future. This is a part of step six in exhibit 14–1. Identifying the ham as the "cause" of the outbreak then is not the final step. One needs to find out where the breakdown occurred in the restaurant. Was the ham undercooked, and why? Did someone with a staphylococcal infection prepare the ham in an unsanitary manner? Is hand washing strictly enforced? Was the ham improperly stored? These and other questions need to be answered before the outbreak investigation can be concluded.

Disease Clusters

Disease clusters were defined earlier in this chapter. To reiterate, a disease cluster is an aggregation of cases of a typically uncommon disease in space or time that is believed not to be due to chance.[4] A *true* disease cluster is expected to have a common cause that is unique for the particular place or time. Often the presumed cause is environmental in origin (e.g., pesticides, hazardous wastes, or radiation). A *suspected* disease cluster may be evaluated to determine if it: (a) is likely due to chance, or (b) represents a collection of undifferentiated diseases (e.g., cancer, congenital anomalies) that may be due to variety of unrelated causes. If either of these circumstances is evident, it is doubtful that a true disease cluster exists. In the latter case, for example, reports of cancer clustering in the workplace are often found to consist of cases of different types of cancer that are not known to have a common cause that can be explained by the particular work environment.

The role that chance can play in generating apparent disease clusters is illustrated in the following example. A Sunday morning newspaper reports the following winning numbers from the Saturday night state lottery: 12-13-14-15-38-44. Notice that the first four numbers are consecutive and appear to have clustered in a nonrandom fashion. Because the lottery process is random, however, we know this "clustering" must be due to chance. In fact, this sequence is as likely an occurrence as any other combination of six lottery numbers. As another example, say you were to take 200 evenly sized marbles, 100 black and 100 white, place them in a large, oversized container, shake them vigorously to be sure they were well mixed, and then dump them on a smooth, unobstructed floor. You would likely find that the overall distribution of the marbles would be well dispersed by color, but there would be some small clusters of black or white marbles that occurred strictly by chance. Something similar can be operating when several cases of brain cancer are reported on the same block in a neighborhood. This distribution might be just a chance occurrence in the overall expected pattern of brain cancer for the entire community, county, or state. The number of cases on the block may be like the cluster of black or white marbles in the overall distribution of marbles on the floor.

Not all suspected disease clusters are due to random variation or undifferentiated diagnoses, however. Several disease clusters have been found to have environmental causes, particularly those discovered in occupational settings. As far back as 1775, Percival Pott, an English physician, noticed a clustering of scrotal cancer cases among young chimney sweeps in England. The habit at the time was for young boys to be lowered into the chimneys naked so they could remove the accumulated ash without ruining their clothes. Due to poor hygienic practices, the soot accumulated in the ridges of their scrota where over the years it increased their rate of scrotal cancer. Today we know the cause of the cancer was benzo(α)pyrene, a potent environmental carcinogen and a component of soot.[7] Some other environmental agents that have been identified from the study of occupational disease clusters include coal dust (black lung disease), asbestos (mesothelioma), vinyl chloride (angiosarcoma of the liver), and dibromochloropropane or DBCP (male infertility).[8, 9]

Examples of documented disease clusters in community settings are rare, one reason being the generally smaller exposures compared to occupational settings. A famous example of a disease cluster in a community setting occurred in Woburn, Massachusetts, where cases of childhood leukemia were linked to certain wells contaminated by industrial chemicals.[10, 11] This still controversial incident became the subject of a popular book and film entitled *A Civil Action*. Another disease cluster of 20 deaths from mesothelioma, a rare form of cancer of the lining of the pleural cavity in the thorax, occurred during a four-year period in a small village in Turkey. The disease was linked to erionite, a fibrous mineral found in high concentrations in the village's soil.[12]

Most of the thousand to two thousand suspected disease clusters that come to the attention of public health authorities in the United States each year are not substantiated even when detailed investigations are conducted. Most of these alleged clusters are reported by members of the public who know of several cases of a given disease in the same neighborhood, community, or workplace and who may be affected with the disease themselves. Usually the reported clusters involve some type of cancer (i.e., **cancer clusters**), and most who report them believe they have specific environmental causes. The sheer volume of reports of suspected disease clusters has led many state health departments, which usually take the lead role, to develop policies regarding their investigation.[13] Most of these policies establish a protocol that, as a minimum, involves: (a) some type of preliminary review to determine the likelihood that a true disease cluster exists; (b) a more formal review by a multidisciplinary committee when warranted; and (c) formal investigation, if deemed appropriate, for reasons related to public health, scientific advancement, public relations, or legal requirements.

Investigating Disease Clusters

Investigating disease clusters can be problematic for a number of reasons.[9] First, the frequency of the disease is typically low so it may be difficult or impossible to use standard statistical methods that have relatively large sample size requirements. Second, as discussed above, the case definition used to represent a disease cluster is often imprecise and may represent several diseases, each with its own specific causes. This would make it very unlikely that one could find a common reason for the cluster. Third, it may be impossible to identify an appropriate population at risk from which to develop incidence rates. This is because the group in which the suspected cluster exists is often poorly defined and may not represent all who are at risk of the disease. If a suspected disease cluster should occur in a neighborhood, for example, does that mean that only those who live in the neighborhood are at risk of the disease? Unless some specific exposure is associated only with that neighborhood, it might be arbitrary to say that the neighborhood is the population at risk. Without incidence rates to compare, one cannot determine if the disease exceeds expected levels (i.e., those of the community, county, state, or nation). Finally, it may be difficult to estimate exposures for diseases like cancer because of the long latency periods between exposure and outcome. Most cancers have latency periods that range from 10 to 20 years. Mesothelioma, referred to above, has a latency period that normally ranges from 25–40 years.[7] In some cases it may be even longer. Most disease clusters that are found to be due to environmental or occupational exposures are those where the exposure is persistently high in the affected population but rare in other populations. Also, the usual relative risk of the disease is extremely high (e.g., 20 or higher).[12]

Public Health Surveillance

Definition and Types of Surveillance

In 1986 the Centers for Disease Control in Atlanta, Georgia, defined epidemiologic surveillance as "the ongoing systematic collection, analysis, and interpretation of health data essential to the planning, implementation, and evaluation of public health practice, closely integrated with the timely dissemination of these data to those who need to know."[14(p.ii)] The agency went on to say that the "final link in the surveillance chain is the application of these data to prevention and control."[14(p.ii)] This comprehensive and well-conceived definition describes what today we refer to as **public health surveillance** (see figure 14–5). The use of "public health" in the definition underscores the fact that surveillance is an integral part of public health practice.[15] The historical roots of modern public health surveillance can be traced back to John Graunt and his "Bills of Mortality" referred to in chapter 2.

There are two basic types of public health surveillance—active and passive. **Active surveillance** requires that the health authority formally responsible for surveillance (e.g., the public health department) obtain the health data being sought directly from various health care providers, such as physi-

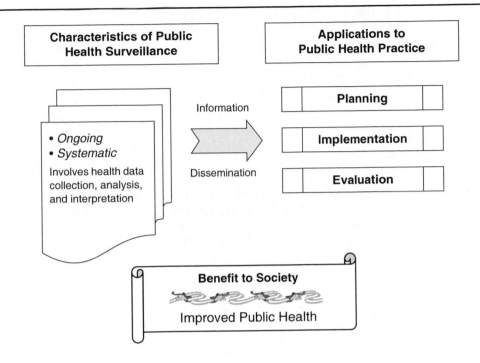

Reference: Centers for Disease Control (1986). *Comprehensive Plan for Epidemiologic Surveillance: Centers for Disease Control, August, 1986.* Atlanta: The Centers.

Figure 14–5 Public health surveillance

cians, hospitals, and laboratories. This requires telephone, e-mail, or personal visits to the reporting sources. Active surveillance must be frequent enough to provide useful data, and it is usually very expensive and time consuming. This is a reason why it is infrequently practiced, and when it is, it is usually practiced for only a limited time to deal with a specific problem or continuously for only one or a small number of diseases. Active surveillance may be helpful in detecting and monitoring **emerging infectious diseases** or **reemerging infectious diseases**,* such as drug-resistant tuberculosis or cholera, respectively, because of their epidemic potential.

Passive surveillance does not use active means to solicit health-related data. Instead, various health care providers usually are required by law to report certain diseases or conditions using prescribed methods designed by the agency formally responsible for surveillance. Systems based on passive

---

* Emerging infectious diseases are infectious diseases, previously unknown or virtually unknown in a population, that have been increasing or threatening to increase in recent years. Reemerging infectious diseases are once familiar infectious diseases in a population that were thought to be decreasing or disappearing but are now on the rise. These diseases need to be monitored closely because they can quickly become established in a population.

surveillance are much less expensive and troublesome to operate than those based on active surveillance, and, hence, most surveillance systems in the U.S. and abroad are passive. Reporting in passive surveillance systems, however, often seriously understates the true incidence of many reportable diseases, especially those that might not be considered very serious by health care practitioners or that might be embarrassing to patients (e.g., influenza and gonorrhea, respectively). In some systems a combination of active and passive strategies may be used.[5]

Another type of surveillance is **sentinel surveillance**. This strategy prearranges for certain health care providers to report all cases of the **sentinel events**, the diseases or conditions that are to be reported under the sentinel surveillance system. The reporting sources are usually a select sample of health care providers who are likely to see the sentinel events and who have agreed to report them to the appropriate health authority.[2] Sentinel events are typically those that alert public health authorities to potential problems (e.g., epidemics, failure of preventive measures) and may require some type of public health response when reported. Emerging and reemerging infectious diseases fit this description. Also, the National Institute for Occupational Safety and Health operates the Sentinel Event Notification System for Occupational Risks (SENSOR) for certain work-related conditions.[16] A shortcoming of a sentinel surveillance system is that the number of cases reported may understate the true number of cases in the population at risk, and, therefore, incidence or attack rates estimated from sentinel surveillance may be negatively biased. An advantage is that the rate of reporting for sentinel events is generally better than that from purely passive surveillance systems.[5]

Data Sources

An essential element of public health surveillance is timely data collection. Some of the types of data used in public health surveillance systems in the United States have been described by the CDC.[2] These include:

- *Mortality data*. These data come primarily from death certificates, including fetal death certificates, which are required under the vital statistics registration system (see exhibit 2–1) and secondarily from medical examiners or coroners, who can usually provide additional details about the circumstances of specific deaths.

- *Morbidity data*. These data come from reports of notifiable diseases (exhibit 2–1), laboratory reports, hospital discharge records, disease registries (chapter 11), and other sources that include information on outpatients, adverse drug reactions, injuries, and occupational illnesses.

- *Health surveys*. These include the National Health and Nutrition Examination Survey (NHANES), the National Health Interview Survey (NHIS), and the Behavioral Risk Factor Surveillance System, which collects information on common risk factors like smoking, drinking, and diet.

- *Disease indicators*. These include morbidity and mortality data on animal diseases that may be transmissible to humans (e.g., bovine spongiform encephalopathy or BSE, commonly referred to as "mad cow disease," which is associated with a variant form of Creutzfeld-Jakob disease in humans), information on the presence of pathogens in certain animals (e.g., plague in rodents), and changes in the distribution of vectors or animals that carry certain diseases (e.g., monitoring birds for mosquito-borne encephalitis).

- *Environmental monitoring.* This includes data generated from the routine local monitoring of food, water, and milk supplies and data collected from monitoring for compliance with state or national legislation, including the Clean Air Act, the Clean Water Act, the Safe Drinking Water Act, the Emergency Planning and Community Right to Know Act, and other state or national legislation.

- *Utilization of certain drugs and biologics.* This information may provide clues to potential or actual outbreaks or epidemics (e.g., increased use of antibiotics).

- *School and employer data.* These include school absenteeism records that may help in monitoring influenza-like diseases in the community and occupational records that can be used to monitor occupational illnesses and injuries. It might be noted that the sources of data on occupational injuries and injury fatalities in the U.S. are rather fragmented and diverse.[17]

Population data normally are combined with surveillance data to generate relevant prevalence, incidence, or mortality rates that can then be used to compare health problems by person, place, or time variables. The major source of population data in the United States is the U.S. Census Bureau, which is located in the Department of Commerce and has been conducting comprehensive counts and profiles of the U.S. population every ten years since 1790.

There are several agencies responsible for public health surveillance in the U.S. The Centers for Disease Control and Prevention, located in the Department of Health and Human Services, is the major agency at the federal level.[18] The major agencies at the state and local levels are usually public health departments or their equivalent, while at the international level it is the World Health Organization. The principal health statistics agency within the federal government is the National Center for Health Statistics (NCHS), located in the CDC. This agency is a major resource for information on the health status of the nation. It is legally responsible for the collection, analysis, and dissemination of a wide range of health-related data. It also provides technical assistance to state and local authorities.[19] A summary of the surveys and data systems administered by the NCHS are presented in appendix C.

Uses of Public Health Surveillance

While the ongoing collection, analysis, interpretation, and dissemination of appropriate health-related data are the bedrock of public health surveillance, these activities have little meaning if the data are not used appropriately.

Stated simply, surveillance systems are designed to be used. As noted in the definition of public health surveillance, data are collected, analyzed, interpreted, and disseminated for *use* in planning, implementing, and evaluating public health programs that are ultimately aimed at preventing and controlling public health problems.[14] According to the CDC, there are five major objectives that can be achieved by using public health surveillance data: (1) assessment of the public health status of a population, (2) establishment of public health priorities, (3) evaluation of public health programs, (4) initiation of health-related research, and (5) identification of health-related problems.[20]

The above purposes are reflected in the following examples of how public health surveillance data are commonly used.

- *Detecting disease outbreaks and clusters.* Ongoing surveillance can provide information on current and endemic levels of diseases, which can be used to determine if an outbreak or epidemic is occurring. Surveillance data, if available for the disease, may also be helpful in evaluating apparent disease clusters to determine if the number of cases in a given place or time exceed what would be expected due to chance alone.

- *Identifying changes or trends in health-related problems or practices.* Routine surveillance can be helpful in uncovering changes, including secular trends or other patterns of disease morbidity or mortality. For example, surveillance data have revealed a secular decline in the age-adjusted cause-specific mortality rate for heart disease in the U.S. over the past three decades.[21] It has also been used to identify changes in a number of health practices, such as the increase in deliveries by cesarean section.[5]

- *Monitoring the effectiveness of prevention and control programs.* A public health program to reduce sexually transmitted diseases, for example, can be compared before and after an intervention using surveillance data on the incidence of sexually transmitted diseases. The limitations of this type of comparison are discussed in chapter 13.

- *Establishing public health programs and priorities.* Analysis of surveillance data provides information on the magnitude of health problems and helps to identify groups at high risk. This information can be valuable to planners and policymakers in determining what programs are needed. For example, an analysis of surveillance data over the years has identified low birth weight as being the factor most closely associated with neonatal deaths.[22] Programs designed to reduce neonatal deaths should therefore focus on factors that may increase the risk of having low birth weight babies.

- *Understanding the natural history of disease.* Over time, public health surveillance can help us better understand the life cycles of specific diseases. It has aided our understanding of a number of public health problems, including AIDS, Lyme disease, tuberculosis, and malaria.

- *Stimulating analytical research.* While hypothesis testing is not an objective of public health surveillance per se, it is frequently a consequence. Description of surveillance data by person, place, and time variables provides information that can be helpful to researchers in generating and testing hypotheses about specific health problems. For example, an international comparison of injury mortality among 11 nations by staff of the NCHS revealed that the death rate from suicide poisoning in Denmark is three times that in the United States.[23] Assuming the reporting procedures are comparable, this could generate several hypotheses and lead to epidemiologic studies to uncover the reasons for this difference.

Characteristics of Effective Surveillance Systems

As stated earlier, public health surveillance is a vital element of public health practice. Ideally, it provides useful information for decision making that helps public health agencies achieve their goals. At the same time, surveillance requires valuable resources and can be expensive and time consuming. Therefore, surveillance systems need to be evaluated on a regular basis to determine if they are fulfilling their intended objectives. Some of the questions that need to be asked are summarized below. These questions are not exhaustive but are provided to give an idea of the characteristics of effective public health surveillance systems and to generate additional ideas about how public health surveillance can be improved.

1. Does the system detect important health events in a reliable and consistent manner?
2. Does the system provide data that are representative of the population served?
3. Is the system easy to use and acceptable to those who use it?
4. Is the reporting and dissemination of health information timely and useful?
5. Is the system efficient in terms of cost and flexibility?
6. Does the system make a qualitative difference in public health practice?

Affirmative answers to these questions would at least indicate that the surveillance system being reviewed is on the right track.

Summary

- Disease outbreaks are epidemics confined to a localized area, such as a town or within a hospital. They usually involve communicable diseases or acute poisonings.
- The primary purpose of investigating a disease outbreak is to identify its cause so as to prevent any further cases and to prevent similar outbreaks in the future.
- The steps involved in outbreak investigations include verifying the existence of an outbreak; confirming the diagnosis of the disease; preparing a case definition and counting cases; characterizing the data by

person, place, and time; formulating and testing hypotheses; and preparing a written report and conducting control and prevention measures. These steps may not always be followed sequentially, and some may be completed simultaneously.

- One of the most revealing steps in outbreak investigation occurs when one characterizes the data by person, place, and time. This can help generate hypotheses about the nature and cause of the outbreak. Especially helpful are spot maps and epidemic curves. The shape and characteristics of epidemic curves can be used to help identify the type of epidemic.

- Common source outbreaks result from a common exposure of a group to a pathogen or toxic substance. They include point source, continuing source, and intermittent source outbreaks. Propagated outbreaks are progressive and spread by direct person-to-person contact or indirectly through vectors, such as mosquitoes. Mixed outbreaks are a combination of common source and propagated outbreaks.

- Disease clusters represent an aggregation of cases of a typically uncommon disease, such as leukemia, in space or time that is believed not to be due to chance. They are suspected of originating from a common exposure, usually environmental in origin. Clustering of cases due to chance or clustering of diseases that have similar signs and symptoms but different etiologies are not considered true disease clusters. Most suspected disease clusters are not substantiated even when field investigations are conducted.

- Investigating disease clusters can be problematic due to: the small number of cases, which are usually below the threshold required for most statistical tests; the mixing of related but etiologically distinct diseases; the difficulty of identifying the appropriate population at risk; and the difficulty of estimating exposures that may have occurred up to two decades earlier.

- Public health surveillance is the ongoing systematic collection, analysis, interpretation, and rapid dissemination of health data essential to public health practice.

- There are two basic types of public health surveillance—active surveillance and passive surveillance. Active surveillance requires that the health authority contact health care providers for the desired health data, while passive surveillance requires that the health care providers provide the health authority with the desired health data. Another type of surveillance is sentinel surveillance, in which the health authority prearranges health data reporting with selected health care providers to help ensure that important health indicators are reported promptly.

- Sources of data for surveillance purposes include: mortality data from death certificates; morbidity data from notifiable disease reports, hospital discharge records, and disease registries; health surveys of populations; school and employer data; and other specialized sources.

- Uses of surveillance data include detecting disease outbreaks and clusters, identifying changes or trends in health-related problems or practices, monitoring the effectiveness of prevention and control programs, establishing health programs and priorities, and stimulating analytical research. Surveillance programs should be evaluated on a regular basis.

New Terms

active surveillance
attack rate
attack rate table
cancer cluster
common source outbreak
continuing source
   outbreak
disease cluster
disease outbreak

emerging infectious
   disease
epidemic curve
index case
intermittent source
   outbreak
mixed outbreak
passive surveillance
point source outbreak

propagated outbreak
public health surveillance
reemerging infectious
   disease
sentinel event
sentinel surveillance
vector
vehicle

Study Questions and Exercises

1. For a given disease with an incubation period of 2–6 days, what specific type of disease outbreak is most likely represented by the epidemic curve below, and why? Also, what is the probable time of exposure for this outbreak?

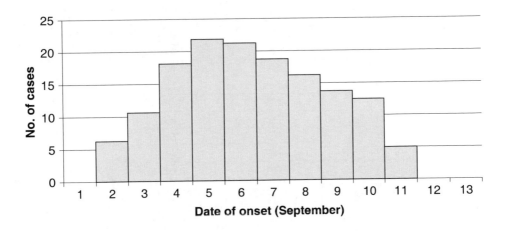

2. For a given disease with an incubation period of 10–18 days, what type of disease outbreak is most likely represented by the epidemic curve on the following page, and why? Also, what is the probable mode of transmission for this outbreak?

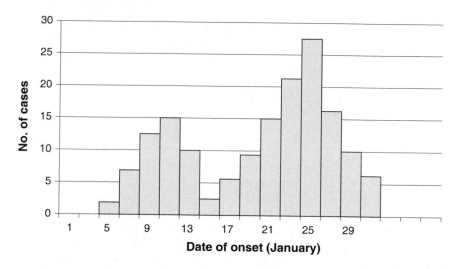

3. Briefly outline how you would investigate an alleged outbreak of viral meningitis on a college campus.

4. On June 1, 2001, 13 people became ill after attending a retirement dinner for a colleague. The symptoms were acute gastritis, vomiting, and fever. Using the food histories in the table below for the 20 individuals attending the dinner, construct an attack rate table and determine the most likely source of the outbreak. Justify your response.

Person	Became Ill?	Ate Beef?	Ate Chicken?	Ate Salad?
1	Yes	Yes	Yes	Yes
2	Yes	Yes	Yes	No
3	Yes	No	Yes	Yes
4	No	Yes	No	No
5	Yes	Yes	No	Yes
6	No	Yes	No	No
7	Yes	Yes	Yes	Yes
8	Yes	Yes	No	Yes
9	Yes	No	Yes	No
10	No	No	Yes	No
11	Yes	Yes	Yes	No
12	No	No	No	Yes
13	No	No	No	No
14	Yes	Yes	Yes	Yes
15	No	No	No	Yes
16	No	No	Yes	No
17	Yes	Yes	No	Yes
18	Yes	Yes	No	Yes
19	Yes	Yes	Yes	No
20	Yes	Yes	Yes	No

5. Assume you are working as the chief epidemiologist at the local county health department. You receive a phone call from a woman who believes there is a cancer cluster in her community. She states that she lives in the northern part of the county in Clayton, a city with a population of about 25,000. She further states that her sister, who lives two blocks away, was recently diagnosed with non-Hodgkin's lymphoma, and a neighbor of her sister recently died of leukemia. She also relates that she knows of at least five other cases of cancer in the community, including a child with a brain tumor, two cases of prostate cancer, an elderly man with malignant melanoma, and a woman with cervical cancer. She suspects that the cause may be a pesticide manufacturing plant that was built just outside the city last year. She demands that the health department investigate immediately. Is it likely the situation described represents a true cancer cluster, and why or why not? Also, as the chief epidemiologist at the health department, how would you respond to the woman's demand for an immediate investigation of the alleged problem?

6. Compare and contrast the relative advantages and disadvantages of active, passive, and sentinel surveillance systems. Include in your analysis a consideration of the six characteristics of effective surveillance systems described in the latter part of this chapter. Also, give an example of a disease or condition that would be most appropriate for each type of surveillance system.

References

1. Reingold, A. L. (1998). Outbreak Investigations—A Perspective. *Emerging Infectious Diseases* 4(1): 21–27.
2. Centers for Disease Control and Prevention (1992). *Principles of Epidemiology: An Introduction to Applied Epidemiology and Biostatistics*, 2nd ed. Atlanta: The Centers.
3. Chin, J., ed. (2000). *Control of Communicable Diseases Manual*, 17th ed. Washington, DC: American Public Health Association.
4. Last, J. M., ed. (1995). *A Dictionary of Epidemiology.* New York: Oxford University Press.
5. Gregg, M. B., ed. (1996). *Field Epidemiology.* New York: Oxford University Press.
6. Kelsey, J. L., Thompson, W. D., and Evans, A. S. (1986). *Methods in Observational Epidemiology.* New York: Oxford University Press.
7. Nadakavukaren, A. (1995). *Our Global Environment: A Health Perspective*, 4th ed. Prospect Heights, IL: Waveland Press.
8. Kolata, G. (1999). Probing Disease Clusters: Easier to Spot Than Prove. *New York Times*, January 31. Available: http://junkscience.com/jan99/kolata.htm (Access date: June 12, 2001.)
9. Brownson, R. C. (1998). Outbreak and Cluster Investigations. In *Applied Epidemiology: Theory to Practice*, R. C. Brownson and D. B. Petitti, eds. New York: Oxford University Press, pp. 71–104.
10. Cutler, J. J., Parker, G. S., Rosen, S., Prenney, B., Healy, R., and Caldwell, G. G. (1986). Childhood Leukemia in Woburn, Massachusetts. *Public Health Reports* 101(2): 201–205.
11. Durant, J. L., Chen, J., Hemond, H. F., and Thilly, W. G. (1995). Elevated Incidence of Childhood Leukemia in Woburn, Massachusetts: NIEHS Superfund Basic Research Program Searches for Causes. *Environmental Health Perspectives* 103 (Supplement 6): 93–98.
12. Neutra, R. R. (1990). Counterpoint from a Cluster Buster. *American Journal of Epidemiology* 132(1): 1–8.
13. Fiore, B. J., Hanrahan, L. P., and Anderson, H. A. (1990). State Health Department Response to Disease Cluster Reports: A Protocol for Investigation. *American Journal of Epidemiology* 132 (Supplement No. 1): S14–S22.
14. Centers for Disease Control (1986). *Comprehensive Plan for Epidemiologic Surveillance: Centers for Disease Control, August, 1986.* Atlanta: The Centers.

15. Thacker, S. B., and Berkelman, R. L. (1988). Public Health Surveillance in the United States. *Epidemiologic Reviews* 10: 164–190.
16. Brownson, R. C., Remington, P. L., and Davis, J. R. (1998). *Chronic Disease Epidemiology and Control*, 2nd ed. Washington, DC: American Public Health Association.
17. Rubens, A. J., Oleckno, W. A., and Papaeliou, L. (1995). Establishing Guidelines for the Identification of Occupational Injuries: A Systematic Appraisal. *Journal of Occupational and Environmental Medicine* 37(2): 151–159.
18. Jekel, J. F., Elmore, J. G., and Katz, D. L. (1996). *Epidemiology, Biostatistics, and Preventive Medicine*. Philadelphia: W. B. Saunders Company.
19. U.S. Department of Health and Human Services, Centers for Disease Control and Prevention, National Center for Health Statistics (1999). *National Center for Health Statistics . . . Monitoring the Nation's Health: Programs and Activities*. DHHS Publication No. (PHS) 99-1200. Hyattsville, MD: The Centers.
20. Centers for Disease Control and Prevention (no date). *Lesson 1: Overview of Public Health Surveillance*. Available: http://www.cdc.gov/epo/surveillancein/overview.htm (Access date: June 13, 2001.)
21. Hoyert, D. L., Kochanek, K. D., and Murphy, S. L. (1999). Deaths: Final Data for 1997. *National Vital Statistics Reports* 47(19). Hyattsville, MD: National Center for Health Statistics.
22. Health Resources and Services Administration, Maternal and Child Health Bureau (1999). *Child Health USA 1999*. Washington, DC: The Bureau.
23. Fingerhut, L. A., Cox, C. S., Warner, M., et al. (1998). International Comparative Analysis of Injury Mortality: Findings from the ICE on Injury Statistics. *Advance Data from Vital and Health Statistics*, No. 303. Hyattsville, MD: National Center for Health Statistics.

Appendix A
Table of Formulas

Formula	Page Number

Accuracy of the Screening Test (9.6)   166

$$\% \text{ Accuracy} = \frac{\text{Number of true positives} + \text{Number of true negatives}}{\text{Total number in the sample}} \times 100$$

Attack Rate (14.1)   284

$$\text{Attack Rate} = \frac{\begin{array}{c}\text{Number of new cases occurring among a specified} \\ \text{population during a given time period}\end{array}}{\text{Population at risk at the beginning of the time period}} \times 10^n$$

Where: $n = 1, 2, 3, 4$, etc.

Attributable Rate or Rate Difference (6.6 b)   111

$$\text{Attributable Rate or Rate Difference} = IR_{P\text{-}T\text{-}e} - IR_{P\text{-}T\text{-}ue}$$

Where: $IR_{P\text{-}T\text{-}e}$ = Person-time incidence rate in the exposed group
$IR_{P\text{-}T\text{-}ue}$ = Person-time incidence rate in the unexposed group

---

Attributable Rate Percent (Table 12–4)   245

$$\text{Attributable Rate Percent} = \frac{IR_{P\text{-}T\text{-}e} - IR_{P\text{-}T\text{-}ue}}{IR_{P\text{-}T\text{-}e}} \times 100$$

Where: $IR_{P\text{-}T\text{-}e}$ = Person-time incidence rate in the exposed group
$IR_{P\text{-}T\text{-}ue}$ = Person-time incidence rate in the unexposed group

---

Attributable Risk (AR) or Risk Difference (6.6 a)   111

$$\text{AR or Risk Difference} = IR_{C\text{-}e} - IR_{C\text{-}ue}$$

Where: $IR_{C\text{-}e}$ = Cumulative incidence rate in the exposed group
$IR_{C\text{-}ue}$ = Cumulative incidence rate in the unexposed group

---

Formula	Page Number

Attributable Risk Percent (AR%) (6.7, 6.8)   112

(6.7)
$$AR\% = \frac{IR_{C\text{-}e} - IR_{C\text{-}ue}}{IR_{C\text{-}e}} \times 100$$

(6.8)
$$AR\% = \frac{RR - 1}{RR} \times 100$$

Where: $IR_{C\text{-}e}$ = Cumulative incidence rate in the exposed group
$IR_{C\text{-}ue}$ = Cumulative incidence rate in the unexposed group
RR = Relative risk

Case Fatality Rate (CFR) (5.8)   79

$$CFR = \frac{\text{Number of deaths from a specific disease during a specified time period}}{\text{Number of cases of the disease during the same time period}} \times 10^n$$

Where: n = 1, 2, 3, 4, etc.

Cause-Specific Mortality Rate (C-S MR) (Figure 5–2)   77

$$\text{C-S MR} = \frac{\text{Number of deaths from a specific cause during a specified time period}}{\text{Mid-interval population}} \times 10^n$$

Where: n = 1, 2, 3, 4, etc.
The usual rate base for the Cause-Specific Mortality Rate is 100,000.

Chi-Square (χ^2) Test of Independence Based on a 2 × 2 Contingency Table (10.4, Table 12–3)   195, 240

$$\chi^2 = \frac{n\,(ad - bc)^2}{(a + b)(c + d)(a + c)(b + d)}$$

Where: a = Number of exposed individuals with the disease
b = Number of exposed individuals without the disease
c = Number of unexposed individuals with the disease
d = Number of unexposed individuals without the disease
n = Total number of individuals in the sample

Cohen's Kappa (Exhibit 9–1)   172

See Exhibit 9–1 for the formula of Cohen's Kappa.

95% Confidence Interval (CI) for Cumulative Incidence Rate (IR_C) and Prevalence Rate (PR) (Exhibit 5–2)   86

$$95\% \text{ CI} = r \pm 1.96 \sqrt{r\,(1 - r)\,/\,n}$$

Where: r = Cumulative incidence rate or prevalence rate stated as a decimal fraction
n = Population at risk (for IR_C) or total population (for PR)

Formula	Page Number

95% Confidence Interval (CI) for Decrease in the Rate Ratio (13.2)   267

Upper Confidence Limit (UCL) = (1 − 95% UCL of Rate Ratio) × 100

Lower Confidence Limit (LCL) = (1 − 95% LCL of Rate Ratio) × 100

95% Confidence Interval (CI) for Mantel-Haenszel Odds Ratio (Figure 11–3)   220

$$95\% \text{ CI} = \exp \{\ln (OR_{MH}) [1 \pm (1.96 / \sqrt{\chi^2_{MH}})]\}$$

Where: exp = Exponential (e) raised to the power represented by the entire expression

In = Natural logarithm

OR_{MH} = Mantel-Haenszel odds ratio

χ^2_{MH} = Mantel-Haenszel chi-square test

95% Confidence Interval (CI) for Odds Ratio (OR) (11.2)   218

$$95\% \text{ CI} = \exp [\ln (OR) \pm 1.96 \sqrt{1/a + 1/b + 1/c + 1/d}]$$

Where: exp = Exponential (e) raised to the power represented by the entire expression

In = Natural logarithm

OR = Odds ratio

a = Number of exposed individuals with the disease

b = Number of exposed individuals without the disease

c = Number of unexposed individuals with the disease

d = Number of unexposed individuals without the disease

95% Confidence Interval (CI) for Odds Ratio Using Matched Analysis (Exhibit 11–1)   215

$$95\% \text{ CI} = \exp [\ln (b / c) \pm 1.96 \sqrt{1 / b + 1 / c}]$$

Where: exp = Exponential (e) raised to the power represented by the entire expression

In = Natural logarithm

b = Number of case-control pairs in which only the cases are exposed

c = Number of case-control pairs in which only the controls are exposed

95% Confidence Interval (CI) for Person-Time Incidence Rate (Exhibit 5–2)   86

$$95\% \text{ CI} = r \pm 1.96 \sqrt{e / T^2}$$

Where: r = Person-time incidence rate stated as a decimal fraction

e = Number of new events

T = Total person-time units at risk

Formula	Page Number

95% Confidence Interval (CI) for Prevalence Rate Ratio and Relative Risk (10.5, 12.1)   195, 240

$$95\% \ CI = \exp \{\ln (Ratio) \pm 1.96\sqrt{[(b/a)/(a+b)] + [(d/c)/(c+d)]}\}$$

Where: exp = Exponential (e) raised to the power represented by the entire expression

ln = Natural logarithm

Ratio = Prevalence rate ratio or relative risk (risk ratio)

a = Number of exposed individuals with the disease

b = Number of exposed individuals without the disease

c = Number of unexposed individuals with the disease

d = Number of unexposed individuals without the disease

95% Confidence Interval (CI) for Rate Difference (12.5)   245

$$95\% \ CI = Rate \ Difference \pm 1.96 \ \sqrt{(a/T_e^2) + (c/T_{ue}^2)}$$

Where: T_e = Total person-time units generated by the exposed group

T_{ue} = Total person-time units generated by the unexposed group

a = Number of exposed subjects who developed the outcome

c = Number of unexposed subjects who developed the outcome

95% Confidence Interval (CI) for Rate Ratio (12.4)   244

$$95\% \ CI = \exp [\ln (Rate \ Ratio) \pm 1.96 \ \sqrt{1/a + 1/c}]$$

Where: exp = Exponential (e) raised to the power represented by the entire expression

ln = Natural logarithm

a = Number of exposed subjects who developed the outcome

c = Number of unexposed subjects who developed the outcome

95% Confidence Interval (CI) for Risk Difference (RD) (12.2)   241

$$95\% \ CI = RD \pm 1.96 \ \sqrt{\{[IR_{C-e} (1 - IR_{C-e})]/(a+b)\} + \{[IR_{C-ue} (1 - IR_{C-ue})]/(c+d)\}}$$

Where: RD = Risk difference

IR_{C-e} = Cumulative incidence rate in the exposed group stated as a decimal fraction

IR_{C-ue} = Cumulative incidence rate in the unexposed group stated as a decimal fraction

a = Number of exposed individuals with the disease

b = Number of exposed individuals without the disease

c = Number of unexposed individuals with the disease

d = Number of unexposed individuals without the disease

Formula	Page Number

95% Confidence Interval (CI) for the Standardized Mortality (or Morbidity) Ratio (Exhibit 6–2)

105

$$95\% \text{ CI} \cong \text{SMR} \pm 1.96 \sqrt{\text{SMR} / \text{EE}}$$

Where: SMR = Standardized mortality (or morbidity) ratio
EE = Total number of expected events

Crude Birth Rate (CBR) (Figure 5–2)

77

$$\text{CBR} = \frac{\text{Number of live births during a specified time period}}{\text{Mid-interval population}} \times 10^n$$

Where: n = 1, 2, 3, 4, etc.
The usual rate base for the Crude Birth Rate is 1,000.

Crude Death Rate (CDR) (Figure 5–2)

77

$$\text{CDR} = \frac{\text{Number of deaths during a specified time period}}{\text{Mid-interval population}} \times 10^n$$

Where: n = 1, 2, 3, 4, etc.
The usual rate base for the Crude Death Rate is 1,000 or 100,000.

Cumulative Incidence Rate (IR_C) (5.1)

62

$$\text{IR}_C = \frac{\text{Number of new events occurring during a specified time period}}{\text{Population at risk}} \times 10^n$$

Where: n = 1, 2, 3, 4, etc.

Estimated Number of Cases Needed When Using Multiple Controls in a Case-Control Study (11.1)

213

$$\text{Number of cases} \cong [k (c + 1)] / 2c$$

Where: k = Original number of cases required based on a 1:1 ratio of controls to cases
c = Number of controls per case that one plans to use

Estimated Sample Size Requirement for Randomized Controlled Trials* (13.1)

256

$$n = \frac{P_C (1 - P_C) + P_E (1 - P_E)}{(P_E - P_C)^2} \times 10.5$$

Where: n = Number of subjects required in each group
P_C = Proportion of outcomes expected in the control group
P_E = Proportion of outcomes expected in the experimental group

*This method assumes the groups are equal in size and the measure of interest is a difference in proportions of the outcome in each group. See text on page 256 for other assumptions.

Formula	Page Number

False Negative Rate (FNR) (Table 9-2) — 167

$$FNR\ (\%) = \frac{\text{Number of false negatives}}{\text{Number of true positives} + \text{Number of false negatives}} \times 100$$

False Positive Rate (FPR) (Table 9-2) — 167

$$FPR\ (\%) = \frac{\text{Number of false positives}}{\text{Number of false positives} + \text{Number of true negatives}} \times 100$$

Fertility Rate (FR) (Figure 5-2) — 77

$$FR = \frac{\text{Number of live births during a specified time period}}{\text{Mid-interval population of women aged 15–44 years}} \times 10^n$$

Where: $n = 1, 2, 3, 4$, etc.

The usual rate base for the Fertility Rate is 1,000.

Fetal Death Rate (FDR) (Figure 5-2) — 77

$$FDR = \frac{\text{Number of fetal deaths after 20 weeks or more of gestation during a specified time period}}{\text{Number of live births} + \text{Number of fetal deaths after 20 weeks or more of gestation}} \times 10^n$$

Where: $n = 1, 2, 3, 4$, etc.

The usual rate base for the Fetal Death Rate is 1,000.

Infant Mortality Rate (IMR) (Figure 5-2) — 77

$$IMR = \frac{\text{Number of deaths in infants aged 0–1 year during a specified time period}}{\text{Number of live births in the same time period}} \times 10^n$$

Where: $n = 1, 2, 3, 4$, etc.

The usual rate base for the Infant Mortality Rate is 1,000.

Kappa (See Cohen's Kappa in Exhibit 9-1.) — 172

Mantel-Haenszel Odds Ratio (OR_{MH}) (11.3) — 219

$$OR_{MH} = \frac{\Sigma\ (a_i\ d_i\ /\ n_i)}{\Sigma\ (b_i\ c_i\ /\ n_i)}$$

Where: a = Number of exposed individuals with the disease

b = Number of exposed individuals without the disease

c = Number of unexposed individuals with the disease

d = Number of unexposed individuals without the disease

n = Total number of individuals in the sample

i = Level of stratification

Formula	Page Number

Mantel-Haenszel Relative Risk (RR$_{MH}$) (12.3) **241**

$$RR_{MH} = \frac{\Sigma \left[a_i \left(c_i + d_i \right) / n_i \right]}{\Sigma \left[c_i \left(a_i + b_i \right) / n_i \right]}$$

Where: a = Number of exposed individuals with the disease
   b = Number of exposed individuals without the disease
   c = Number of unexposed individuals with the disease
   d = Number of unexposed individuals without the disease
   n = Total number of individuals in the sample
   i = Level of stratification

Maternal Mortality Rate (MMR) (Figure 5–2) **77**

$$MMR = \frac{\text{Number of deaths due to childbirth during a specified time period}}{\text{Number of live births in the same time period}} \times 10^n$$

Where: $n = 1, 2, 3, 4$, etc.
The usual rate base for the Maternal Mortality Rate is 100,000.

Negative Predictive Value (NPV) (9.4) **165**

$$\% \, NPV = \frac{\text{Number of true negatives}}{\text{Number of false negatives} + \text{Number of true negatives}} \times 100$$

Neonatal Mortality Rate (NMR) (Figure 5–2) **77**

$$NMR = \frac{\text{Number of deaths in infants aged less than 28 days during a specified time period}}{\text{Number of live births in the same time period}} \times 10^n$$

Where: $n = 1, 2, 3, 4$, etc.
The usual rate base for the Neonatal Mortality Rate is 1,000.

Odds Ratio (OR) (6.5) **109**

$$OR = ad / bc$$

Where: a = Number of exposed individuals with the disease
   b = Number of exposed individuals without the disease
   c = Number of unexposed individuals with the disease
   d = Number of unexposed individuals without the disease

Odds Ratio for Matched Case-Control Studies (Exhibit 11–1) **215**

$$OR = b / c$$

Where: b = Number of case-control pairs in which only the cases are exposed
   c = Number of case-control pairs in which only the controls are exposed

Formula	Page Number

Percent Relative Effect (6.3 a and b)   107

For a ratio > 1:
(6.3 a)   % Increased Change = (Ratio − 1) × 100

For a ratio < 1:
(6.3 b)   % Decreased Change = (1 − Ratio) × 100

Where: ratio = Relative risk (risk ratio), rate ratio, odds ratio, or prevalence rate ratio

Perinatal Mortality Rate (PMR) (Figure 5–2)   77

$$PMR = \frac{\text{Number of fetal deaths after 28 weeks or more of gestation} + \text{Infant deaths within 7 days of birth during a specified time period}}{\text{Number of live births} + \text{Number of fetal deaths after 28 weeks or more of gestation}} \times 10^n$$

Where: n = 1, 2, 3, 4, etc.
The usual rate base for the Perinatal Mortality Rate is 1,000.

Period Prevalence Rate (Period PR) (5.6)   71

$$\text{Period PR} = \frac{\text{Number of persons with a specific disease or attribute anytime during a specified time period}}{\text{Total defined population during the specified time period}} \times 10^n$$

Where: n = 1, 2, 3, 4, etc.

Person-Time Chi-Square Test of Independence (χ^2_{P-T}) (Table 12–4)   245

$$\chi^2_{P-T} = \frac{\{a - [T_e\,(a + c)] / T\}^2}{T_e\,[T_{ue}\,(a + c)] / T^2}$$

Where: T = Total person-time units generated by the study sample
T_e = Total person-time units generated by the exposed group
T_{ue} = Total person-time units generated by the unexposed group
a = Number of exposed subjects who developed the outcome
c = Number of unexposed subjects who developed the outcome

Person-Time Incidence Rate (IR_{P-T}) (5.2, 5.7)   65, 75

$$(5.2) \quad IR_{P-T} = \frac{\text{Number of new events occurring during a specified time period}}{\text{Total person-time units at risk}} \times 10^n$$

$$(5.7) \quad IR_{P-T} = \frac{\text{Point PR}}{D\,(1 - \text{Point PR})}$$

Where: n = 1, 2, 3, 4, etc.
Point PR = Point prevalence rate
D = Average duration of the disease from diagnosis to recovery or death

Formula	Page Number

Point Prevalence Rate (Point PR) (5.5)   **71**

$$\text{Point PR} = \frac{\text{Number of persons with a specific disease or attribute at a specific point in time}}{\text{Total defined population at the same time}} \times 10^n$$

Where: n = 1, 2, 3, 4, etc.

Population Attributable Rate (Table 12–4)   **245**

$$\text{Population Attributable Rate} = IR_{P\text{-}T} - IR_{P\text{-}T\text{-ue}}$$

Where: $IR_{P\text{-}T}$ = Person-time incidence rate in the population
$IR_{P\text{-}T\text{-ue}}$ = Person-time incidence rate in the unexposed group

Population Attributable Rate Percent (Table 12–4)   **245**

$$\text{Population Attributable Rate Percent} = \frac{IR_{P\text{-}T} - IR_{P\text{-}T\text{-ue}}}{IR_{P\text{-}T}} \times 100$$

Where: $IR_{P\text{-}T}$ = Person-time incidence rate in the population
$IR_{P\text{-}T\text{-ue}}$ = Person-time incidence rate in the unexposed group

Population Attributable Risk (Pop AR) (6.9)   **114**

$$\text{Pop AR} = IR_{C\text{-}p} - IR_{C\text{-ue}}$$

Where: $IR_{C\text{-}p}$ = Cumulative incidence rate in the population
$IR_{C\text{-ue}}$ = Cumulative incidence rate in the unexposed group

Population Attributable Risk Percent (Pop AR%) (6.10 a and b)   **115**

(6.10 a) $$\text{Pop AR\%} = \frac{IR_{C\text{-}p} - IR_{C\text{-ue}}}{IR_{C\text{-}p}} \times 100$$

(6.10 b) $$\text{Pop AR\%} = \frac{P_e\,(RR - 1)}{P_e\,(RR - 1) + 1} \times 100$$

Where: $IR_{C\text{-}p}$ = Cumulative incidence rate in the population
$IR_{C\text{-ue}}$ = Cumulative incidence rate in the unexposed group
P_e = Proportion of the exposed individuals in the population
RR = Relative risk

Positive Predictive Value (PPV) (9.3)   **165**

$$\%\ \text{PPV} = \frac{\text{Number of true positives}}{\text{Number of true positives} + \text{Number of false positives}} \times 100$$

Formula	Page Number

Prevalence Rate (PR) Derived from Screening Tests (9.5)   165

$$PR = \frac{\text{Number of true positives} + \text{Number of false negatives}}{\text{Total number in the sample}} \times 100$$

Prevalence Rate Difference (PRD) (10.3)   194

$$PRD = PR_e - PR_{ue}$$

Where: PR_e = Prevalence rate among the exposed subjects

PR_{ue} = Prevalence rate among the unexposed subjects

Prevalence Rate Ratio (or Prevalence Ratio) (PRR) (10.2)   194

$$PRR = PR_e / PR_{ue}$$

Where: PR_e = Prevalence rate among the exposed subjects

PR_{ue} = Prevalence rate among the unexposed subjects

Proportionate Mortality Ratio (PMR) (Figure 5–2)   77

$$PMR = \frac{\text{Number of deaths from a specific cause during a specified time period}}{\text{Total number of deaths in the same time period}} \times 10^n$$

Where: n = 1, 2, 3, 4, etc.

The usual rate base for the Proportionate Mortality Ratio is 100.

Rate Ratio (6.4)   108

$$\text{Rate Ratio} = \frac{IR_{P\text{-}T\text{-}e}}{IR_{P\text{-}T\text{-}ue}}$$

Where: $IR_{P\text{-}T\text{-}e}$ = Person-time incidence rate in the exposed group

$IR_{P\text{-}T\text{-}ue}$ = Person-time incidence rate in the unexposed group

Relationship of Cumulative Incidence Rate (IR_C) and Person-Time Incidence Rate ($IR_{P\text{-}T}$) (5.4 a and b)   68

(5.4 a) $IR_C \cong IR_{P\text{-}T} \times Y$

(5.4 b) $IR_{P\text{-}T} \cong IR_C / Y$

Where: IR_C = Cumulative incidence rate

$IR_{P\text{-}T}$ = Person-time incidence rate

Y = Length of the study period (usually in years)

These formulas only apply when the cumulative incidence rate is relatively low, and the length of the study period is relatively short.

Formula	Page Number

Relative Risk (RR) Derived from a Regression Equation (10.1)   **188**

$$RR \cong 1 + (b/a)$$

Given the regression equation: $Y = a + bX$

Where: a = Intercept
  b = Slope
  Y = Dependent variable (outcome variable)
  X = Independent variable (exposure variable)

Relative Risk (RR) (6.2)   **106**

$$RR = \frac{IR_{C\text{-}e}}{IR_{C\text{-}ue}}$$

Where: $IR_{C\text{-}e}$ = Cumulative incidence rate in the exposed group
  $IR_{C\text{-}ue}$ = Cumulative incidence rate in the unexposed group

---

Sensitivity of a Screening Test (9.1)   **163**

$$\% \text{ Sensitivity} = \frac{\text{Number of true positives}}{\text{Number of true positives} + \text{Number of false negatives}} \times 100$$

Specificity of a Screening Test (9.2)   **163**

$$\% \text{ Specificity} = \frac{\text{Number of true negatives}}{\text{Number of false positives} + \text{Number of true negatives}} \times 100$$

Standardized Mortality (or Morbidity) Ratio (SMR) (6.1)   **101**

$$SMR = \frac{\text{Total number of observed events in the comparison population}}{\text{Total number of expected events in the same population}}$$

Survival Rate (SR) (5.9)   **79**

$$SR = \frac{\text{Number of newly diagnosed patients with a given disease} - \text{Number of deaths observed among the patients in a specified time period}}{\text{Number of newly diagnosed patients with the disease in the same time period}} \times 10^n$$

Where: n = 1, 2, 3, 4, etc.

Test of Significance for Dependent Rates (z) (6.11)   **117**

$$z = (r_S - r_L)\sqrt{n/(r_L - r_L^2)}$$

Where: z = z-score with a standard deviation of 1 and a mean of 0
  r_S = Rate calculated from the smaller population
  r_L = Rate calculated from the larger population
  n = Size of the smaller population

Formula	Page Number

Test of Significance for Mantel-Haenszel Odds Ratio (χ^2_{MH}) (Figure 11–3)   **220**
(one degree of freedom)

$$\chi^2_{MH} = \frac{\{\Sigma\, a_i - \Sigma\, [(a_i + c_i)\,(a_i + b_i)\,/\,n_i]\}^2}{\Sigma\,(a_i + c_i)\,(b_i + d_i)\,(a_i + b_i)\,(c_i + d_i)\,/\,n_i^2\,(n_i - 1)}$$

Where: a = Number of exposed individuals with the disease
b = Number of exposed individuals without the disease
c = Number of unexposed individuals with the disease
d = Number of unexposed individuals without the disease
n = Total number of individuals in the sample
i = Level of stratification

Test of Significance for Odds Ratio for Matched Case-Control Studies (McNemar's Chi-square Test) (χ^2) (Exhibit 11–1)   **215**
(one degree of freedom)

$$\chi^2 = \frac{(b - c)^2}{(b + c)}$$

Where: b = Number of case-control pairs in which only the cases are exposed
c = Number of case-control pairs in which only the controls are exposed

Total Person-Time Units at Risk (T) (5.3)   **66**

$$T = \Sigma t_i$$

Where: t_i = Each individual's person-time units at risk

Years of Potential Life Lost (YPLL) (5.10)   **81**

$$YPLL = \Sigma\,(E - a_i)$$

Where: E = Chosen endpoint, which is an age in years not considered to represent premature death (e.g., 65, 75)
a_i = Individual age at death prior to the endpoint

Years of Potential Life Lost Rate (YPLL Rate) (5.11)   **81**

$$YPLL\ Rate = \frac{YPLL}{Number\ of\ people\ in\ the\ population\ below\ the\ selected\ endpoint} \times 10^n$$

Where: n = 1, 2, 3, 4, etc.
YPLL = Years of potential life lost in a given population during a specified time period

Appendix B
A Brief Introduction to Epi Info

Epi Info is a versatile database and set of statistical programs designed for public health professionals. The most recent version of Epi Info is Epi Info™ 2000, which operates on the Microsoft Windows operating system. Previous versions of Epi Info were designed to be used with DOS.

Epi Info was developed by the Centers for Disease Control and Prevention (CDC) and can be used to conduct disease outbreak investigations, manage databases for public health surveillance, and perform a variety of statistical calculations, including sample size determination and power, measures of association, confidence intervals, and tests of statistical significance. Epi Info 2000 will produce tables, graphs, and maps and perform more advanced statistical procedures, including logistic regression and survival analysis. With Epi Info users can quickly develop study questionnaires, design specific databases, and analyze data.

The most amazing feature of Epi Info 2000, however, is that it is completely free of charge. The manual and application programs may be downloaded from the following website:

http://www.cdc.gov/epiinfo

The CDC also provides free technical support for users, and this support is accessible through e-mail, telephone, or fax. Specific information about Epi Info 2000, including downloading instructions and how to obtain technical support, is available at the website noted above.

Appendix C
Summary of Surveys and Data Systems from the National Center for Health Statistics

Name	Data Source/Methods	Planned Sample	Planned Periodicity
Vital Statistics Cooperative Program (VSCP)	• State vital registration	• All births, deaths, and fetal deaths • Counts of marriages and divorces	Annual
Linked Birth/Infant Death Program	• Birth and death certificates	• All U.S. births and infant deaths	Annual
National Death Index (NDI)	• State registration death certificates	• All deaths	Annual
National Maternal and Infant Health Survey (NMIHS)	• Follow back—state vital records • Interviews—mothers • Hospital medical records • Prenatal care providers	• 10,000 live births • 4,000 fetal deaths • 6,000 infant deaths • Oversample Blacks	Every 8 years, with longitudinal follow-up
National Mortality Follow-Back Survey (NMFS)	• Follow back—state death records • Telephone and/or personal interviews with informants • Hospital medical records • Medical examiner/coroner records	• 23,000 deaths of persons ages 15 years and over	Every 7 years
National Survey of Family Growth (NSFG)	• Personal interviews	• 14,000 women 15–44 years of age sampled to complete over 10,000 interviews • Oversample Blacks and Hispanics	3 and 4 years (2000 & 2003)

(continued)

Name	Data Source/Methods	Planned Sample	Planned Periodicity
National Health Interview Survey	• Personal interviews	• 40,000 households • Oversample Blacks and Hispanics	Annual
Access to Care Survey (ACS)	• Follow-up sample identified in 1993 NHIS • Telephone interviews • Sample of persons without telephones interviewed in person	Sample formed from responding NHIS households in the last 2 quarters of 1993 composed of: • 4,000 general population respondents • 3,000 respondents identified as having experienced access problems • 1,400 respondents identified as having asthma or ischemic heart disease	Targeted population study
National Health Interview Survey on Disability (NHIS-D)	• Personal interviews	• Phase 1 screens 90,000 households • Phase 2 is a follow-up of those persons with moderate to severe disabilities, approximately 20,000 per year	Special 2-year study
Second Supplement on Aging (SOA II)	• Personal interviews • Administrative match data: Medicare, NDI, and cause of death files	• 9,447 persons aged 70 and over at the time of phase 2 of NHIS-D (1994–1996)	Cross-sectional survey, serves as a baseline to the LSOA II
Second Longitudinal Study of Aging (LSOA II)	• Telephone interviews • Administrative match data: NDI, cause of death, and HCFA Medicare files	• 9,447 persons age 70 and over at the time of phase 2 of NHIS-D (1994–1996)	Baseline plus 3 follow-up waves, each at 2-year intervals
National Health and Nutrition Examination Survey (NHANES)	• Personal interviews • Physical examinations • Laboratory tests • Nutritional assessment	• ~5,000 persons, all ages • Oversample adolescents • Oversample Blacks and Mexican Americans	Annual with capability for longitudinal follow-up

(continued)

Name	Data Source/Methods	Planned Sample	Planned Periodicity
NHANES I Epidemiologic Follow-Up Study (NHEFS)	• Longitudinal follow-up—NHANES I cohort • Personal and telephone interviews • Medical records—hospitals and nursing homes • Death certificates	• 14,407 persons aged 25–74 years from 1971–75 NHANES I sample • Oversample persons in poverty areas, women of childbearing age and elderly	Special cohort study
National Hospital Discharge Survey (NHDS)	• Hospital records • Computerized data sources	• 542 hospitals • 250,000 discharges	Annual
National Survey of Ambulatory Surgery (NSAS)	• Abstract forms completed by facility staff	• 750 facilities • 120,000 surgery visits	Annual through 1996; periodic thereafter
National Ambulatory Medical Care Survey (NAMCS)	• Encounter forms completed by physicians practicing in private offices	• 3,000 physicians in office-based practices • 30,000 patient visits	Annual
National Hospital Ambulatory Medical Care Survey (NHAMCS)	• Encounter forms completed by physicians and other hospital staff	• 600 hospitals • 50,000 patient visits	Annual
National Nursing Home Survey (NNHS)	• Long-term care providers	• 1,500 nursing homes • 9,000 NH residents • 9,000 NH discharges	Historically every 4–10 years; converting to bi-annual cycle
National Home and Hospice Care Survey (NHHCS)	• Home health agencies and hospices	• 1,350 home health agencies and hospices • 6,000 current patients • 6,000 discharged patients	Annual through 1996, bi-annual thereafter. Small mail survey conducted in 1997.

(continued)

Name	Data Source/Methods	Planned Sample	Planned Periodicity
National Health Provider Inventory (NHPI)	• Health care facilities • State licensing agencies • Professional associations	• All facilities in covered categories	Periodic
National Employer Health Insurance Survey (NEHIS)	• Business establishments, organizations, and governments • Computer-assisted telephone interviewing	• Stratified national sample of establishments to include all sizes of businesses, both private and public • 81,000 establishments screened to conduct 39,000 interviews	One-time survey
National Immunization Survey (NIS)	• Telephone interviews • Data from NHIS personal interviews used to assess bias associated with telephone interviewing and adjust accordingly • Provider record check component	• 800,000 households screened to find NIS sample of households, with children 19–35 months • 400 completed NIS interviews in each of 78 nonoverlapping areas • Option allows for additional data collection on other topics from up to 400,000 of the households screened for NIS sample	Continuous with quarterly 12-month moving averages
State and Local Area Integrated Telephone Surveys (SLAITS)	• Telephone interviews • Data from NHIS and CPS personal interviews used to assess bias associated with telephone interviewing and adjust accordingly • Piggyback NIS sample	• 1,000–2,000 in each state sampled, possible oversamples • Up to 14 states in 2 years • Add states in subsequent years as funding permits	One-time pilot study of various modules as developed pending additional funding

Source: Adapted from U.S. Department of Health and Human Services, Centers for Disease Control and Prevention, National Center for Health Statistics (1999). *National Center for Health Statistics . . . Monitoring the Nation's Health: Programs and Activities.* DHHS Publication No. (PHS) 99-1200. Hyattsville, MD: The Centers.

Appendix D
Resources in Epidemiology

Major Journals Publishing Epidemiologic Studies

American Journal of Epidemiology
American Journal of Public Health
American Journal of Preventive Medicine
Annals of Epidemiology
Annual Review of Public Health
British Medical Journal
Canadian Journal of Public Health
Cancer Causes and Control
Controlled Clinical Trials
Epidemiologic Reviews
Epidemiology
Epidemiology and Infection
European Journal of Epidemiology
Infection Control and Hospital Epidemiology
International Journal of Epidemiology
Journal of the American Medical Association
Journal of Community Health
Journal of Epidemiology and Community Health
Journal of Public Health Medicine
Lancet
New England Journal of Medicine
Pan-American Journal of Public Health
Public Health
Public Health Reports

Other Useful Publications

The Epidemiology Monitor
(e-mail: *epimon@aol.com*)

Morbidity and Mortality Weekly Report
(*http://www.cdc.gov/mmwr/*)

Helpful Internet Sites

Selected Health Organizations

Centers for Disease Control and Prevention: *http://www.cdc.gov*
National Cancer Institute: *http://www.nci.nih.gov*
Pan American Health Organization: *http://www.paho.org*
U.S. Census Bureau: *http://www.census.gov*
World Health Organization: *http://www.who.int/home-page*

Epidemic Investigation

Anatomy of an Epidemic (Descriptions, Maps, etc.)
http://library.thinkquest.org/11170

EXCITE (Tools for Teachers)
http://www.cdc.gov/excite/index.htm

Comprehensive Information on Epidemiology

Epidemiology Supercourse (Lectures on Epidemiology)
http://www.pitt.edu/~super1

Epidemiology for the Uninitiated (Primer on Epidemiology)
http://www.bmj.com/epidem/epid.html

Appendix E
Selected Answers to Chapter Study Questions and Exercises

Chapter Two

1. G, K, D, F, I, B, H, C, J, E, A

Chapter Four

1. E
2. G
3. A
4. D
5. F
6. C
7. H
8. A
9. D
10. B

Chapter Five

1. 1.7 per 10,000 (cumulative incidence rate)

2. 1.7 per 100

3. 6.7 per 1,000 person-years
   (95% CI = 5.2 per 1,000 person-years–8.2 per 1,000 person-years)

4. 3.4 per 10,000 and 4.6 per 10,000

5. 227 YPLL and 10.5 per 1,000

6. a. Crude death rate
   b. Cumulative incidence rate
   c. Survival rate
   d. Proportionate mortality ratio
   e. Neonatal mortality rate
   f. Cause-specific mortality rate
   g. Period prevalence rate
   h. Case fatality rate

Chapter Six

3. a. 2.8 (cigarette smoking) and 3.1 (hypertension)
   b. 180% (cigarette smoking) and 210% (hypertension)
   c. 64.2% (cigarette smoking) and 67.7% (hypertension)
   d. 29.3% (cigarette smoking) and 26.8% (hypertension)

4. Not significantly different, $p > 0.05$

Chapter Eight

1. D
2. B
3. A
4. B
5. C
6. D
7. A
8. C
9. B
10. A

Chapter Nine

1. Sensitivity = 84.5%
   Specificity = 96.3%
   Positive Predictive Value = 86.1%
   Negative Predictive Value = 95.8%
   Accuracy of the Screening Test = 93.7%

2. a. F
   b. C
   c. A
   d. G
   e. E
   f. C
   g. D
   h. B

3. a. F
   b. F
   c. T
   d. F
   e. F
   f. F
   g. T

Chapter Ten

3. 2.0 (95% CI = 1.8–2.2)

Chapter Eleven

2. OR = 2.3, χ^2 = 12.4, p < 0.001, 95% CI = 1.4–3.7
3. OR = 3.1 (calcium deficient) and OR = 1.9 (calcium sufficient)
   χ^2 = 7.3, p < 0.01 (calcium deficient) and χ^2 = 4.6, p < 0.05
   (calcium sufficient)
4. OR = 1.6 (95% CI = 0.8–3.1) and χ^2 = 2.2, p > 0.05 (note: matched
   pair analysis)

Chapter Twelve

3. Rate ratio = 2.5 (95% CI = 1.2–5.2)
4. a. F
    b. F
    c. T
    d. F
    e. T

Chapter Thirteen

2. Percent relative effect = 40% (95% CI = 10%–60%)
4. a. F
    b. F
    c. F
    d. T
    e. F
    f. T
    g. T
    h. F
    i. T
    j. T
    k. F
    l. T

Chapter Fourteen

1. Common source, continuing source outbreak
   Probable time of exposure is August 31–September 5

2. Propagated outbreak
   Probable mode of transmission is person to person

4. Most likely source of the outbreak is beef (RR = 3.0, χ^2 = 6.3, p < 0.05;
   AR = 56%; AR% = 66%)

Glossary

absolute risk   The probability that a disease will occur in a given time period. It is commonly referred to simply as risk and is measured by the cumulative incidence rate.

accuracy   A measure of the degree to which something is correct. Epidemiologic findings are accurate to the extent that they are free of errors. Accuracy has two major components—validity and precision. Also see **validity; precision.**

accuracy of the screening test   A general measure of the extent to which the results of a screening test are valid. The accuracy of the screening test usually is calculated as a percent by dividing the number of individuals who are classified correctly by the screening test (i.e., true positives plus true negatives) by the total number of individuals tested and multiplying the result by 100. The accuracy of the screening test is a weighted average of the test's sensitivity and specificity.

active immunity   A type of immunity that results when the body produces its own antibodies in reaction to an infection or a vaccine. Also see **passive immunity.**

active surveillance   Surveillance that requires the health authority responsible for surveillance to obtain the health data being sought directly from various health care providers, such as physicians, hospitals, and laboratories. Also see **public health surveillance; passive surveillance.**

adjusted odds ratio   An odds ratio that has been statistically adjusted for one or more confounding factors. A common example is the Mantel-Haenszel odds ratio (OR_{MH}).

adjusted rate   A summary rate that has been statistically modified to remove the effect of one or more confounding factors, such as differences in age, sex, or racial/ethnic distributions between the populations being compared.

age adjustment   A statistical procedure that controls for differences in age distributions when comparing crude morbidity or mortality rates between populations. Because different age distributions can distort the magnitude of the crude rates, age adjustment is often necessary. It provides a way of making fair, unbiased comparisons between summary rates. Also known as *age standardization.*

age standardization   A synonym for **age adjustment.**

alpha level (α)   The chance of a type I error that an investigator is willing to take when testing a hypothesis. Common alpha levels are 0.05 and 0.01. Also see **p-value.**

analytic cross-sectional study   A cross-sectional study that tests one or more predetermined hypotheses about associations between exposure and outcome. Also see **cross-sectional study.**

analytic ecological study   An ecological study that tests one or more predetermined hypotheses about associations between exposure and outcome. Also see **ecological study.**

analytic epidemiology   An aspect of epidemiology concerned with understanding the causes or determinants of morbidity or mortality. This branch of epidemiology relies on observational studies to test hypotheses directed at identifying and confirming suspected risk factors for disease. Also see **descriptive epidemiology; experimental epidemiology.**

analytic study   A type of observational epidemiologic study that tests one or more predetermined hypotheses about associations between exposure and outcome. There are six common types of analytic studies—ecological studies, cross-sectional studies, case-control studies, prospective cohort studies, retrospective cohort studies, and hybrid studies. Also see **descriptive study; experimental study.**

antecedent cause of death   A term used on death certificates. It refers to any disease or condition that led to the immediate cause of death.

antibody   A protein substance or globulin derived from B and T lymphocytes that is formed as a defensive response to a specific antigen. Also see **antigen.**

antigen   A foreign substance, such as an infectious organism, that stimulates antibody production when it enters the body. Also see **antibody.**

attack rate   A cumulative incidence rate applied to a narrowly but well-defined population being observed over a limited time period, such as during a disease outbreak.

attack rate table   A table of attack rates among individuals exposed and unexposed to potential causes of a disease outbreak. Attack rate tables typically are used in retrospective cohort analyses of disease outbreaks where several exposures are examined simultaneously.

attributable rate   The amount of the person-time incidence rate of a disease among the exposed group that can be attributed to the exposure. Attributable rate assumes the exposure is a cause of the disease. Also see **attributable risk.**

attributable rate percent   The percent of the person-time incidence rate of a disease among the exposed group that can be attributed to the exposure. The attributable rate percent assumes the exposure is a cause of the disease. Also see **attributable risk percent.**

attributable risk   The amount of the absolute risk of a disease among the exposed group that can be attributed to the exposure. Attributable risk assumes the exposure is a cause of the disease. Also see **attributable rate.**

attributable risk percent   The percent of the absolute risk of a disease among the exposed group that can be attributed to the exposure. The attributable risk percent assumes the exposure is a cause of the disease. Also see **attributable rate percent.**

Berkson's bias   A type of selection bias, named after Dr. Joseph Berkson, that can occur in hospital-based case-control studies when the combination of the study exposure and outcome increases the chance that exposed cases will be admitted to the hospital. This can result in an artificially higher rate of exposure among hospitalized cases than controls.

beta level (β)   The probability of making a type II error when testing a hypothesis.

bias   Nonrandom (systematic) error in a study that can lead to erroneous results. In epidemiologic studies bias can cause overestimation of the measure of association (positive bias) or underestimation of the measure of association (negative bias). The two major categories of bias are selection bias and measurement bias.

Bills of Mortality   A phrase used for the weekly and annual recording of births and deaths in England in the sixteenth and seventeenth centuries. John Graunt used the Bills of Mortality in a 1662 landmark publication that is now considered the forerunner of modern vital statistics.

biological plausibility   A criterion for judging if an association is causal, based on Hill's postulates. This criterion asks whether or not the association makes biological sense given what is known about the exposure and outcome.

biomarker A cellular or molecular indicator of exposure to an environmental agent, such as elevated liver enzymes or the presence of toxic residues in the blood, urine, hair, or other body specimens.

blinding A procedure that keeps the investigators and/or the subjects unaware of subject classifications in analytic or experimental studies. The purpose of blinding is to minimize the bias that can result from knowing how the subjects are classified by exposure or outcome. Also see **single-blinded study; double-blinded study; triple-blinded study.**

cancer cluster The occurrence of a group of diagnostically distinct cancer cases in space or time whose distribution is believed not to be due to chance. Also see **disease cluster.**

carrier An individual who has no overt signs or symptoms of a communicable disease but nevertheless harbors the causative agent, which can be transmitted to others. For example, Typhoid Mary was a carrier of typhoid fever, which she unwittingly transmitted to others.

carryover effects The residual effects of an intervention that can occur in a crossover study during the period after the intervention has been completed.

case fatality rate The rate at which cases die from a given disease within a specified time period. The case fatality rate is both an indicator of the seriousness of a disease and a measure of the prognosis for those with the disease. The case fatality rate for diagnosed cases of AIDS is estimated to be about 85% within five years in the absence of specific treatment.

case finding In the context of screening for disease, case finding is screening that is requested and supervised by a health care provider during a patient visit for other reasons. Also known as *opportunistic screening.*

case report A type of descriptive study that presents a detailed description of an individual patient in order to characterize and understand a specific disease or syndrome. This type of study is common in clinical epidemiology, although in the strictest sense it is not an epidemiologic study.

case series A type of descriptive study that is an extension of the case report. It describes the characteristics of a group or cluster of individuals with the same disease or symptoms in an attempt to quantify various aspects of the group and thus present a relatively complete profile of the illness. Technically, a case series is not an epidemiologic study, although it is commonly used in clinical epidemiology and can suggest hypotheses about causation that can lead to further study.

case-control study A type of analytic epidemiologic study in which the subjects are selected according to outcome status before exposure status is determined. Well-designed case-control studies select new cases (those with the disease) and comparable controls (those without the disease) and then determine their prior exposure status, thereby maintaining a correct temporal sequence between exposure and outcome, which is a requirement for establishing causal associations.

causal association A statistical association in which a change in the exposure produces a corresponding change in the outcome. A causal association is an association that cannot be explained by sampling error, bias, or confounding.

cause A factor that produces a change in another factor. Also see **necessary cause; sufficient cause.**

cause-specific mortality rate A measure of the risk of death due to a specific cause, such as the breast cancer mortality rate.

chi-square test of independence A statistical test of significance commonly used to determine if two nominal variables (e.g., exposure and outcome status) are associated by comparing observed and expected frequencies in a contingency table.

clinical epidemiology   The application of epidemiologic principles and methods to clinical decision making, such as diagnosis, prognosis, and treatment of disease. Clinical epidemiology is patient oriented, while classical epidemiology is population oriented.

clinical significance   A level of statistical significance that is meaningful from a public health or clinical point of view. Also known as *practical significance*.

clinical trial   A randomized controlled trial in a clinical setting.

coefficient of determination   In simple linear regression, the coefficient of determination is the proportion of the variance in the dependent variable (e.g., the outcome measure) that is explained by the independent variable (e.g., the exposure measure). The coefficient of determination is measured by the square of the correlation coefficient (r), which is a measure of the degree of linear relationship between the variables. When there are multiple independent variables, as in multiple linear regression, the coefficient of determination is the proportion of the variance in the dependent variable that is explained by all the independent variables considered simultaneously. It is measured by the square of the multiple correlation coefficient (R).

Cohen's kappa   A statistic used to measure the proportion of nonrandom agreement between two or more observers of the same phenomenon. The kappa statistic ranges from zero to one with higher values indicating better agreement.

cohort   A group of individuals who are followed over time (e.g., in a retrospective or prospective cohort study).

common source outbreak   An outbreak that results from the exposure of a susceptible group of people to a common agent of disease (e.g., pathogenic organism, toxic substance). Also see **propagated outbreak.**

communicable disease   A disease that can be transmitted directly or indirectly to a susceptible person through contact, inhalation, or ingestion. Also known as an *infectious disease*.

community trial   An experimental or quasi-experimental epidemiologic study where the units of analysis are groups of people or communities. Typically, one community receives an intervention and another community serves as a control group.

comparison population   The smaller or less stable of the two populations being compared when indirect rate adjustment is being used.

confidence interval   The probable range in which a population parameter lies based on a random sample of the population. The most commonly reported confidence interval is the 95% confidence interval. It represents the range of values in which one can be 95% confident that the population parameter lies. In epidemiology confidence intervals are commonly calculated for rates and measures of association.

confidence level   The level of certainty that the population parameter lies within a stated confidence interval. In a 95% confidence interval the level of certainty or confidence level is 95%. Thus, one can be 95% confident that the population parameter lies within the stated interval.

confidence limits   The start and the end of the range represented by a confidence interval. For example, 4.2 and 6.5 represent the lower and upper confidence limits, respectively, for the following confidence interval: 95% CI = 4.2–6.5.

confounder   A synonym for **confounding factor.**

confounding   A distortion in the degree of association between a study exposure and outcome due to a mixing of effects between the exposure and an incidental factor known as a confounding factor or confounder. Four criteria are necessary for confounding to occur: (1) the incidental factor must be associated with the study exposure, (2) it must be an independent risk factor for the study outcome, (3) it must not be an intermediate step in a causal chain between the exposure and outcome, and (4) it must be unequally distributed between the study and the comparison groups.

confounding factor   An incidental factor that distorts an apparent association between an exposure and outcome in an epidemiologic study. The effect of a confounding factor, also known as a confounder, can partially or totally explain the effect of an exposure on an outcome. Four criteria, which are listed under confounding, must be met for an incidental factor to be considered a confounding factor. Also see **confounding.**

consistency of the association   A criterion for judging if an association is causal, based on Hill's postulates. An association is said to be consistent when multiple investigators studying a problem among different populations at different times in different places using different methodologies obtain similar results.

continuing source outbreak   A type of common source outbreak where the exposure to the common agent of disease is prolonged beyond a brief period, and the exposure is not simultaneous among those exposed. Continuing source outbreaks are expected to last longer than the time range of the incubation period of the disease because the exposure period is protracted, and not all are exposed at the same time. Also see **point source outbreak; intermittent source outbreak.**

contributory cause   A causative factor that is neither necessary nor sufficient to cause disease. Sedentary lifestyle is a contributory cause of coronary heart disease. Most causes of chronic diseases are contributory causes.

convenience sample   A sample of study subjects selected for expedience. Convenience samples are usually chosen because they are readily available, but they may not be representative of the target population from which they were selected.

correct temporal sequence   A criterion for judging if an association is causal, based on Hill's postulates. This criterion states that in order for an exposure to cause an outcome it must precede the outcome. Of all the criteria used to judge whether an association is causal or not, this is the only one that is considered absolutely essential.

crossover   A subject in the experimental group of a randomized controlled trial who does not complete the assigned intervention or a subject in the control group who seeks the intervention being tested. Crossovers represent violations of the study protocol and can lead to erroneous conclusions about the efficacy of an intervention.

crossover design   A variation of the traditional randomized controlled trial in which the intervention is applied at different times to each subject; that is, after a specified period of time the original experimental group becomes the control group, and the original control group becomes the experimental group. Also see **randomized controlled trial.**

cross-sectional study   An observational epidemiologic study in which exposure and outcome status are assessed simultaneously, that is, at the same point in time or during a brief period of time. Cross-sectional studies can be either descriptive (exploratory) or analytic, depending on whether or not a predetermined hypothesis is being tested.

crude birth rate   The proportion of live births occurring in a defined population during a specified time period. The crude birth rate is a good indicator of population growth.

crude death rate   A measure of the risk of death from all causes in a defined population during a specified time period.

crude odds ratio   The overall odds ratio without regard to specific classification variables, such as age, sex, or race/ethnicity.

crude prevalence rate   The overall prevalence rate without regard to the exposure status of the group or population being studied.

crude rate   An overall or summary rate for a defined population. It is determined by dividing the total number of events of interest for a given time period by the entire defined population and multiplying the result by a selected rate base. Common examples include the crude death rate and the crude birth rate, although any overall morbidity or mortality rate is considered a crude rate. Also see **specific rate.**

cumulative incidence rate   A measure of the risk of disease development (or other health event) in a defined population during a specified time period. The cumulative incidence rate is usually calculated by dividing the number of new events in a population by those at risk of the event at the beginning of the specified time period (i.e., the initial population at risk) and multiplying the result by a selected rate base.

cyclic pattern   Periodic, often predictable, increases in the frequency of a particular cause of morbidity or mortality in a specified population. For example, there is a seasonal variation in the frequency of influenza, which peaks in the late fall and winter months.

dependent rates   Rates in which some of the events in the numerator of one rate are also included in the numerator of the other rate. This occurs when one rate is based on a subgroup of a population used to calculate the other rate (e.g., rate in Minnesota and rate in United States) or when the rates are based on the same population but during overlapping time periods (e.g., 2001 and 2000–2002).

dependent variable   The outcome variable or effect that is influenced or predicted by other independent variables in a study. In epidemiology, the dependent variable is typically outcome status, which is presumed to be dependent on exposure status, the independent variable. Also see **independent variable.**

descriptive epidemiology   An aspect of epidemiology concerned with describing the variations in the distribution of morbidity or mortality by person, place, or time variables. This branch of epidemiology involves observation and description of what exists in a population and does not test predetermined hypotheses. Also see **analytic epidemiology; experimental epidemiology.**

descriptive study   An observational epidemiologic study that has no predetermined hypothesis. A descriptive study simply describes what exists in a population by person, place, or time variables. These studies are useful in demonstrating trends and generating hypotheses about disease causation. There are four common types of descriptive studies—case reports, case series, exploratory ecological studies, and descriptive cross-sectional studies. Only the latter two, however, are true epidemiologic studies. Also see **analytic study; experimental study.**

diagnostic suspicion bias   A form of measurement bias that can occur when knowledge of the subjects' exposure status influences how the outcome is diagnosed.

differential misclassification   A type of measurement bias that occurs when subjects in a study are incorrectly classified with respect to exposure or outcome status in an unequal manner. In other words, there is an unequal frequency of incorrect classifications on exposure status between the outcome groups or on outcome status between the exposure groups. Differential misclassification can lead to over- or underestimation of the measure of association. Also see **nondifferential misclassification.**

direct causal association   A causal association in which the cause leads directly to the effect without any intervening steps. For example, fire is a direct cause of burns, and *Yersinia pestis* is a direct cause of bubonic plague. Also see **indirect causal association.**

direct cause   A cause that leads directly to an effect without any intervening steps.

direct method   A method of rate adjustment used when the specific rates (e.g., age-specific rates) in each population being compared are stable and available. Also see **indirect method.**

disease   A physiological or psychological dysfunction. Also see **morbidity.**

disease cluster   The occurrence of a group of cases, usually of a relatively uncommon disease (e.g., leukemia), in space or time, whose distribution is believed not to be due to chance.

disease iceberg concept   An analogy that explains the clinician's often distorted view of the severity or frequency of certain diseases in a population, due to the fact that only a small portion of those who have the disease seek treatment. This term derives from the fact that four-fifths of an iceberg is normally submerged or out of view.

disease outbreak   An epidemic confined to a localized area, such a town or within an institutional setting such as a day-care center or prison. Disease outbreak is often used synonymously with epidemic.

disease registry   See **population-based disease registry.**

dose-response relationship   A criterion for judging if an association is causal, based on Hill's postulates. This is a relationship where increasing levels of exposure (dose) are associated with increases in the magnitude or frequency of the effect (response). For example, there is a dose-response relationship between alcohol consumption and driving ability and between smoking and lung cancer.

double-blinded study   A study in which neither the subjects nor the investigators are aware of the subjects' exposure status in prospectively designed studies or outcome status in retrospectively designed studies. Double-blinded studies are the standard for randomized controlled trials. Also see **blinding.**

e   See **exp.**

ecological fallacy   An error of reasoning that occurs when associations among groups of people are used to draw conclusions about associations among individuals that may not necessarily exist. Ecological fallacies can occur when ecological studies reveal associations between exposure and outcome, and it is inferred from this that the same associations exist among individuals.

ecological model   A model that attempts to explain disease causation as an imbalance of the interaction among host, agent, and environmental factors. Also known as the *epidemiologic triangle*.

ecological study   An observational epidemiologic study in which the units of analysis are groups of people versus individuals and where summary measures of exposure and outcome are used to determine associations. Ecological studies can be descriptive (i.e., exploratory ecological studies) or analytic. The analytic ecological studies include multiple-group comparison studies, time-trend studies, and mixed studies.

ecological unit   An aggregate of individuals that comprises a unit of analysis in an ecological study. Typically ecological units represent groups defined by geographical areas, such as states or countries, or by time periods.

effect modification   A real effect that occurs in a study when a third factor influences the direction or magnitude of a causal association between a study exposure and outcome. For example, cigarette smoking modifies the effect of radon exposure on the development of lung cancer. Individuals exposed to radon who smoke cigarettes have a much higher risk of lung cancer than individuals exposed to radon who do not smoke cigarettes. Thus, cigarette smoking is an effect modifier of the risk of lung cancer due to radon exposure. Also known as *interaction*.

effect size   The size of the association one would like to detect in a study if the association exists. In randomized controlled trials, the effect size can be calculated by subtracting the proportion of outcomes expected in the control group from the proportion of outcomes expected the experimental group (i.e., $P_E - P_C$).

effective sample size   The remaining sample size after losses from a study (i.e., due to death, withdrawal, loss to follow-up, etc.).

effectiveness   A measure of the benefits of a treatment, procedure, or service among those to whom it is offered, whether or not they use it. Effectiveness is often tested in community trials.

efficacy   A measure of the benefits of a treatment, procedure, or service among those who use it compared to those who do not. Efficacy is normally tested in randomized controlled trials.

eligibility criteria   The criteria used to define who is to be included and excluded from a study. In randomized controlled trials, the goal of the eligibility criteria is to optimize the conditions for successful testing of the efficacy of an intervention. Also see **inclusion criteria; exclusion criteria.**

emerging infectious disease   An infectious disease previously unknown or virtually unknown in a population that has been increasing or threatening to increase in recent years. Also see **reemerging infectious disease.**

end point   A study outcome in a randomized controlled trial.

endemic   The constant presence or usual frequency of a specific disease in a given population.

epidemic   Circumstances where there is a clear increase in the number of cases of a disease compared to that which is normally expected for the particular time and place.

epidemic curve   A graphic representation of the distribution of disease cases by time of onset in the form of a histogram. Epidemic curves are commonly used in the investigation of disease outbreaks and may provide clues to the source or mode of transmission of the disease.

epidemiology   The study of the distribution, determinants, and deterrents of morbidity or mortality in human populations.

evaluation study   A study designed to evaluate the impact of a health-related program, project, or campaign on a community.

exclusion criteria   The criteria used to define who is to be excluded from a study, for example, in a randomized controlled trial.

exp   The exponential or e, which is the base used in natural logarithms. The value of exp is approximately 2.7183. The expression exp (x) is equivalent to e^x; thus, exp (2) is e^2, which is 2.7183^2 or approximately 7.3892. Also see **ln.**

experimental epidemiology   An aspect of epidemiology concerned with identifying the causes or determinants of morbidity or mortality in human populations using experimental methods. Also see **descriptive epidemiology; analytic epidemiology.**

experimental evidence   A criterion for judging if an association is causal, based on Hill's postulates. Confirmation of an association by a randomized controlled trial or randomized community trial provides strong evidence that an association is causal.

experimental population   A practical representation of the reference population for a randomized controlled trial. If the reference population is adult males, the experimental population will be an available subset of adult males (e.g., a sample of adult males in Cook County, Illinois).

experimental study   An epidemiologic study in which the investigators have direct control over the study conditions. Experimental studies employ some type of intervention to determine its effect on a given outcome. There are two major types of planned experimental studies in epidemiology—randomized controlled trials and community trials. Also see **observational study.**

exploratory case-control study   A descriptive case-control study in which there is no predetermined hypothesis about the association between exposure and outcome. Exploratory case-control studies can be useful in identifying potential risk factors and possible causes of epidemics.

exposure   The potential risk factor in an epidemiologic study, whether that factor represents an actual exposure (e.g., environmental tobacco smoke), a behavior (e.g., sedentary lifestyle), or an individual attribute (e.g., age). Also see **outcome.**

exposure status   A term for classifying individuals or groups according to their level of exposure to a potential risk factor. Exposure status may be dichotomous (i.e., present or absent) or may represent several levels, such as heavy, moderate, and light drinkers. Also see **outcome status.**

exposure suspicion bias   A form of measurement bias that can occur when knowledge of the subjects' outcome status influences how exposure is assessed.

external comparison group   In the context of a cohort study, an external comparison group is a group outside the original cohort that serves as a control group for comparison purposes. External comparison groups are often composed of general population samples in the same geographic area with similar demographic characteristics as the original cohort.

external validity   The degree to which the results of a study are relevant for populations other than the target population. Also known as *generalizability.*

factorial design   A variation of the traditional randomized controlled trial which is intended to answer two or more research questions at the same time. In this type of study the subjects are randomized into experimental and control groups and then these groups are randomized again to test additional study hypotheses. Also see **randomized controlled trial.**

false negative   A negative test result where the individual being tested has the attribute for which testing is being done. In the context of screening for disease, a false negative is one who tests negative on the screening test but really has the disease.

false negative rate   The percent of those with the disease who are falsely classified as not having the disease based on a screening test.

false positive   A positive test result where the individual being testing does not have the attribute for which testing is being done. In the context of screening for disease, a false positive is one who tests positive on the screening test but really does not have the disease.

false positive rate   The percent of those without the disease who are falsely classified as having the disease based on a screening test.

fertility rate   The number of live births occurring in a population during a specified time period in relation to the number of women 15–44 years of age during the same time period. Like the crude birth rate, the fertility rate is a good indicator of population growth.

fetal death rate   The number of fetal deaths after 20 weeks or more of gestation during a specified time period in relation to the number of live births plus fetal deaths after 20 weeks or more of gestation during the same time period.

force of morbidity   A term sometimes used to refer to the person-time incidence rate.

frequency matching   A form of matching that seeks to make study and comparison groups similar with respect to the frequency of extraneous variables. For example, in a case-control study that uses frequency matching for gender, if 40% of the case group are females, then the investigator seeks to obtain 40% females in the control group. Frequency matching tends to reduce but not eliminate confounding.

generalizability   A synonym for **external validity.**

gold standard A diagnostic test that is widely accepted as being the best available. For example, the angiogram is the gold standard for diagnosing coronary heart disease. Gold standard is also used in a general sense as the best in its class, such as when the randomized controlled trial is referred to as the gold standard of epidemiologic studies.

health A state of well-being and positive functioning and not just the absence of disease.

healthy worker effect A form of selection bias that can arise when health outcomes among workers are compared to those among general population samples. The comparison is usually more favorable for the workers. The healthy worker effect is due to the fact that workers tend to be healthier as a group, and hence less susceptible to morbidity and premature mortality, than the general population. This is because workers must have a certain level of health to work, while the general population includes those who are unable to work because of health problems.

herd immunity The resistance of a group or population to the spread of a disease due to the fact that a high proportion of the group is immune to the disease.

Hill's postulates A set of criteria developed by Austin Bradford Hill in 1965 to determine whether or not a statistical association is likely to represent a causal association. Some of these criteria are: correct temporal sequence, strength of the association, consistency of the association, dose-response relationship, biological plausibility, and experimental evidence.

historical cohort study See **retrospective cohort study.**

historical prospective cohort study An epidemiologic study that combines features of retrospective and prospective cohort studies. This type of study identifies a historical cohort and then follows it up into the future.

hospital controls Subjects comprising the control group of a hospital-based case-control study. Hospital controls are selected from hospitalized patients without the study disease.

hospital-based case-control study A case-control study in which the subjects are selected among patients admitted to one or more clinical facilities, usually, but not necessarily, hospitals.

hybrid study An analytic epidemiologic study that combines features of two or more epidemiologic study designs. Some of the common types of hybrid studies are: nested case-control studies, nested case-cohort studies, panel studies, and repeated surveys.

immediate cause of death A term used on death certificates. It is the disease or condition that directly led to death.

immunity See **active immunity; passive immunity; herd immunity.**

incidence The number of new events (e.g., cases of disease) occurring in a defined population during a specified time period. It is also sometimes referred to as the incidence number or incident number.

incidence density A term sometimes used to refer to the person-time incidence rate.

incidence rate The rate at which new events occur in a defined population. There are two basic types of incidence rates—cumulative incidence rates and person-time incidence rates.

inclusion criteria The criteria used to define who is to be included in a study, for example, in a randomized controlled trial.

incubation period The time between the invasion of an infectious agent and the development of the first signs or symptoms of a communicable disease.

independent rates Rates that do not include any of the same events in their numerators.

independent variable   A variable that is expected to influence or predict the out-come (dependent) variable in a study. In epidemiology, the independent variable is typically exposure status, which is used to predict outcome status, the dependent variable. Also see **dependent variable.**

index case   The first case of a disease in a defined group to come to the attention of investigators during a disease outbreak. Often the index case is the one who intro-duced the causative agent to the group.

indirect causal association   An association in which the cause leads to the effect through one or more intervening steps. For example, sharing syringes can cause HIV infection, which causes AIDS. Therefore, sharing syringes is an indirect cause of AIDS. Also see **direct causal association.**

indirect cause   A cause that leads to the effect through one or more intervening steps.

indirect method   A method of rate adjustment used when one or more of the spe-cific rates (e.g., age-specific rates) in one of the populations being compared is either unstable or unavailable. Also see **direct method.**

induction period   See **latency period.**

infant mortality rate   The number of deaths among infants up to one year of age during a specified time period in relation to the number of live births during the same time period. It is often used as an indicator of the health status of a population.

infectious disease   See **communicable disease.**

information bias   A synonym for **measurement bias.**

initial population at risk   The number of susceptible individuals in a defined pop-ulation who are disease-free at the beginning of a specified time period. Also see **cumulative incidence rate.**

intention-to-treat analysis   The analysis of the results of a randomized con-trolled trial based on the original assignments to experimental and control groups at the time of randomization, whether or not all the subjects complied with the study protocol.

interaction   The combined effect of two or more independent variables on a depen-dent variable. For example, interaction occurs when two risk factors together increase or decrease the magnitude of an outcome compared to only one of the factors. For practical purposes, interaction can be considered synonymous with effect modification. Also see **effect modification.**

intermittent source outbreak   A common source outbreak where the exposure to the causative agent is irregular. An intermittent source outbreak might occur, for example, when a contaminated food is served on different days over the course of a week.

internal comparison group   In the context of a cohort study, an internal compari-son group represents those in the cohort who are unexposed to the study expo-sure. This group serves as a control group.

internal validity   The degree to which the results of a study are not due to bias or confounding.

interobserver variability   A measure of the extent of disagreement between two or more observers of the same phenomenon. For example, when two laboratory tech-nicians interpret the same results of a laboratory test differently, interobserver vari-ability has occurred.

intervention study   A synonym for **experimental study.** This name derives from the fact that in experimental studies the investigators intervene in the lives of the subjects by manipulating the conditions of exposure.

intervention trial   A type of randomized controlled trial that focuses on high-risk individuals with the purpose of testing an intervention to see if disease develop-ment can be forestalled. Also see **preventive trial; therapeutic trial.**

interviewer bias A type of measurement bias that can occur when the interviewers' awareness of the subjects' outcome status influences how they solicit, record, or interpret information on the subjects' exposure status or vice versa.

intraobserver variability A measure of the degree of inconsistency in the conclusions drawn by a single observer regarding the same phenomenon at different times. For example, if a radiologist reads an x-ray as positive for disease on one day but negative for disease on another day, intraobserver variability has occurred.

kappa See **Cohen's kappa.**

latency period The time it takes for a noncommunicable disease to develop once the causes are in place. Also known as *induction period.*

lead time The extra time acquired to treat a disease because of earlier than usual detection. Lead time can be gained when a new screening test is able to detect a disease in an earlier stage of development (e.g., during the stage of presymptomatic disease).

lead time bias A type of bias that occurs when survival time is overestimated due to an early diagnosis that does not improve prognosis. Lead time bias can occur when comparing survival times for two groups in which the disease has been diagnosed at different stages in its natural history (e.g., at the stage of presymptomatic disease, using a screening test in one group, and at the stage of clinical disease, using a physical examination in the other group).

length bias A type of bias that occurs when there is a higher proportion of individuals with slowly progressing disease in one group compared to another group. Because individuals with slowly progressing disease tend to have a better prognosis, and hence a longer survival time, this type of bias can lead to overestimation of the efficacy of screening programs, since screening is more likely to detect those with slowly progressing than rapidly progressing diseases.

levels of prevention The levels at which disease can be prevented or controlled. There are three levels of prevention—primary, secondary, and tertiary. Primary prevention seeks to prevent new cases of disease from developing in a population. Secondary prevention seeks to reduce the number of existing cases of disease in a population. Finally, tertiary prevention seeks to limit disability and improve functioning resulting from disease and its complications.

lifetime prevalence rate The proportion of individuals in a defined population who have had a given disease or attribute anytime in their lives.

ln The logarithm in the base e, or simply, the natural logarithm. In the expression exp $(x) = Y$, x is the natural logarithm of Y; that is, x is the power that e must be raised to get Y. In the expression ln $(x) = Y$, x is the value of e raised to a power of Y. Also see **exp.**

logistic regression See **multiple logistic regression.**

lower confidence limit The beginning (lowest) value of a confidence interval.

loss to follow-up bias A form of selection bias that can occur in longitudinal studies when significant losses to follow-up result in a sample that is systematically different from the original in terms of exposure frequency or outcome susceptibility.

lower confidence limit The beginning (lowest) value of a confidence interval.

Mantel-Haenszel odds ratio An adjusted odds ratio that represents a type of weighted average of stratum-specific odds ratios where the strata are the levels of a potential confounder and the weights depend on the number of observations in each stratum. The Mantel-Haenszel odds ratio may be used when confounding is present but should not be used when effect modification is expected, since it can obscure the effect, which needs to be described and explained in a study.

Mantel-Haenszel relative risk An adjusted relative risk that represents a type of weighted average of stratum-specific relative risks where the strata are the levels of a potential confounder and the weights depend on the number of observations in each stratum. The Mantel-Haenszel relative risk may be used when confounding is present but should not be used when effect modification is expected, since it can obscure the effect, which needs to be described and explained in a study.

masking   See **blinding.**

mass screening   Screening for disease, which is aimed at large population groups that vary widely in their risk of the disease. Also see **selective screening.**

matched case-control study   A case-control study that uses pair matching; that is, individual cases are paired with individual controls during the selection process to control for potential confounding. Matched studies are analyzed differently than unmatched studies.

matching   A procedure that attempts to produce study and comparison groups that are similar with regard to extraneous or potentially confounding factors. Also see **frequency matching; pair matching.**

maternal mortality rate   The number of deaths due to childbirth during a specified time period in relation to the number of live births during the same time period.

measure of association   A measure that indicates the strength or impact of the relationship between an exposure and outcome in an epidemiologic study. Ratio measures of association (e.g., relative risk or rate ratio) indicate the strength of a relationship, while difference measures (e.g., attributable risk or attributable rate) indicate the impact of a relationship.

measurement bias   Systematic (nonrandom) error that arises from inaccurate measurements or misclassification of subjects with regard to exposure or outcome status.

membership bias   A type of selection bias that results from the fact that those who belong to organized groups (e.g., the military, athletic associations, civic groups, religious organizations) tend to differ systematically with regard to their health status from the general population. In general, members of organized groups tend to be healthier and less susceptible to morbidity and premature mortality than members of the general population, which include those too ill to participate in groups.

meta-analysis   A method of statistically pooling the results of several studies on the same topic in order to identify overall trends and to develop policy.

method variability   The variability in the results of a measure due to the measure itself. Method variability is a property of an unreliable measure. For example, a screening test that under similar conditions shows positive results on some occasions and negative results on other occasions suffers from method variability.

mixed outbreak   A combination of common source and propagated outbreaks. Often a mixed outbreak begins with a common source exposure that is followed by person-to-person spread of the disease.

morbidity   Any departure from physiological or psychological well-being, whether objective or subjective. It is commonly used interchangeably with disease and refers to nonfatal conditions.

mortality   Deaths in a population.

multifactorial etiology   A term referring to multiple, interrelated causes or determinants of disease. Diseases that have multiple causes, such as heart disease, are said to have a multifactorial etiology.

multiphasic screening   Screening for disease that uses a variety of screening tests to detect several diseases or conditions at the same time. Health fairs, for example, may use multiphasic screening to test for possible diabetes, hypertension, hearing impairment, and other potential disorders at the same time.

multiple logistic regression   A type of regression analysis in which the dependent variable is dichotomous (e.g., present or absent) and the independent variables are nominal or continuous. This method is popular in analyzing data from case-control and other epidemiologic studies because adjusted odds ratios can be derived easily from the regression coefficients, which are part of the regression equations.

multivariable method   One of several statistical methods used to analyze the effects of more than one independent variable on a dependent variable (e.g., multiple logistic regression).

natural experiment   An unplanned type of experimental study. This is a relatively rare situation in nature where the levels of exposure to a presumed cause differ among a population in a way that is relatively unaffected by extraneous factors so that the situation resembles a planned experiment.

natural history of disease   The potentially predictable life cycle of a disease from onset to final outcome. The natural history of disease has four stages—stage of susceptibility, stage of presymptomatic disease, stage of clinical disease, and stage of diminished capacity.

natural logarithm   See **ln.**

necessary and sufficient cause   A cause that is required to produce the outcome and is able to cause the outcome by itself. For example, mercury exposure is a necessary and sufficient cause of mercury poisoning.

necessary but not sufficient cause   A cause that is required to produce the outcome but is not able to cause the outcome by itself. Other causes are necessary for the outcome to occur. *Mycobacterium tuberculosis* is necessary to produce tuberculosis, but it is not sufficient.

necessary cause   A cause that is always required for a particular outcome to occur.

negative bias   Bias that results in an underestimation of the magnitude of the measure of association between an exposure and outcome.

negative confounder   A confounding factor that leads to underestimation of the magnitude of the measure of association between an exposure and outcome.

negative predictive value   A measure of the percent of people who test negative on a screening test and really do not have the disease.

neonatal mortality rate   The number of deaths among infants less than 28 days old during a specified time period in relation to the number of live births during the same time period.

nested case-cohort study   A variation of the nested case-control study in which controls are selected randomly from all members of the cohort at the beginning of the study. Those subjects who later become cases can be sorted out during the analysis phase. Also see **nested case-control study.**

nested case-control study   A case-control study derived from the subjects of a cohort study. This type of hybrid study has the advantage of minimizing selection bias since the cases and controls come from the same well-defined population.

Neyman's bias   See **prevalence-incidence bias.**

noncausal association   A statistical association between an exposure and outcome that is usually due to confounding. The association exists because the exposure is associated with a cause of the outcome. For example, there is a noncausal association between alcohol consumption and lung cancer that is due to confounding by cigarette smoking.

noncommunicable disease   A disease that cannot be transmitted to others, either directly or indirectly. Also known as a *noninfectious disease*.

nondifferential misclassification   A type of measurement bias that occurs when subjects in a study are incorrectly classified with respect to exposure or outcome status in a uniform manner. In other words, there is an equal frequency of incorrect classifications with regard to exposure status between the outcome groups or with regard to outcome status between the exposure groups. Nondifferential misclassification generally results in a dilution of the magnitude of the measure of association, that is, toward no association. Also see **differential misclassification.**

noninfectious disease   See **noncommunicable disease.**

not necessary and not sufficient cause   A cause that is not required to produce the outcome and when present is not able to cause the outcome by itself. Hence, there are other causes of the outcome. A not necessary and not sufficient cause is known as a contributory cause. For example, stress is a contributory cause of heart disease.

not necessary but sufficient cause   A cause that is not required to produce the outcome but when present is able to cause the outcome by itself. This means that there are other causes of the outcome. For example, dehydration is not necessary but is sufficient to cause headaches.

not statistically significant   An indication that an apparent association is likely due to sampling error. An association is usually considered not statistically significant when the p-value is greater than 0.05 ($p > 0.05$).

notifiable disease   A disease or condition that must be reported to the appropriate health authority by law whenever it is diagnosed. Also known as a *reportable disease.*

null value   The value of a measure of association that represents no association. For example, the null value for a relative risk is one, and the null value for a risk difference is zero.

observation bias   A synonym for **measurement bias.**

observational study   An epidemiologic study in which the investigators do not control the exposure status of the subjects. Observational studies include descriptive and analytic studies. Also see **experimental study.**

observer variability   A general term referring to either interobserver or intraobserver variability. Also see **interobserver variability; intraobserver variability.**

odds   The probability of an event occurring relative to it not occurring. For example, if 10 people get a disease when exposed to a particular risk factor and only 5 get the disease when not exposed to the factor, the odds of getting the disease are 10 to 5 or 2 to 1.

odds ratio   The ratio of two odds. In a case-control study, the odds ratio may be expressed as the odds of exposure among the cases to the odds of exposure among the controls.

opportunistic screening   A synonym for **case finding.**

outcome   The disease or other health-related problem that is being investigated in an epidemiologic study. Also see **exposure.**

outcome status   A term for classifying subjects in an epidemiologic study by whether or not they have the disease or other health-related problem under investigation. Outcome status is usually dichotomous (i.e., present or absent), but it can be measured using several levels, such as severe, moderate, mild, and no disease. Also see **exposure status.**

pair matching   A form of matching in which each subject in the study group is paired with a similar subject in the comparison group with regard to the variables for which matching is sought.

pandemic   An epidemic on grand scale causing illness or death over an extensive area, generally crossing international borders and afflicting large numbers of people. A pandemic of plague, for example, occurred in Western Europe between 1347 and 1351.

panel study   A type of hybrid study that combines features of the cross-sectional and prospective cohort designs. Panel studies can be viewed as a series of cross-sectional studies conducted on the same subjects (the panel) during successive time intervals.

passive immunity A type of immunity that occurs when one receives antibodies from another host. It may be conferred by injection of a serum, placental transfer, or breast-feeding. The immunity is immediate and occurs without the body producing its own antibodies. Also see **active immunity.**

passive surveillance Surveillance in which various health care providers are required by law to report certain diseases or conditions using prescribed methods designed by the agency responsible for surveillance. Also see **public health surveillance; active surveillance.**

Pearson correlation coefficient (r or Pearson's r) A statistical measure of the magnitude of the linear relationship between two continuous variables. Pearson's r ranges from -1 to $+1$, where -1 indicates a perfect inverse relationship, 0 indicates no relationship, and $+1$ indicates a perfect positive relationship.

percent relative effect The percent change in a ratio measure of association from the baseline value of one. For example, a relative risk of 3.2 represents an increased risk of 220%, and a relative risk of 0.7 represents a decreased risk of 30%.

perinatal mortality rate The number of fetal deaths after 28 weeks or more of gestation plus the number of infant deaths within 7 days of birth during a specified time period in relation to the number of live births plus the number of fetal deaths after 28 weeks or more of gestation during the same time period.

period prevalence rate The proportion of a defined population that has had a given disease or attribute, regardless of outcome, at any time during a specified time period. The period prevalence rate measures disease prevalence over a span of time.

person-time chi-square ($\chi_{P\text{-}T}^2$) A chi-square test that is used to determine the statistical significance of the rate ratio. It is known as the person-time chi-square because the rate ratio is based on person-time incidence rates.

person-time incidence rate The rate at which new events (e.g., cases of a disease) are occurring in a population. It is calculated by dividing the number of new events during a specified time period by the total person-time units at risk of the event. The person-time incidence rate is frequently employed in cohort studies where different individuals may be at risk of the event for different lengths of time. Also known as *incidence density, force of morbidity,* or simply *incidence rate.*

person-time units Units of measure that combine the number of persons at risk of a specified outcome with their time at risk (e.g., person-years). Total person-time units are calculated by summing each individual's time at risk in a population and comprise the denominators used in calculating person-time incidence rates.

placebo An inert substance or treatment that is made to appear like the intervention in a randomized controlled trial. A placebo has no known therapeutic effect. Also see **placebo-controlled trial.**

placebo effect The tendency for those receiving a treatment to experience beneficial effects even when the treatment has no known therapeutic value.

placebo-controlled trial A randomized controlled trial in which the control group receives a placebo. Many drug trials are placebo-controlled.

plague An infectious disease, primarily of historical importance, that is caused by *Yersinia pestis*, a bacterium that is transmitted by the bite of the infected rat flea. Plague can have three clinical forms—bubonic, septicemic, and pneumonic.

point estimate An estimated population parameter calculated from a sample of a population.

point prevalence rate The proportion of a defined population that has a specific disease or attribute at a point in time, usually represented by a particular day or specific date. The point prevalence rate measures disease prevalence at a specific time.

point source outbreak   A type of common source outbreak where the duration of exposure to the common agent of disease is relatively brief and virtually simultaneous among those exposed. Point source outbreaks are relatively short-lived and normally conclude within a time frame equal to the range of the incubation period of the disease. Also see **continuing source outbreak; intermittent source outbreak.**

population at risk   The people in a defined population who are susceptible to the event under investigation. In practice, it is usually represented either by the number of susceptible individuals in the defined population who are event-free at the beginning of the specified time period or by the average or mid-interval population during the specified time period.

population attributable risk   The amount of absolute risk of a disease in a population that can be attributed to the exposure. The population attributable risk assumes the exposure is a cause of the disease. It is also referred as the population excess risk attributable to the exposure.

population attributable risk percent   The percent of the absolute risk of a disease in a population that can be attributed to a specific exposure. The population attributable risk percent assumes the exposure is a cause of the disease.

population controls   Subjects comprising the control group of a population-based case-control study. These subjects are usually selected randomly from the general population without the study disease.

population-based case-control study   A case-control study in which the subjects are selected from the total or a representative sample of a defined population.

population-based disease registry   An ongoing system that collects and registers all cases of a particular disease or class of diseases as they develop in a defined population (e.g., a cancer registry). Not all disease registries, however, are population-based.

positive bias   Bias that results in an overestimation of the magnitude of the measure of association between an exposure and outcome.

positive confounder   A confounding factor that leads to overestimation of the magnitude of the measure of association between an exposure and outcome.

positive predictive value   A measure of the percent of people who test positive on a screening test and really have the disease.

potential confounder   A factor that may distort (i.e., confound) an association between a study exposure and outcome. Since in practice one rarely knows if all criteria for confounding are met, any factors suspected of meeting one or more of the criteria for confounding should be considered potential confounders. Also see **confounding.**

power   In the context of statistics, power is the probability of detecting an association if one really exists. Power is calculated by subtracting beta (type II error) from one (i.e., power = $1 - \beta$).

practical significance   A synonym for **clinical significance.**

precision   The component of accuracy that is concerned with the consistency or stability of the results. The results of small samples are more likely to be imprecise because of a greater chance of sampling error, for example.

precision of a screening test   The reliability of a screening test, that is, the degree to which it provides consistent results from one application to the next.

predisposing or enabling factor   A factor that can increase susceptibility or facilitate a specific outcome. The term is often used to refer to a risk factor. For example, advanced age is a predisposing factor for Alzheimer's disease. Also, poor nutrition is an enabling factor for tuberculosis.

prevalence The number of cases of a given disease or other attribute (e.g., drug use, obesity) that exists in a defined population at a specified time. It is also sometimes referred to as the prevalence number.

prevalence rate The proportion of a defined population that has a specific disease or attribute during a specified time. There are three basic types of prevalence rates—point prevalence rate, period prevalence rate, and lifetime prevalence rate.

prevalence rate difference The difference between the prevalence rate in the exposed group and the prevalence rate in the unexposed group in an epidemiologic study.

prevalence rate ratio A measure of association commonly used in cross-sectional studies. The prevalence rate ratio (PRR) is the ratio of the prevalence rate in the exposed group to the prevalence rate in the unexposed group.

prevalence ratio A synonym for **prevalence rate ratio.**

prevalence study A term sometimes used to refer to a cross-sectional study because prevalence rates are the usual measures calculated.

prevalence-incidence bias A form of selection bias that can occur when asymptomatic, mild, clinically resolved, or fatal cases are inadvertently excluded from the case group in a study because the cases are examined sometime after the disease process has begun (i.e., looking at prevalent versus incident cases). This bias exists if the association would have been different had the missed cases been included in the sample. Also known as *Neyman's bias.*

preventive trial A type of randomized controlled trial that focuses on individuals without the study disease in order to determine if a particular intervention reduces the risk of the disease. Also known as a *prophylactic trial.* Also see **intervention trial; therapeutic trial.**

primary prevention See **levels of prevention.**

primary source A source of data collected firsthand by the investigator (i.e., original data).

probability sample A type of sample in which everyone in the target population has a known probability of being selected.

propagated outbreak A progressive outbreak that is usually due to direct person-to-person transmission of the disease (e.g., via touching, sneezing, coughing, or sexual relations) or by indirect transmission through a vector. Also see **common source outbreak.**

proportionate mortality ratio The ratio of the number of deaths due to a specific cause to the total number of deaths occurring in a population during a specified time period. The proportionate mortality ratio is a measure of how important a particular cause of death is in relation to all deaths in the population. Unlike the cause-specific mortality rate, it is not a measure of the risk of death.

prospective cohort study An analytic epidemiologic study that classifies subjects without the study disease according to exposure status and then follows them into the future to determine if the rate of development of the study disease is significantly different in the exposed and unexposed groups.

protocol See **study protocol.**

public health surveillance The ongoing systematic collection, analysis, interpretation, and dissemination of health data essential to the planning, implementation, and evaluation of public health practice. Also see **active surveillance; passive surveillance; sentinel surveillance.**

p-value The probability that a given result is due to sampling error. The lower the p-value, the less likely sampling error accounts for an observed association. By convention, associations are considered statistically significant when the corresponding p-value is equal to or less than 0.05 and not significant when the p-value is greater than 0.05.

quasi-experimental study   A study where the investigator does not have full control over the assignment or timing of the intervention but where the study is still conducted as if it were an experiment. Nonrandomized community trials are quasi-experimental studies.

random allocation   See **randomization.**

random error   A nonsystematic type of error that occurs by chance. For example, sampling error is a type of random error.

randomization   The assignment of subjects to different study groups (e.g., experimental and control groups) using random means. Randomization assures that the subjects have the same probability of being assigned to any of the study groups. Also known as *random allocation.*

randomized controlled trial   An experimental epidemiologic study designed to test the efficacy of an intervention on a group of volunteers. It involves random allocation of subjects into experimental and control groups for comparison purposes. The unit of analysis in this type of study is the individual. Randomized controlled trials include preventive trials, intervention trials, and therapeutic trials. Also see **clinical trial.**

rare disease assumption   The assumption that the study outcome is rare. This assumption normally is required when one uses the odds ratio to estimate the relative risk or rate ratio. A cumulative incidence rate of less than 2 per 100 is good rule of thumb for what constitutes a "rare" outcome.

rate adjustment   A statistical procedure that controls for differences in the distribution of factors, such as age, that may confound a comparison of crude morbidity or mortality rates between populations. It provides a way of making fair, unbiased comparisons between population summary rates. Also known as *rate standardization.* Also see **age adjustment.**

rate base   A unit of measure routinely used in expressing incidence, prevalence, and mortality rates. It is used to assure that the reported rate is always expressed as a value equal to or greater than one for a given population size. The rate base is 10 raised to a power of 2, 3, 4, etc. (e.g., 100, 1,000, 10,000, etc.) and is used to avoid fractional rates. For example, an incidence rate of 0.20 is expressed as 20 per 100 using a rate base of 100 ($0.20 \times 100 = 20$ per 100) or 200 per 1,000 using a rate base of 1,000.

rate difference   The difference between the person-time incidence rates in the exposed and unexposed groups in an epidemiologic study. The rate difference is a measure of association between an exposure and outcome.

rate ratio   The ratio of the person-time incidence rate in the exposed group to the person-time incidence rate in the unexposed group in an epidemiologic study. The rate ratio is a measure of association between an exposure and outcome.

rate standardization   A synonym for **rate adjustment.**

recall bias   A form of measurement bias that can occur in case-control and cross-sectional studies because of differential recall about past exposure status between those who have the disease and those who do not. In general, cases tend to recall past exposures more accurately than noncases.

reemerging infectious disease   A once familiar infectious disease that was thought to be decreasing or disappearing in a population but is now on the rise. Also see **emerging infectious disease.**

reference population   The population to which the investigator hopes to generalize the findings of a randomized controlled trial.

regression equation A mathematical expression that describes the relationship between a dependent and one or more independent variables. A regression equation allows investigators to predict the effect of the independent variable(s) on the dependent variable. A regression equation is sometimes referred to as a prediction equation or a regression model.

regression line The line that best describes the relationship between a dependent and an independent variable. A regression line can be obtained by performing a simple linear regression analysis. It represents the line that best fits the data in a scatter plot.

relative risk The ratio of the absolute risk of a disease among the exposed group to the absolute risk of the disease among the unexposed group in an epidemiologic study. The relative risk is a measure of association between an exposure and outcome. Also known as the *risk ratio*.

reliability The degree of consistency or stability of a measure from one use to the next. A measure that gives consistent results under similar circumstances shows a high degree of reliability.

repeated surveys A type of hybrid study where successive cross-sectional studies are performed over time on the same study population, but each sample is selected independently. Therefore, while the samples may be representative of the study population, the actual subjects may not be the same from one survey to the next.

reportable disease A synonym for **notifiable disease.**

response bias A form of selection bias that can occur because of systematic differences in those who participate in studies and those who do not. For example, questionnaires in magazines or on the Internet may produce a response bias.

restriction A procedure that limits the subjects of a study to only those with certain characteristics (e.g., white males). Restriction commonly is used as a method of controlling for potential confounders in a study. A study restricted to males only, for example, cannot be confounded by differences in sex.

retrospective cohort study An analytic epidemiologic study in which the study sample (cohort) represents an historical group assembled using available data sources. In this study design the subjects are classified according to exposure status at the time the cohort existed and followed up to the present to determine if the rate of development of the study disease is significantly different in the exposed and unexposed groups. Also known as a *historical cohort study.*

risk The probability that a specific event will occur in a given time frame. The risk of disease occurrence is measured by the cumulative incidence rate.

risk difference The difference between the absolute risk in the exposed and unexposed groups in an epidemiologic study. The risk difference is a measure of association between an exposure and outcome.

risk factor A behavior, environmental exposure, or inherent human characteristic that is associated with an increased probability of a particular health-related outcome (i.e., disease). For example, a high serum cholesterol level is a risk factor for coronary heart disease.

risk ratio A synonym for **relative risk.**

sample See **study sample.**

sampling error The random variation that can result when using sample statistics to estimate population parameters.

scatter plot The pattern of points that results when two quantitative variables are plotted on a graph. Each point formed by the intersection of the values of the two variables represents one unit in the analysis. The pattern of the points is indicative of the degree and direction of the relationship between the variables. For example, the more the points cluster along a straight line, the stronger the relationship. Also known as a *scatter diagram.*

screening for disease detection   A relatively quick means of identifying individuals who may have a given disease and who should therefore undergo diagnostic testing for confirmation.

screening level   The cutoff point at which the result of a screening test is considered positive. Below the cutoff point the test is considered negative. For example, a blood glucose screening test for diabetes may set the cutoff point at 110 milligrams per deciliter.

secondary prevention   See **levels of prevention.**

secondary source   A source of data that has not been collected firsthand. It is a non-original source of data collected by someone else (i.e., secondhand data).

secular trend   A long-term change in the rate of morbidity or mortality for a given disease in a specified population. For example, the mortality rate for septicemia in the U.S. showed a steady increase between 1951 and 1988, representing a secular trend.

selection bias   Systematic error that results from the way in which the subjects are selected or retained in a study. This error can occur when the characteristics of the subjects selected for a study differ systematically from those in the target population or when the study and comparison groups are selected from different populations.

selective screening   Screening for disease that is applied to groups at high risk of the disease. Also known as *targeted screening.* Also see **mass screening.**

sensitivity   The ability of a screening test to identify correctly those who have the disease. Sensitivity is measured as the percent of those with the disease who test positive for the disease on a screening test.

sentinel event   A disease or condition that alerts public health authorities to a potential public health problem (e.g., epidemic, failure of preventive measures) and that may require some type of public health response when reported.

sentinel surveillance   Surveillance that pre-arranges for certain health care providers to report all cases of certain predetermined diseases or conditions that may require a public health response (sentinel events). The reporting sources are usually a select sample of health care providers that are likely to see the events and that have agreed to report them to the appropriate authorities. Also see **sentinel event; public health surveillance.**

short-term fluctuation   A relatively brief, unexpected increase in the frequency of a particular disease in a defined population (e.g., an epidemic).

single-blinded study   A study in which the subjects are kept unaware of their group assignment, although the investigators are aware. Also see **blinding.**

source population   The population from which the cases are selected for a case-control study. In general, the controls also should be selected from the source population.

specific rate   A rate for a distinct subgroup within a defined population. The most commonly reported specific rates are those based on age, sex, or race/ethnicity (i.e., age-specific rates, sex-specific rates, and race/ethnicity-specific rates).

specificity   The ability of a screening test to identify correctly those who do not have the disease. Specificity is measured as the percent of those without the disease who test negative for the disease on a screening test.

spot map   A map showing the geographical location of each case of a disease or other attribute. It is frequently used in disease outbreak investigations to discover where cases aggregate, thus suggesting possible causes of the outbreak.

spurious association   A false association generally caused by sampling error or bias.

standard population   A population used for comparison purposes in rate adjustment. It is a stable population whose distribution with regard to the factors being controlled (e.g., age, sex, or race/ethnicity) is known. The standard population may be an actual or a derived population.

standardized morbidity ratio   When used in reference to indirect rate adjustment, it is the ratio of the number of observed cases in the comparison population to the number of expected cases based on the specific rates in the standard population.

standardized mortality ratio   When used in reference to indirect rate adjustment, it is the ratio of the number of observed deaths in the comparison population to the number of expected deaths based on the specific rates in the standard population.

statistically significant   An indication that sampling error is an unlikely explanation for an observed association. An association is usually considered statistically significant when the p-value is less than or equal to 0.05 ($p \leq 0.05$).

steady-state conditions   Conditions where a population is stable, and the incidence and prevalence rates under consideration are unchanging.

stratification   A procedure used in the analysis phase of an epidemiologic study to control for confounding or to detect effect modification. Stratification involves separating a sample into two or more subgroups according to specified levels of a third variable. For example, the results of a study of the effects of cigarette smoking on the development of cerebrovascular disease might be stratified by blood pressure levels to control for potential confounding by blood pressure or to examine whether or not different blood pressure levels modify the effect of cigarette smoking on cerebrovascular disease.

stratified randomization   A randomization technique sometimes used in randomized controlled trials when the sample size is relatively small. This technique increases the probability that the experimental and control groups will be similar with regard to the stratified factor(s). Stratified randomization involves three basic steps: (1) separation of the sample into appropriate strata, (2) random allocation of subjects in each stratum into experimental and control groups, and (3) compilation of the stratum-specific experimental and control groups into final experimental and control groups.

stratum-specific odds ratio   An odds ratio that is specific to a stratification subgroup and thus is free of the confounding effect of the variable used in the stratification. For example, with stratification by sex the odds ratio for males is free of confounding by sex as is the odds ratio for females. There are also other stratum-specific measures of association (e.g., stratum-specific relative risk).

strength of the association   A criterion for judging if an association is causal, based on Hill's postulates. This refers to the fact that, in general, the stronger an association is between an exposure and outcome, the more likely it is a causal association. For example, when the relative risk or rate ratio is very high it is unlikely that the association can be explained by unrecognized or subtle sources of bias or confounding.

study protocol   The written plan and procedures to be followed in a study.

study sample   The subjects included in an epidemiologic study. A study sample may be selected in different ways and may or may not be representative of a larger population. In a randomized controlled trial the study sample consists of volunteers from the experimental population who have met the eligibility criteria for participation in the study.

subclinical disease   A disease that is fully developed but produces no symptoms in the host (i.e., asymptomatic disease). Subclinical disease can be communicable or noncommunicable.

subject variability   The variability in the results of a measure that occurs due to changes taking place in the subject being observed. For example, a screening test for hypertension may produce different results in the same individual at different times of the day due to physiological changes in the body.

sufficient cause   A cause that by itself is able to produce a particular outcome. Most diseases, however, are due to multiple causes.

survival analysis   A method of analyzing data from studies involving follow-up that is especially useful when the follow-up periods for subjects vary widely or when the subjects enter the study at different times. In survival analysis one plots the time it took for each subject to develop the study outcome on a survival curve that provides data on the percent survival for any given time period, median survival time for a group, and other useful information.

survival rate   A measure of the probability that cases of a given disease will survive for a specified period of time. Like the case fatality rate, it is an indicator of the prognosis for those with the disease. An example is the five-year survival rate for breast cancer.

systematic error   A nonrandom flaw in study design, conduct, or analysis that can have the effect of either uniformly increasing or decreasing the magnitude of the measure of association between a study exposure and outcome. Bias and confounding are the two primary reasons for systematic error.

target population   The population to which an investigator hopes to generalize study findings.

targeted screening   A synonym for **selective screening.**

temporal pattern of disease   The change in the frequency or rate of a cause of morbidity or mortality over time. Temporal patterns include short-term fluctuations, cyclic patterns, and secular trends.

tertiary prevention   See **levels of prevention.**

test of heterogeneity   A statistical test used in the process of stratification to examine the probability that differences in stratum-specific measures of association (e.g., odds ratios or relative risks) are statistically different.

therapeutic trial   A type of randomized controlled trial that focuses on patients with existing disease or disability in order to test interventions that might improve the condition or the patients' quality of life. Also see **preventive trial; intervention trial.**

threshold   A level of exposure that must be reached before effects become apparent. Below the threshold level there are no observed effects.

triple-blinded study   A study in which the subjects, the investigators, and those analyzing the data are unaware of the subjects' group assignments. Also see **blinding.**

true negative   A negative test result where the individual being tested does not have the attribute for which testing is being done. In the context of screening for disease, a true negative is one who tests negative on the screening test and really does not have the disease.

true negative rate   The percent of people without the disease who are classified correctly as not having the disease based on a screening test. This is the same as specificity.

true positive   A positive test result where the individual being tested has the attribute for which testing is being done. In the context of screening for disease, a true positive is one who tests positive on the screening test and really has the disease.

true positive rate   The percent of people with the disease who are classified correctly as having the disease based on a screening test. This is the same as sensitivity.

type I error   The error of finding an association when none exists. The probability of this type of error is measured by the p-value or alpha level.

type II error   The error of failing to detect an association when one exists. The probability of this type of error is measured by the beta level.

underlying cause of death A term used on death certificates. It is the cause or injury that initiated the chain of events that ultimately produced death. It is the official cause of death used in mortality statistics in the United States.

unit of analysis The object of study or what is being studied. The unit of analysis is usually the individual, but it can also be a group of people defined by a geographical area or a time period (i.e., an ecological unit).

unmatched case-control study A case-control study design in which pair matching is not used; that is, individual cases are not pair matched to individual controls during the selection process. Frequency matching, however, may be used.

upper confidence limit The ending (highest) value of a confidence interval.

validity The component of accuracy that is concerned with the degree of systematic error in a study. There are two types of validity: internal validity and external validity.

validity of a screening test The degree to which a screening test does what it is designed to do (i.e., detect those who have a given disease and those who do not).

vector An animate source, such as a fly, mosquito, or rodent, that is capable of transmitting an agent of disease to a susceptible host. The vector serves as an intermediary in disease transmission, and the mechanism of transmission is considered indirect. A vector may be infected with the disease organism or may be a mechanical carrier. Some limit the term vector to nonvertebrate species only, although it is common practice to apply it to small vertebrate animals as well (e.g., rats, skunks, and bats).

vehicle An inanimate substance or object, such as food, water, bedding, or surgical equipment, that is capable of transmitting an agent of disease to a susceptible host. The vehicle serves as an intermediary in disease transmission, and the mechanism of transmission is considered indirect. A vehicle may or may not support growth of the agent.

vital event A registered life event such as a birth, death, marriage, divorce, or serious disease. In the U.S. vital events must be reported by law.

vital record A completed registration form or certificate of birth, death, marriage, divorce, etc. Also see **vital event.**

vital statistics Information derived from registered life events, such as births, deaths, marriages, divorces, and certain diseases.

vital statistics registration system A system for the collection of vital records. In the U.S. vital records are filed with a local vital statistics registrar, forwarded to the state registrar for vital statistics, and then to the Centers for Disease Control and Prevention.

volunteer bias A form of selection bias that can occur because those who volunteer for studies tend to be systematically different from those who do not. Volunteer bias is a form of response bias.

washout period A stage in a crossover design of a randomized controlled trial during which the effects of a previously applied intervention are believed to wear off. Normally, the control condition is assigned after the washout period.

years of potential life lost (YPLL) A measure of the impact of premature death on a population. It is calculated by adding together the total years of potential life lost before a given age (e.g., 65 years), and thus gives more weight to deaths that occur at younger ages. Years of potential life lost is useful in establishing public health priorities.

yield In the context of screening programs, yield is the number of new cases diagnosed and treated as a result of screening.

YPLL rate For a given population and time period, the YPLL rate is the number of years of potential life lost prior a specified age in relation to all those in the population below the specified age.

z-score A transformed score based on a standardized normal distribution with a mean of zero and a standard deviation of one. A z-score of 2.0 is two standard deviations above the mean, and a z-score of –2.0 is two standard deviations below the mean.

Index